CASE DISCUSSIONS in SURGERY

with Questions and Answers

A Key to Success in Surgical Clinical Examinations

CASE DISCUSSIONS in SURGERY

with Questions and Answers

A Key to Success in Surgical Clinical Examinations

Sudhir Kumar Jain
MS, MBA(HCA), FRCS, FICS, FIAS
Professor and Senior Consultant
Department of Surgery
Maulana Azad Medical College
and associated Lok Nayak Hospital
New Delhi

Raman Tanwar MS, FMAS
MCh Urology Registrar
PGIMER and Dr RML Hospital
New Delhi

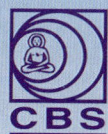

CBS

CBS Publishers & Distributors Pvt Ltd

New Delhi • Bengaluru • Chennai • Kochi • Mumbai • Pune
Hyderabad • Kolkata • Nagpur • Patna • Vijayawada

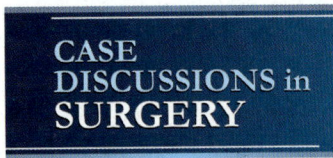

ISBN: 978-81-239-2592-9

Copyright © Authors and Publisher

First Edition: 2015

Published by Satish Kumar Jain and Produced by Varun Jain for

CBS Publishers & Distributors Pvt Ltd
4819/XI Prahlad Street, 24 Ansari Road, Daryaganj, New Delhi 110 002, India.
Ph: 23289259, 23266861, 23266867   Fax: 011-23243014   Website: www.cbspd.com
e-mail: delhi@cbspd.com; cbspubs@airtelmail.in.

Corporate Office: 204 FIE, Industrial Area, Patparganj, Delhi 110 092
Ph: 4934 4934   Fax: 4934 4935   e-mail: publishing@cbspd.com; publicity@cbspd.com

Branches

- **Bengaluru:** Seema House 2975, 17th Cross, K.R. Road,
  Banasankari 2nd Stage, Bengaluru 560 070, Karnataka
  Ph: +91-80-26771678/79   Fax: +91-80-26771680   e-mail: bangalore@cbspd.com
- **Chennai:** 7, Subbaraya Street, Shenoy Nagar, Chennai 600 030, Tamil Nadu
  Ph: +91-44-26260666, 26208620   Fax: +91-44-42032115   e-mail: chennai@cbspd.com
- **Kochi:** 36/14 Kalluvilakam, Lissie Hospital Road, Kochi 682 018, Kerala
  Ph: +91-484-4059061-65   Fax: +91-484-4059065   e-mail: kochi@cbspd.com
- **Mumbai:** 83-C, Dr E Moses Road, Worli, Mumbai-400018, Maharashtra
  Ph: +91-22-24902340/41   Fax: +91-22-24902342   e-mail: mumbai@cbspd.com
- **Pune:** Bhuruk Prestige, Sr. No. 52/12/2+1+3/2 Narhe, Haveli
  (Near Katraj-Dehu Road Bypass), Pune 411 041, Maharashtra
  Ph: +91-20-64704058/59, 32392277   Fax: +91-20-24300160   e-mail: pune@cbspd.com

Representatives

- **Hyderabad** 0-9885175004
- **Nagpur** 0-9021734563
- **Vijayawada** 0-9000660880
- **Kolkata** 0-9831437309, 0-9051152362
- **Patna** 0-9334159340

Printed at: HT Media Ltd., Noida

to

our families

who have supported us in every possible way

and made us what we are.

Our teachers who instilled in us the capability

to perform, teach and write.

Our patients and students who teach us daily

List of Contributors

Aparajita Mitra
MCh Senior Resident
Department of Pediatric Surgery
All India Institute of Medical Sciences, New Delhi
Contributed to the chapters "Common Neck Swellings" and "Cleft Lip and Palate"

Raman Tanwar
MCh Senior Resident
Department of Urology
Post Graduate Institute of Medical Education and Research and Dr RML Hospital, New Delhi

Sudhir Kumar Jain
Professor and Senior Consultant
Department of Surgery
Maulana Azad Medical College
and associated Lok Nayak Hospital, New Delhi

Vivek Manchanda
Assistant Professor
Department of Pediatric Surgery
Chacha Nehru Bal Chikitsalaya, New Delhi
Contributed the chapters "Pediatric Inguinal Hernias" and "Cleft Lip and Palate"

Preface

The longest of journeys begin with a single step. Learning the art and craft of surgery is also a long journey. It often takes a lifetime and still perfection seems distant, but there have been many a men who have been the torchbearers and shown that it is possible. The first step to embarking upon this journey is to accumulate knowledge of what is most commonly encountered. Case discussions are one of the easiest ways to make the first step interesting and complete. In this book lie the common situations that a young surgeon or student of the surgical discipline would daily encounter and the answers to what shall come naturally to the mind in the form of doubts and questions. It is these questions that are subsequently put forward during the exit examination as well and determine the ability of the student to guide the patient successfully towards recovery. The content within this book represents internationally accepted guidelines and widely practiced treatment standards that have been abridged and simplified so that they can be reproduced and understood. The book also represents the gist of discussions that we have had with the students as members of the surgical faculty and the methodology by which we manage our patients. The text within the book has been supplemented with clinical pictures and figures to make the clinical situation more comprehensible.

With our growing experience in book writing and addressing issues relevant to students we have tried to be precise and provide facts based on standard teaching, adding to it our own experience and methodology of investigating and managing the cases herein. An attempt has been made to go into a reasonable depth of management of each case making this a useful book not only for undergraduate and postgraduate medical students but also for students appearing in post-doctoral exit exams. The book is enriched with crisp content and close ended. Single answer questions have been avoided to prevent duplication of text. Since this is the first edition, we understand that it will raise many more questions that have not been answered herein. We are hopeful that a rich correspondence with readers like you will help to solve these queries and improve the book further. We aim to supplement this book with more pictures, videos and experiences via the online medium and social media to keep the contents dynamic and up-to-date. We hope that this book will be a helpful companion in this long journey of learning surgery and the first step will be pleasing and effortless. Wishing you all the best!

Sudhir Kumar Jain
Raman Tanwar

Acknowledgements

Our deepest regards and thanks to our parents and families for being the pillars of our foundation and their blessings. Our heartfelt thanks to our wives Dr Deepti Jain, and Dr Kirti Vijay Rathore and our parents for their constant support during the course of this work. We would like to thank our teachers who have been a guiding light for us and our students who have helped us learn and grow on a daily basis. We express our gratitude towards our patients for vesting their faith in us and helping us to understand the subject beyond what books could express.

We are grateful for the support of Mr SK Jain, Chairman and Managing Director; Mr YN Arjuna, Vice President—Publishing, Editorial and Publicity, and his entire team at CBSPD comprising Mrs Ritu Chawla, Mr Tarun Rajput, Mr Neeraj Prasad and Mr Sunil Dutt. It is only due to the untiring team work that the difficult task of bringing out this book has been achieved.

Sudhir Kumar Jain

Raman Tanwar

Contents

Head and Neck

Section 1

Cleft Lip and Palate

In a case of cleft lip and palate, the history given by the parents and rarely the patient (if the patient grows old enough) is that of the obvious defect. Other secondary symptoms are difficulty in speech and inability to pronounce certain sounds effectively, hearing defects, ear infections, delayed tooth development and other facial developmental defects. It is essential to ask for other components of associated syndromes like Pierre Robin sequence where glossoptosis may be present. History of maternal disease especially epilepsy, the antenatal care received and history of drug intake by mother should be well documented in the history. Associated defects should be looked for in other areas in head and neck, brain, heart and extremities. Associated syndromes make it essential to subject the patient to a thorough physical examination of other possible associations.

The final diagnosis is depicted and classified using any of the standard classification systems:

LAHSHAL

- Complete cleft: Capital L/A/S/H
- Incomplete cleft: Lower case l/a/s/h
- Microform clefts: Asterisk
- To be read like an X-ray, i.e. right side letters denote left side cleft

Kernahan's Striped Y

- 1, 4—lip
- 2, 5—alveolus
- 3, 6—premaxilla
- 7, 8—hard palate
- 9—soft palate
- Degree of stippling corresponds to the degree of clefting

Modifications of Kernahan's Classification

- *Millard's modification:* Two triangles are added above 1 and 4 to denote the nasal deformity and nasal floor.

How does cleft lip and palate develop?

Cleft lip and palate arise as a result of fusion abnormalities of the facial processes (Fig. 1.1). About 15% of clefts have syndromic association and more than 170 syndromes have known association with facial clefts. Few to name are median cleft lip in trisomy D syndrome and cleft lip with pits on lower lip in van der Woude syndrome. Although no single gene has been identified, candidate loci have been found in chromosomes 1, 2, 4, 6, 11, 14, 17 and 19.

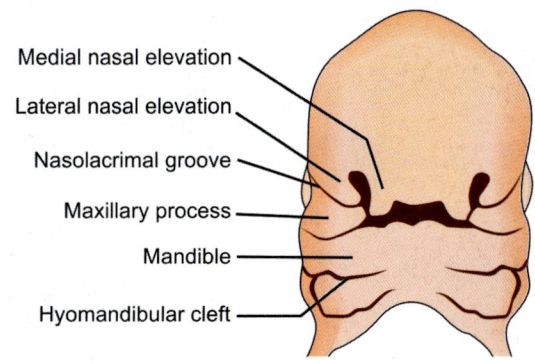

Medial nasal elevation
Lateral nasal elevation
Nasolacrimal groove
Maxillary process
Mandible
Hyomandibular cleft

Fig. 1.1: Development of the face

Clefts are also associated with maternal smoking and use of certain drugs like phenytoin, steroids, diazepam, retinoic acid and folate antagonists in pregnancy. Vitamin supplementation in first 4 months of gestation has shown protective effects.

What is the incidence and prevalence pattern of cleft lip and palate (Figs 1.2 and 1.3)?

Cleft lip is a fairly common congenital defect with an incidence of 1 in 500 to 1 in 1500, exhibiting

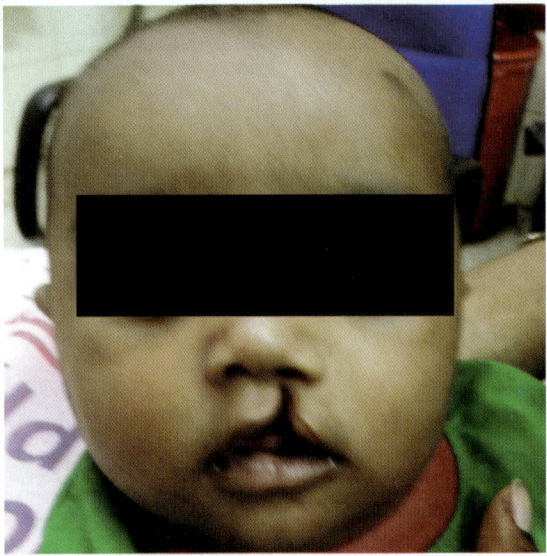

Fig. 1.2: Unilateral cleft lip

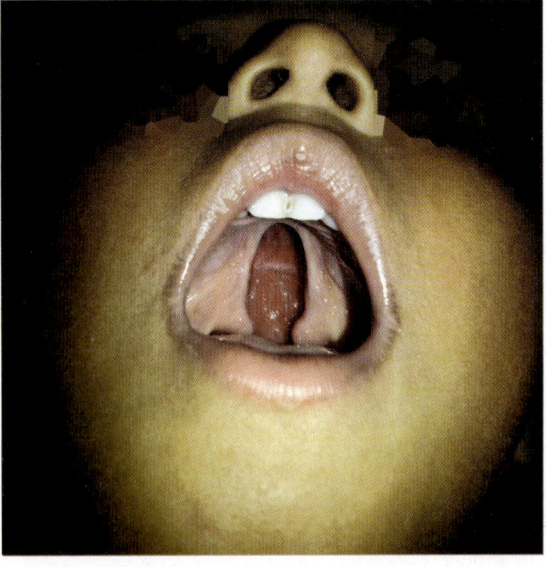

Fig. 1.3: Isolated cleft palate

racial differences likely resulting from differences in facial tissue thickness. It is more common on the left side. In India, the incidence is nearly 1 in 800 live births. Isolated cleft palate occurs in 1 in 1000 live births. Isolated cleft lip occurs in 15% (left more common than right 3:2) of the cases, cleft lip and palate combined in 45% (more common in males) and isolated cleft palate in 40% (more common in females) of the cases.

What are the anatomical abbrevations in cleft defects?

Anatomical defects in cleft lip are centred around the three muscular rings of Delaire, namely the nasolabial muscle ring which circumvents the nasal aperture, the labiomental muscular ring which is present around the lower lip and chin and the bilabial muscle ring around the oral aperture.

In unilateral cleft lip nasolabial and bilabial muscle rings are disrupted on one side leading to the displacement of nasal skin onto the lip along with retraction of the nasal skin, whereas in bilateral cleft lip, muscle rings on both the sides are disrupted leading to a protusive premaxilla and prolabium along with flaring of the nose.

The palate is formed in two stages, namely the primary palate and secondary palate. The primary palate consists of the structures anterior to the incisive foramen including the alveolus, premaxilla and upper four incisors. The secondary palate includes structures which lie behind the incisive foramen. The soft palate consists of muscles, namely tensor palati, levator palati, palatopharyngeus, palatoglossus, and musculus uvulae which are oriented transversely in a normal palate. In the presence of cleft palate the orientation becomes anteroposterior and the muscles are inserted into the posterior edge of the hard palate. When the defect is complete the nasal septum and vomer bone are completely separate from the palatine processes. In an incomplete cleft palate the palate remains attached to the nasal septum and vomer but the palatine processes fail to fuse in the midline.

How will you manage of a case of cleft lip and palate?

Management of the condition depends upon the time at which it is diagnosed. In the antenatal period diagnosis by antenatal ultrasound is possible which will help to prognosticate parents, and undergo counselling with the cleft team (that is ultimately going to manage the condition) and genetic counselling regarding the chances of future offspring having the anomaly. A high resolution ultrasonography can help visualise unilateral/bilateral cleft lip after 18 weeks. Isolated cleft palate cannot be diagnosed by antenatal scan.

In the early neonatal period other syndromic associations must be ruled out apart from maintaining adequate airway (specially in children with Pierre Robin syndrome) and feeding advice. The baby is nursed in a prone position to secure the airway. Some patients may require labio-glossopexy (surgical fixation of tongue to the lower lip) to avoid tounge fall and airway problems. Breastfeeding is not possible as negative suction cannot be created in the mouth due to defects in the lip and/or palate. Palatal obturators are available to cover the palatal defect but are cumbersome to use. Special long nipples with wide bore and *'diva'* with long snout are available for feeding directly into the pharynx so that the nasal regurgitation is prevented. The *'bowl and spoon'* feed in propped up position can also be used. For very wide and misaligned cleft lips neonatal orthopaedic implants are available to help the maxillary processes align themselves and reduce the tension on final repair.

Various techniques have been described to repair the cleft lip and palate. They are sequentially done and aimed at obtaining a normal appearance followed by normal speech and subsequently normal dentation and facial growth in that order of preference. Apart from the surgery it is important to address hearing at 12 months using brainstem audiometry or tympanometry, and rule of sensorineural hearing defects (which can be associated in these patients and Eustachian tube dysfunction which often leads to middle ear infections in these patients. The dental team or facial surgery team must be referred to address the orthodontic issues like delayed eruption and tooth development, alteration in shape and number of teeth and other morphological abnor-malities. Speech is also affected in these patients and it should be assessed at 18 months to explore the need of speech therapy or secondary palatal surgery as detailed below.

When should the repair be advised?

The cleft lip is repaired at age of 3–4 months as per *'Rule of 10'* given by Millard, which suggests that the baby be 10 weeks old, weigh 10 pounds and has 10 grams of haemoglobin, to reduce the anaesthesia risk. The cleft palate is repaired at age of 9 months to 15 months. Early surgery improves the results for acceptable speech. Intervening cleft alveolus is traditionally repaired at age of 5 to 8 years with bone graft. Table 1.1 summarizes the current recommendations regarding timing of repair.

Table 1.1: Timing of repair		
Condition	*Timing*	*Side*
Isolated cleft lip	5–6 months	Unilateral
	4–5 months	Bilateral
Isolated cleft palate	16 months	Soft palate only
	SOFT palate at 6 months	Soft and hard palate
	HARD palate at 15–18 months	
Cleft lip and palate	Cleft lip and soft palate at 5–6 months	Unilateral
	Hard palate and gum pad with/without lip revision at 15–18 months	
	Cleft lip and soft palate at 4–5 months	Bilateral
	Hard palate and gum pad with/without lip revision at 15–18 months	

What are the surgical principles of cleft lip repair?

Aim of the procedure is:

1. Lengthening of the lip along the philtral line
2. Reconstruction of the orbicularis muscle across the cleft
3. Rotation of the displaced nasal base medially
4. Lengthening of the columella
5. Reconstruction of the labial sulcus.

Numerous techniques have been described. The most widely practised are:

1. Millard's rotation advancement flap
2. Tennison's advancement flap
3. Randall's technique

Technique (Millard's procedure)

The Millard's procedure accomplishes rotation of medial flap 'A' and advancement of lateral flap 'B' into the defect thus created. The rotation of flap 'A' accomplishes the creation of cupid's bow and freeing the flap 'C' to form nasal sill and advancement of flap 'B' achieves filling the defect thus created to increase the length of the columella and also rotation of nasal ala for creation of nasal orifice.

The points are marked as shown in Fig. 1.4. (1) Median point on cupid's bow, (2) edge of cupid's bow on normal side, (3) end of cupid's bow on affected side, (4) nasal ala on normal side (5) nasal septum, (6) oral commissure on normal side, (7) oral commissure on affected side, (8) point on affected side to form end of cupid's bow, (9) high point on nasal sill to form tip of advancement flap, (10) nasal ala on affected side, (11 and 12) the line extended along ala to encircle the alar cartilage (X), the back-cut on the rotation flap so that the length 3–5–x is equal to the columella (i.e. 2–5). The incisions are given as shown. The flaps 'A' and 'C' are rotated and the flap 'B' is advanced and the tissues approximated in three layers—muscle, mucosal and skin layers.

For bilateral clefts, the repair may be done either in one stage or in metachronous fashion. If the cleft is too wide and the pre-maxilla is

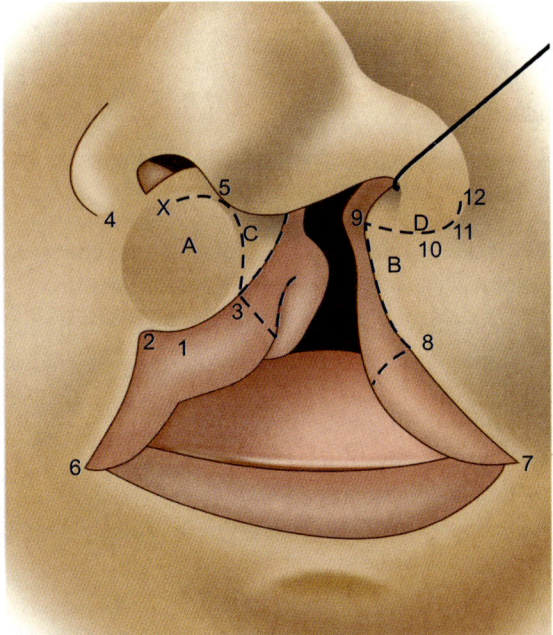

Fig. 1.4: Preoperative marking for clip lip repair

protruding, the tension free repair may not be possible. In such patients, the simple lip adhesion is done at 8–10 weeks of age followed by definitive procedure after 2–3 months when the pre-maxilla comes in line with the rest of maxilla. Any of the described technique may be used.

What are the surgical principles of cleft palate repair?

Aim of the procedure is:

1. Do soft palatal muscular reconstruction
2. Perform two layers (nasal and oral) closure of palate (both hard and soft palate)
3. Perform lengthening of the palate

Among the various techniques described, the representative ones are:

1. Straight line closure like von Langenbeck repair
2. Y-V lengthening like Veau-Wardill-Kilner repair
3. Z-plasty like Furlow repair.

Technique (Veau-Wardill-Kilner Procedure)

1. Injection of adrenal (1:100,000 dilution) reduces the bleeding during the procedure.
2. The incision is made along the junction of nasal and oral mucosa.
3. The subperiosteal flaps are raised, saving the greater palatine vessels (which form the pedicle of the flaps).
4. The release incisions are made laterally along the posterior alveolar ridge.
5. The two incisions are joined to complete a Y-shaped incision.
6. The levator and tensor palatini muscles inserted abnormally in the palatal shelves are freed.
7. The nasal mucosa is approximated in midline.
8. The soft palate muscles are approximated in midline.
9. The oral mucosal flaps are approximated in midline while pushing the palate back (lengthening the palate by closure in a V-fashion).
10. Hemostasis is secured.

What is the role of alveolar bone grafting?

The procedure is done at age of 5–8 years to support the permanent dentition. It also helps to unify the maxilla into a single unit and close oro-nasal fistula. The procedure is done using autologous bone grafts. Some centres have tried grafting at age of

1 year with favourable long-term results in terms of favourable facial growth, improved maxillary arch forms and decreased need for maxillary osteotomies and bone grafting at a later age.

What are the indications of secondary surgery?

The secondary surgery may be needed for scar revision, vermilion realignment, philtral lengthening, nasal base rotation, and correction of nasal tip cartilages. These are to be done before the child goes to school. A complete septorhinoplasty may be needed post-puberty for correction of deviated nasal septum and scar revision.

In cleft palate patients, the secondary surgery may be required for palatal fistulae with an incidence of 10–20% in best of hands. The fistulae occur most commonly at the junction of hard and soft palate or that of primary and secondary palate. The local tissue may be used or a pedicled tongue flap may be needed.

For residual velopharyngeal incompetence, manifested by nasal regurgitation or air leak in speech, pharyngoplasty may be indicated. The maxillary growth is affected in patients with cleft, with restricted anterior and transverse growth. The correction may require Le Fort I osteotomy in up to 30% patients after puberty.

Overall cleft lip and palate require a long-term follow-up and are a collection of surgeries and not just a single surgery for primary repair. Participation of a team of specialists should be considered when managing such a case.

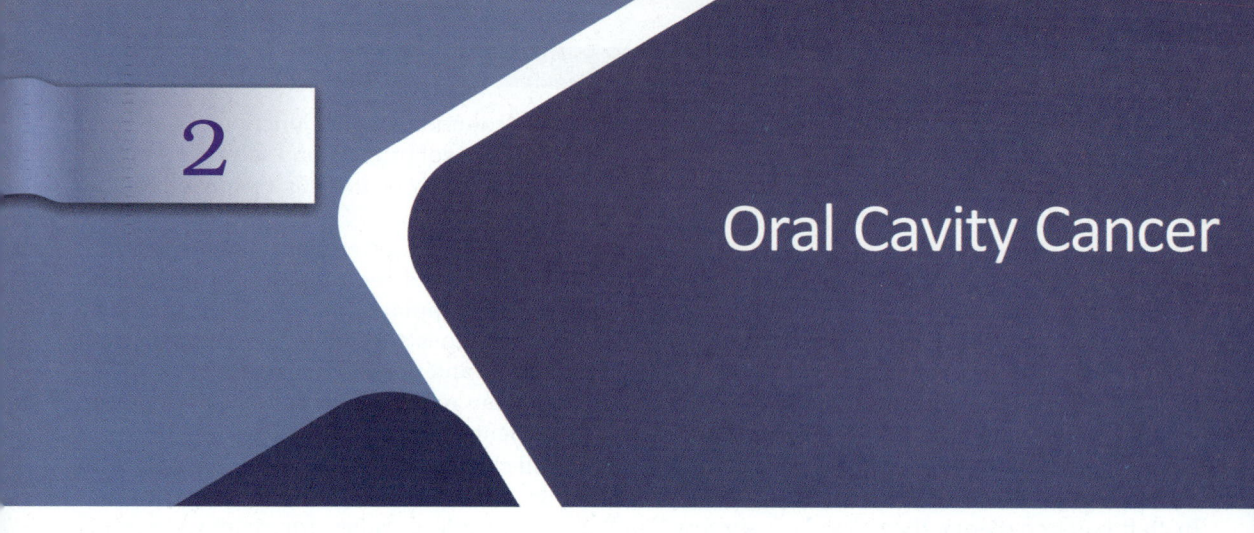

1. What is the incidence of oral cavity cancer?

Oral cavity cancer is 12th most common overall and the 8th most common malignancy in males. It accounts for 30% of head and neck cancers in India. Buccal mucosa cancer is very common in India and constitutes 42% of all oral cavity cancers in contrast to the USA where it forms only 5% of all oral cancers. High incidence of buccal mucosa cancer is due to habit of chewing betel nut with tobacco and keeping a quad in the oral cavity for a long time.

2. Describe the extent of oral cavity and what structures it includes?

Oral Cavity Extends

- Anteriorly from of skin to vermilion border of the lips.
- Posteriorly to the junction of the hard and soft palates above, and the line of circumvallate papillae below. It includes the following structures:
  - Lip mucosa extending from vermilion border
  - Anterior 2/3 of tongue
  - Buccal mucosa
  - Floor of mouth
  - Lower gingiva
  - Retromolar trigone
  - Upper gingiva
  - Hard palate

3. What is the lymph drainage of oral cavity?

Recent studies have shown that lymphatic spread from oral cavity cancer to the neck occurs due to embolic spread rather than through permeation of lymphatic channels. This concept raises a question mark on concept of en block dissection of primary tumour and lymph bearing area. Lymph spread occurs in a stepwise fashion and lower cervical and posterior cervical lymph nodes are rarely involved in oral cavity cancer

- First station nodes: Buccinator, jugulo-digastric, submandibular and submental.
- Second station nodes: Parotid, jugular and the upper and lower posterior cervical nodes.

4. What factors affect lymph node involvement in oral cavity cancer?

Larger tumor, more posterior location of tumour and the less well differentiated tumour are more likely to have lymph node metastasis.

5. What is the aetiology and risk factors for oral cavity carcinoma?

- *Tobacco consumption:* 90% of oral cavity cancers can be directly attributed to smoking. The relative risk of oral cavity cancer is seven times in comparison to non-smokers.
- *Use of alcohol:* Alcohol acts as an irritant, solvent for carcinogen and promoter for carcinogenesis. Risk of developing oral cavity cancer is six times in comparison to non-drinkers. The risk of developing oral cavity cancer is 38 times more for patients who consume both alcohol and tobacco.
- Use of alcohol and tobacco produces a field defect due to chronic carcinogen exposure.
- The entire mucosa of upper aero-digestive tract is at risk.

- Use of the areca (betel) nut
- Leucoplakia (Fig. 2.1)
- Erythroplakia
- Submucous fibrosis
- Consumption of foods rich in nitrites and nitrosamines
- Retroviruses, adenoviruses or the Epstein-Barr virus
- Herpes viruses (HSV) and the human papilloma-viruses (HPV)
- The risk of second malignancy after successful treatment of oral carcinoma is 3.7% every year and increases to 24% at 10 years.

6. Describe the pathology.

A. More than 90% are squamous cell carcinoma.

Macroscopically the squamous cell carcinoma can be:

1. Exophytic type
2. Ulcerative
3. Combination of both.

The exophytic growths are less aggressive.

B. Microscopic types:
- Basaloid type
- Verrucous type present as exophytic growth and has a more favourable prognosis with less chances of metastasis.
- Sarcomatoid type presents as bulky poly-poidal rapidly growing mass and has a very poor prognosis.
- Poorly differentiated carcinoma

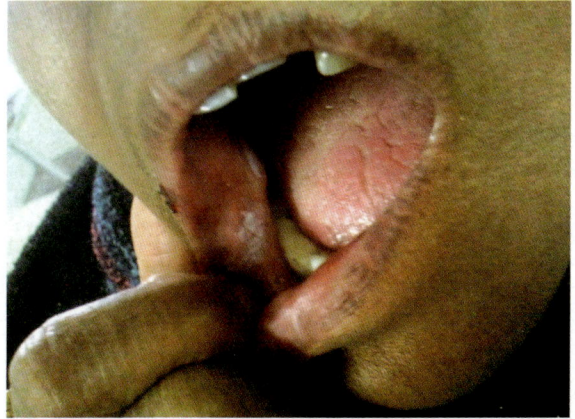

Fig. 2.1: White patch suggestive of leukoplakia of the cheek

7. What is leucoplakia?

Leucoplakia can be defined as white patch in the oral cavity which cannot be rubbed off and cannot be attributed to any other pathology. It is basically a clinical diagnosis.

Average malignant transformation rate is 3 to 6% but it increases from 15 to 31% specially for the nodular or speckled type of leukoplakia.

Prevention of Leucoplakia and malignant transformation

- Frequent consumption of fresh fruit and vege-tables reduces the risk (0.5–0.7) of developing oral cancer
- β-carotene and vitamin E can produce regression of oral leucoplakia.

8. Describe the Staging of oral cavity carcinoma.

TNM Classification

- Primary tumor (T)
  - TX: Primary tumour cannot be assessed
  - T0: No evidence of primary tumour
  - Tis: Carcinoma *in situ*
  - T1: Tumour 2 cm or less in greatest dimension
  - T2: Tumour more than 2 cm but not more than 4 cm in greatest dimension
  - T3: Tumour more than 4 cm in greatest dimension but less than 6 cm
  - T4: Tumour invades adjacent structures, e.g. mandible, skin.
- Regional lymph nodes (N)
  - Nx: Regional lymph nodes cannot be assessed
  - N0: No regional lymph node metastasis
  - N1: Metastasis in a single ipsilateral lymph node, 3 cm or less in greatest dimension
  - N2: Metastasis in a single ipsilateral lymph node, more than 3 cm but not more than 6 cm in greatest dimension; or in multiple ipsilateral lymph nodes, not more than 6 cm in greatest dimension; or in bilateral or contralateral lymph nodes, not more than 6 cm in greatest dimension

    N3: Metastasis in a lymph node more than 6 cm in greatest dimension
- Distant metastasis (M)

  Mx: Distant metastasis not assessed

  M0: No distant metastasis

  M1: Distant metastasis present

AJCC Stage Groupings

Stage 0:   Tis, N0, M0

Stage I: T1, N0, M0

Stage II: T2, N0, M0

Stage III: T3, N0, M0; T1, N1, M0; T2, N1, M0;
             T3, N1, M0

Stage IVA: T4, N0, M0; T4, N1, M0; Any T, N2,
             M0

Stage IVB: Any T, N3, M0

Stage IVC: Any T, Any N, M1

9. How do these tumours spread?

1. *Local spread*: Local spread to adjacent structures like soft tissue, bones, neurovascular structures.
2. *Lymph nodes spread*: First halt is lymph nodes in the supraomohyoidal triangle.
3. Distant metastasis is rare and occurs in advanced cases or in recurrent cases. They generally occur in lungs or bones.

10. How does mandible get involved in oral cavity carcinoma?

It generally starts through dental socket or through dental pulp and reaches the root of tooth. From root of tooth cancellous portion of mandible is involved. After this spread occurs through mandibular canal.

11. What are the various clinical features?

a. Indurated ulcer in the floor of mouth that bleeds on touch lasting for more than 4 weeks.
b. Non-healing ulcer for more than 4 weeks
c. Slurring of speech
d. Tooth extraction socket that fails to heal
e. Persistent gingival inflammation
f. Loosening of tooth
g. Trismus or ankylosis
h. Pain is a late feature
i. Orocutaneous fistula
j. Lymph nodes in the neck
k. Weight loss
l. Painless neck lump

How is preoperative clinical examination in a case of oral cavity carcinoma done?

1. Complete examination of oral cavity along with status of oral hygiene and teeth.
2. Presence of precancerous lesions like submucous fibrosis and leucoplakia is noted.
3. Tumour itself is described in detail, e.g. size of tumour, type (ulcerative, proliferative or infiltrative), involvement of adjacent structures, e.g. skin, bone, lymph nodes, trismus are all documented. (Transoral biditial examination).
4. Neck is carefully examined for lymph node enlargement.

What are the investigations needed in case of oral cavity cancer?

1. Punch biopsy from primary lesion and fine needle aspiration cytology from palpable lymph nodes. If the lesion appears to be verrucous type, then a biopsy by knife needs to be taken.
2. Imaging: Oblique and occlusive views of the mandible and ortho-pantogram (OPG) to rule out mandible involvement specially antral or alveolar involvement. CT scan is useful in doubtful cases of mandible involvement or to rule out extension of disease in infra-temporal fossa. Indications of CT are:
   a. Patient with trismus.
   b. For antral tumours.
   c. Assessment of pterygoid fossa
   d. To evaluate metastatic disease of neck
   e. Clinically negative neck
   f. Patients with large nodes
   Abdominal ultrasonography is done to rule out liver metastasis. Chest X-ray is done for pulmonary metastasis.
   MRI is useful in knowing the extent of soft tissue involvement or perineural involvement.

What are the treatment options in patients of oral cancer?

- Surgery alone
- Radiation therapy alone
- Combination of these.

Stagewise Treatment

Treatment for T1 and T2 lesions: Surgery and radiotherapy give equally good results. Any of the two methods can be utilised. Combined modality is not necessary. Choice of treatment depends upon skill and experience of clinician treating the case and the facilities available at the institution.

Radiotherapy (RT): Prior to starting radiotherapy all broken and loose teeth need to be removed and wound after teeth removal should be allowed to heal. Broken teeth should be removed before RT as the teeth become brittle after RT and there are chances of osteonecrosis of the jaw. RT is given by telecobalt machine in the dose of 6000 cg delivered in 6 weeks. For further boost at the primary site radioactive iridium wire can be implanted (brachytherapy). Advantages of RT are good cosmetic and functional results. Drawbacks of RT are dental problems, dryness of mouth due to radiotherapy induced atrophy of salivary glands and post-irradiation fibrosis leading to delayed trismus.

Surgery

It involves wide excision of lesion carried out intraorally. Raw area can be covered by split skin graft. Benefit to patient is short duration of treatment in comparison to RT. Drawbacks include shrinkage and fibrosis of graft in postoperative period leading to fibrosis and trismus. Sometimes it may be difficult to obtain a clear margin at the base.

Surgery is preferable over radiotherapy in following situations:

a. If there is concomitant submucus fibrosis
b. In presence of mandibular involvement
c. Verrucous carcinoma as it is relatively radio resistant due to less vascularity.
d. T1 lesion as a result of surgery are functionally better.
e. If there is history of previous irradiation
f. Multiple primary tumours
g. Extensive premalignant changes in surrounding areas
h. Adenocarcinoma or melanoma
i. Lesions in lower gingivo-buccal sulcus

Laser Excision

This is a recent alternative for early oral cavity cancer in which carbon dioxide or diode laser is used. The tumour can be excised with a wide margin and clear base. The resultant raw area is left open to heal by epithelisation. There is minimum blood loss and postoperative pain. A more satisfactory histopathological examination of laser excised tissue can be carried out in comparison to cautery excised tissue. An advantage of laser therapy includes very short treatment time, no dental problem, no dryness of mouth and no trismus.

Surgery for T3 and T4 Lesions

Surgery is primary modality of treatment for T3 and T4 lesions as RT is not curative in these cases. RT is only used as palliative treatment for unresectable and recurrent lesions.

Criteria for unresectability are:

1. Involvement of tonsil, hard palate or soft palate.
2. Extensive involvement of skin in the form of fungation.
3. Involvement of pterygoid muscles or infra-temporal fossa.
4. Lymph nodes involvement which are fixed.
5. Patient unfit to undergo major resection and reconstructive procedures as surgery is likely to last for more than 6 hours.

Extent of Surgery in T3 and T4 Lesions

In order to achieve curative resection a wide margin with 2 cm of healthy mucosa should be excised along with the tumour. If it is difficult to obtain clear wide margin superiorly upper teeth are removed along with mucosa of upper alveolus and alveolar bone. The mucosal flap is sutured to the mucoperiosteum of the hard palate. To obtain clear margin posteriorly tonsil can be removed. The resected margin should include all pre-cancerous lesions. It is essential that pathologist should comment on status of cut margins.

Mandibular Involvement in Buccal Mucosa Cancer

Routes of mandibular involvement

1. Direct invasion of mandible by primary tumour
2. Mandible can be involved from occlusive surface, periodontal membrane and the dental canal.
3. Once it reaches the mandibular canal it spreads widely within bone.
4. Infra-temporal fossa can be involved through the peri-neural lymphatic.
5. In elderly patients' vertical height of horizontal ramus of mandible is less as these patients are edentulous, so that mandibular canal comes near the occlusive surface and near the lower border thus there is early mandibular involvement without much chances of marginal mandibulectomy.

Types of mandibular resection in oral cavity cancer

1. **The segmental resection of mandible** is carried out in following situations:
   a. The clinical and radiological involvement of mandible.

b. To facilitate wide margin resection.

c. To facilitate reconstruction.

d. In lesions involving full thickness of cheek

As disease rarely involves the posterior segment of ascending ramus, so it is possible to perform a segmental resection of mandible without removing a L-shaped piece of bone comprising head, neck, posterior border and insertion of medial pterygoid muscle.

Marginal Mandibulectomy

In this procedure the alveolar part is removed preserving the lower border. It results in loss of teeth but without malocclusion and loss of facial contour. It is a good operation for lesions of the floor of the mouth or tongue. The line of excision extends below the mylohyoid muscle thus en block excision of the floor of the mouth is achieved. Marginal mandibulectomy has a little role in T3 or T4 lesions as in these cases one is likely to cut through the involved soft tissue.

Extent of Lymph Node Dissection

In cases of node negative cancer supra-omohyoid dissection is done which involves removal of nodes from level 1 to level 3. The specimen is submitted for frozen section. A complete neck dissection is done only if lymph node shows metastatic disease on frozen section. The classical radical neck dissection is preserved for extensive neck disease, i.e. large or multiple nodes, fixed nodes, nodes in the lower third of the deep cervical chain, nodes in the posterior triangle and recurrence in the neck after RT.

Chemotherapy

Effective chemotherapy drugs are methotrexate, 5-fluorouracil (5 FU), cisplatin and bleomycin. Chemotherapy may have a role in palliative settings, or given as neoadjuvant chemotherapy or as an adjuvant therapy after surgery.

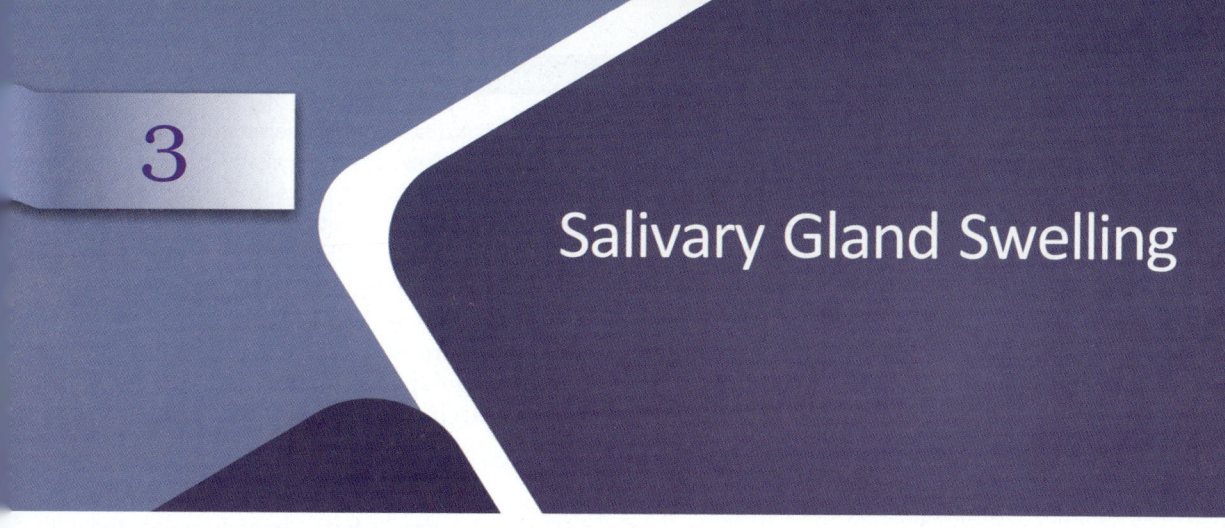

Salivary Gland Swelling

Salient Anatomical Features

The parotid gland is largest salivary gland.

Dimensions

1. On an average 5.8 cm in the cranio-caudal dimension.
2. 3.4 cm in the ventral-dorsal dimension.
3. The average weight of 14–28 gm.
4. Shape is irregular, wedge shaped, and unilobular.
5. The parotid has 5 processes (3 superficial and 2 deep), which makes it very difficult to surgically removal all parotid tissue.

What are the boundaries of the parotid compartment?

Parotid gland lies in musculoskeletal framework or recess which is bounded by:
- Anterior surface of mastoid on posterior aspect.
- Postero-superiorly it is bounded by convex surface of external acoustic meatus.
- Anteriorly by posterior border of mandibular ramus and antero-superiorly by head of mandible articulating in mandibular fossa.
- Medial wall of fossa is completed by posterior belly of diagastric, and muscles originating from styloid process, i.e. stylohyoid, styloglossus and stylopharyngeus. Stylohyoid are seen early during usual surgical exposure.

What are the contents of the parotid compartment?

Contents of parotid compartment are:
1. Parotid gland,
2. CN VII and its branches,
3. Sensory and autonomic nerves,
4. External carotid artery and its branches,
5. Retromandibular (posterior facial) vein, and parotid lymphatics.

Lobes of Parotid

1. Superficial lobe: 80% of the gland overlies the Masseter and mandible and is known as superficial lobe.
2. The remaining 20% deep lobe of the gland extends medially through the stylomandibular tunnel formed by the posterior edge of the mandibular ramus (ventral), sternodiedo-maotoid sternocleidomastoid and posterior belly of the digastric (dorsal), and the stylomandibular ligament (deep and dorsal). In addition, the stylomandibular ligament separates the parotid from the submandibular gland. This portion of the gland lies in the prestyloid compartment of the parapharyngeal space. Thus, a deep parotid tumour can push the tonsillar fossa and soft palate anteromedially.

What is parapharyngeal space?

The parapharyngeal space is of shape of inverted pyramid.
1. Base at the skull base and its apex at the greater cornu of the hyoid bone,
2. Medial boundary by the pharyngeal wall and lateral boundary by the mandibular ramus and medial pterygoid muscle.
3. This space is divided into pre- and post- styloid compartments by a line connecting the styloid process and medial pterygoid plate.

4. Deep lobe parotid tumours occupy the presty-loid compartment and tend to push the carotid sheath laterally.
5. Paragangliomas and nerve sheath tumours usually occupy the poststyloid compartment and tend to push the carotid sheath medially.
6. Parotid tumours that involve the parapharyngeal space are referred to as dumb-bell tumours.

The tail of the parotid overlies the upper ¼th of the sternocleidomastoid muscle and extends toward the mastoid process.

What is anatomical reason of pain during mastication in Parotitis?

Patients with parotitis frequently have pain with mastication because the gland becomes trapped between the mandible and mastoid process upon opening of the mouth.

Discuss anatomy of Stensen's duct (Parotid Duct).

a. Stensen's duct (parotid duct) arises from the anterior border of the parotid
b. Runs parallels to the zygomatic arch, about 1.5 cm (approximately 1 finger breadth) below the inferior margin of the arch.
c. Runs superficial to the masseter muscle.
d. Turns medially 90 degrees at the level of the second maxillary molar to pierce the buccinator muscle where it opens onto the oral cavity.
e. Using surface landmarks, Stensen's duct lies midway between the zygomatic arch and corner of the mouth along a line between the upper lip philtrum and the tragus.
f. The buccal branch of CN VII runs with the parotid duct. The duct measures 4–6 cm in length and 5 mm in diameter.

An accessory parotid gland and duct are noted in 20% of people. The accessory gland is typically found overlying the masseter, and the accessory duct typically lies cranial to Stensen's duct.

Describe anatomy of parotid fascia.

The parotid is invested in its own fascia (capsule), which is continuous with the superficial layer of deep cervical fascia.

The parotid fascia consists of:
1. *Superficial layer:* Extends from the masseter and SCM to the zygoma, and
2. *Deep layer:* Extends from the fascia of the posterior belly of the digastric muscle, and forms the stylomandibular membrane separating the parotid and submandibular glands.

The parotid fascia sends septa into the glandular tissue, which prevents the possibility of separating the glandular tissue from its investing fascia. The attachments of the parotid fascia include:
1. Anterior—mandible
2. Inferior—stylomandibular ligament
3. Posterior—styloid process

Of note, parotid tissue can herniate through the stylomandibular membrane. Thus, deep parotid tumours can present as parapharyngeal masses.

Discuss anatomical facts about seventh cranial nerve.

a. Cranial nerve VII is intimately associated with the parotid gland, dividing it into 2 surgical zones (the superficial and deep lobes).
b. CN VII exits the skull base via the stylo-mastoid foramen (styloid process—medial, mastoid process—lateral).
c. It immediately gives off three motor branches upon exiting the foramen:
   1. To stylohyoid muscle
   2. To post-auricular muscle
   3. To posterior belly of digastric

After exiting the foramen, CN VII turns laterally to enter the parotid gland at its posterior margin. The nerve then branches at the pes anserinus (Fig. 3.1) (goose's foot) approximately 1.3 cm from the stylomastoid foramen. The nerve then gives rise to 2 divisions:
1. Temperofacial (upper)
2. Cervicofacial (lower)

Followed by 5 terminal branches:
1. Temporal
2. Zygomatic
3. Buccal

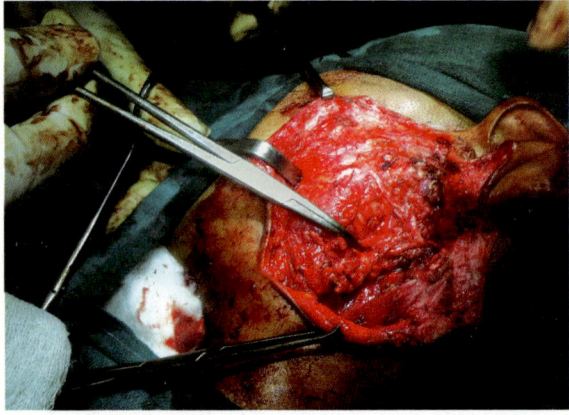

Fig. 3.1: Superficial parotidectomy showing the main facial nerve trunk and its branches

4. Marginal mandibular

5. Cervical

Of note, branches of CN VII are more superficial at the anterior border of the parotid gland, and are therefore, more prone to injury there.

How to localise CN VII during parotid surgery?

The following is a list of important surgical landmarks:

1. *Tragal pointer:* Points to the main trunk of CN VII which lies 1–1.5 cm deep and inferior to the pointer.
2. *Tympanomastoid suture:* This is traced medially and the main trunk of VII is encountered 6–8 mm deep to the suture line.
3. Posterior belly of digastric muscle is followed up to the stylomastoid foramen; the trunk of VII is just superior and posterior to the cephalic margin of the muscle.
4. Styloid process is 5–8 mm deep to the tympanomastoid suture; the trunk of VII lies on the posterolateral aspect of the styloid near its base.

Furthermore, if above mentioned methods do not work, then retrograde dissection is employed to trace one of the terminal branches proximally:

1. Buccal branch—runs with the parotid duct either superiorly or inferiorly.
2. Temporal branch—crosses the zygomatic arch parallel with the superficial temporal artery and vein.
3. Marginal mandibular branch—runs along the inferior border of the parotid superficial to the retromandibular vein.

As a last resort, one can perform a mastoidectomy to identify the nerve at the stylomastoid foramen or to identify the intra-temporal mastoid course of VII. The stylomastoid foramen is the single most constant landmark.

The great auricular nerve courses from deep to superficial around the posterior border of the sternocleidomastoid (SCM), then turns up superiorly, posterior to the external Jugular vein. This nerve arises from the cervical plexus and provides sensation to the posterior pinna and lobule. It is the first nerve encountered in parotid surgery. It usually lies lateral to the parotid fascia and deep to the platysma. The nerve can be safely divided during parotidectomy without any consequences.

What is the autonomic nerve innervation of parotid gland?

The glossopharyngeal nerve (ninth cranial nerve) provides visceral secretory innervations to the parotid gland. The nerve carries pre-ganglionic parasympathetic fibers from the inferior salivary ganglion in the medulla through jugular foramen. These fibers travel along the lesser petrosal nerve in the middle crania fossa and come out through foramen ovale to synapse in the otic ganglion. Post ganglion parasympathetic fibers exit from the otic ganglion to join the auriculotemporal nerve in the infra-temporal fossa. These fibers supply the parotid gland for secretion of saliva. The post-ganglionic sympathetic fibers arise from superior cervical ganglion and supply the salivary glands, sweat glands and cutaneous blood vessels through external carotid plexus.

Desrcibe anatomy of Auriculotemporal nerve and Frey's syndrome

The Auriculotemporal nerve, a branch of mandibular nerve, runs anterior to the external acoustic meatus and parallel to the superficial temporal artery and vein. It carries parasympathetic post-ganglionic fibers from the otic ganglion to the parotid gland. The injury to this nerve intra-operatively can lead to aberrant parasympathetic innervation to the skin overlying the parotid gland area resulting in Frey's syndrome (i.e. gustatory sweating). This nerve may be resected intentionally to avoid Frey's syndrome.

In addition, the auriculotemporal nerve provides sensory innervation to the parotid capsule, and the skin of the auricle and temporal region. This nerve is also responsible for referred pain from parotitis to the auricle, EAM, TMJ, and temples because of common innervation.

The most superficial portion of the parotid makes up the neural compartment, containing CN VII, the auriculotemporal nerve, and the great auricular nerve.

What is the arterial supply to the parotid?

The arterial compartment sits in the deep portion of the gland and contains the external carotid, internal maxillary, and superficial temporal arteries. The superficial temporal supplies the temperoparietal fascial flap which can be used to reconstruct defects left in the parotid bed after total parotidectomy for malignancy. The transverse facial artery which is branch of superficial temporal artery gives arterial supply to the parotid gland, Stensen's duct, and the masseter muscle. This transverse facial artery runs between the zygomatic arch and Stensen's duct.

How is the venous system arranged in the parotid?

The venous compartment lies in the middle of the parotid, deep to CN VII. Venous drainage is by the retromandibular vein, which is situated deep to the facial nerve. This vein runs lateral to the carotid artery, and emerges at the inferior pole of the parotid gland. The retromandibular vein joins:

1. The postauricular vein to form the external jugular
2. The anterior facial vein to form the common facial vein, which empties into the internal jugular.

Lymphatic drainage is with para-parotid and intra-parotid nodes. The para-parotid nodes are more in number and drain the temporal region, scalp, and auricle. The intra-parotid nodes receives drainage from the posterior nasopharynx, soft palate, and ear. The parotid lymphatics ultimately drain into the superficial and deep cervical lymph nodes.

What are common symptoms of salivary gland disease?

Symptoms indicative of salivary gland disorders are generally non-specific. Patients usually complain of:

1. Swelling,
2. Pain,
3. Xerostomia,
4. Foul taste, and
5. *Sialorrhoea*, or excessive salivation.

Describe relevant points in history.

The autoimmune disorder known as *Sjögren's syndrome*, for example, is common in menopausal women, while *mumps*, parotid swelling due to paramyxoviral infection usually occurs in children between the ages of 4 and 10 years.

Drug history of the patient should also be considered, as salivary function is often affected by drug usage. Xerostomia can be due to the use of diuretics, antihypertensive drugs, anticholinergics, antidepressants (particularly tricyclics), and antihistaminics.

The medical history of the patient can provide helpful hints to the current condition of the salivary glands. The many conditions of these glands is often associated with certain systemic disorders such as:

1. Diabetes mellitus,
2. Arteriosclerosis,
3. Hormonal imbalances,
4. Neurologic disorders.

Either xerostomia or sialorrhoea may be due to following:

1. Factors affecting the medullary salivary center,
2. Autonomic outflow pathway,
3. Salivary gland function itself, and
4. Fluid and electrolyte balance.

Patients who are chronically dehydrated or malnourished from bulimia or anorexia or during chemotherapy are at risk for developing parotitis.

Xerostomia can be side effect of radiation therapy to the head and neck and a history of prior radiation should be taken during these initial steps of evaluation.

Swelling and pain during meals followed by a reduction in symptoms after meals may indicate stone in the duct leading to stenosis.

Examination (Fig. 3.2)

Examination of parotid gland should involve:

1. Examination of parotid gland and duct
2. Examination of relevant structures like facial nerve, TM joint and auricle

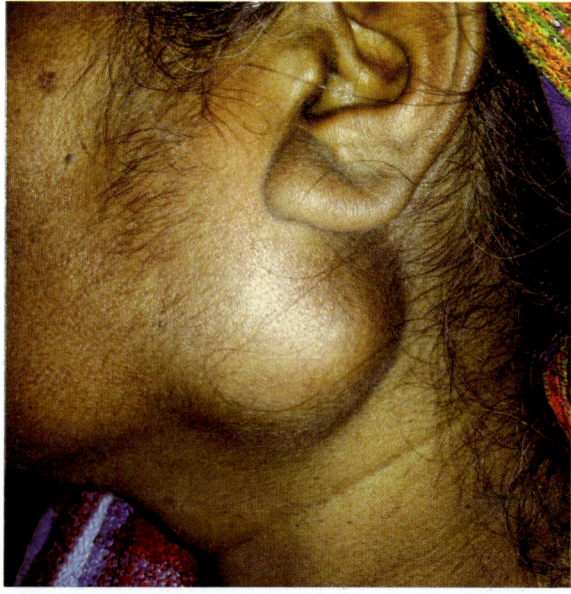

Fig. 3.2: Clinical picture of a benign pleomorphic adenoma of the left parotid

3. Examination of oral cavity
4. Examination of cervical lymph nodes

The superficial location of the parotid gland permits thorough inspection and palpation for a complete physical examination. Initial inspection involves the careful intra-oral and extra-oral examination, and should be performed in a systematic manner so as not to miss any important finding.

What are the features which suggest that a particular swelling is arising from parotid gland?

1. Location in the parotid region or fossa (boundaries of which have been described above)
2. Obliteration of retromandibular sulcus or groove.
3. Upward displacement of ear lobule.
4. Origin from skin, bone or masseter muscle has been excluded.

When does parotid gland become palpable?

Normal parotid gland is not palpable as its consistency is softer than the surrounding tissue. On the contrary normal submandibular gland is easily palpable as its consistency is harder than the surrounding tissue. When the parotid gland becomes harder or firmer due to any pathology, e.g. Sjögren disease, it becomes palpable even without enlargement.

How to state the diagnosis of parotid enlargement?

a. Is it a parotid swelling? Reason described above.
b. Is it unilateral or bilateral enlargement?
c. Type of pathology (acute or chronic/recurrent)
d. Is it a diffuse enlargement of whole of the parotid gland or is it a localized parotid lump?
e. What is the consistency of parotid lump (soft/firm/hard)?
f. Is the swelling intermittent with relation to meal and gush of saliva?
g. Are there any features of inflammation, e.g. tender swelling? Inflammatory features are seen in stone disease, parotitis or adenolymphoma (as there are degenerative changes with inflammation)
h. Are there other salivary glands or lacrimal glands involved?

What features suggest that parotid enlargement may be malignant (Fig. 3.3)?

a. Enlargement is hard in consistency with history of rapid growth in a previously static swelling.

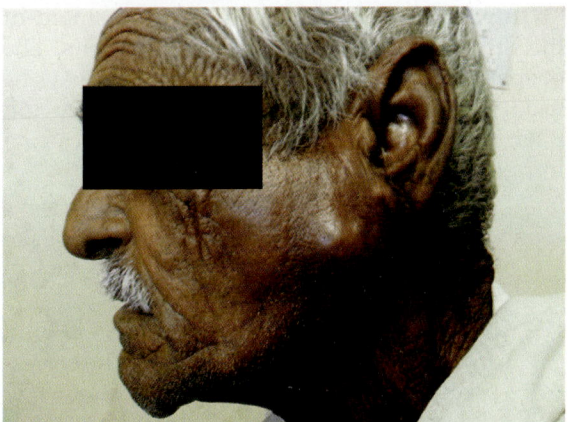

Fig. 3.3: Clinical picture of a parotid malignancy involving the overlying skin

b. Swelling is fixed to underlying structure, e.g. masseter muscle or bone.
c. Involvement of overlying skin (Fig. 3.3).
d. Facial nerve paresis which may initially be indicated by twitching in the area if the patient attempts to contract that particular group of muscle.
e. Restricted mouth opening indicating involvement of TM joint.
f. Palpable cervical lymph nodes.

Describe the scheme of examination.

1. The patient should sit three to four feet away and directly facing the examiner.
2. The examiner should inspect symmetry, color, possible pulsation and discharging sinuses on both sides of the patient.
3. Surface of swelling (smooth or irregular)
4. Margins of the swelling (well defined or diffuse)
5. Retro-mandibular sulcus maintained or obliterated
6. Position of ear lobule: Is it lifted up or not?
7. Symmetry of the face
8. Prominent veins over swelling
9. Signs of facial nerve palsy
10. *Mouth opening:* Adequate mouth opening or not? Mouth opening may be restricted due to involvement of TM joint. Adequate mouth opening is one in which patient is able to open mouth equivalent to width of his or her two fingers.

Intra-oral inspection includes assessment of the duct orifices and possible obstructions. The proper lighting with a headlight should always be used when inspecting within the oral cavity and pharynx. Following points should be noted during intra-oral examination:

A. The openings of Stensen's and Wharton's ducts can be inspected intra-orally opposite the second upper molar and at the root of the tongue, respectively.

B. Drying off the mucosa around the ducts with an air blower and then pressing on the corresponding glands will allow the examiner to assess the flow or lack of flow of saliva.

C. Sialolithiasis can sometimes be found by careful intraoral palpation.

D. Dental hygiene and the presence of periodontal disease should also be noted since deficient oral maintenance is a major predisposing factor to various infectious diseases.

E. Bimanual assessment should be performed whenever possible with the palmar aspect of the fingertips to determine the presence of deep lobe.

F. If the tonsil is shifted towards mid-line, it also indicates involvement of deep lobe.

What is the differential diagnosis of parotid swelling (non-parotid causes)?

a. Hypertrophy of masseter muscle
b. Dental cyst
c. Branchial cyst
d. Myxoma of masseter
e. Neuroma of facial nerve
f. Temporal artery aneurysm
g. Mandibular tumour
h. Mastoiditis
i. Parotid lymphadenitis
j. Subaceous cyst

Discuss aetiology of parotid enlargement.

Parotid enlargement can be due to the following etiology:

1. Congenital
2. Infective
3. Inflammatory
4. Lympho-epithelial conditions
5. Neoplastic

Common conditions giving rise to parotid enlargement are:

Acute infectious disorders which can be due to:

• Bacterial or viral aetiology
• Actinomycosis
• Chronic granulomatous disease like tuberculosis or sarcoidosis
• Tuberculosis
• Chronic viral infection
  – HIV-SGD
  – Hepatitis
  – CMV infection
• Metabolic disorders
  – Sjögren's syndrome
  – Thyroid disease
  – Diabetes (uncontrolled)
  – Alcoholism
  – Malnutrition
  – Eating disorders (anorexia, bulimia)

Classification of salivary gland tumours (WHO classification 1991, simplified)

• Adenoma
  – Pleomorphic adenoma
  – Warthin tumour
• Carcinoma
  – Acinic cell tumour
  – Mucoepidermoid carcinoma
  – Adenoid cystic carcinoma
  – Adenocarcinoma
  – Squamous cell carcinoma
  – Undifferentiated carcinoma
  – Carcinoma in pleomorphic adenoma
• Non-epithelial tumours
  – Hemangioma
  – Lymphangioma
  – Neurofibroma
  – Neurilemoma
• Malignant lymphoma
• Unclassified and allied conditions

What are causes of bilateral parotid enlargement?

a. Acute which is less than 3 weeks duration.
b. Chronic which is more than 3 weeks duration.

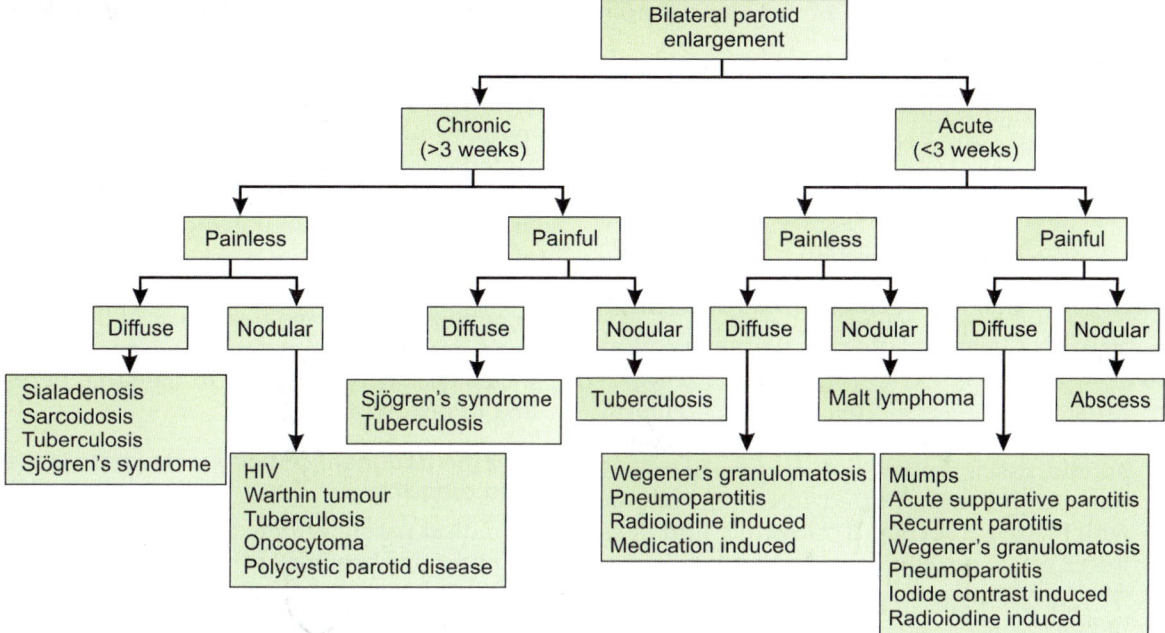

Both acute or chronic enlargement can be painful or painless. Enlargement of parotid gland can be localised to one part of parotid or diffuse.

Investigations of Salivary Gland Tumours

- CT and MRI are equally helpful in case of parotid or submandibular tumour. These imaging modalities will accurately delineate the tumours and will confirm that they are actually arising from salivary gland. These investigations will also confirm if the swelling is well localised (suggestive of benign disease) or diffuse and invasive (suggestive of malignancy). These investigations will define the relation of tumour with surrounding structures thus help in planning future surgery. As the parotid is high in fat contents it has low attenuation values. Imaging can give following important information:

  - Relation of vessels to tumour and their patency.
  - Differentiation of vessels from lymph nodes (lymph nodes enhance less than vessel).
  - Differentiation from benign and malignant lesions (benign have pushing border and malignant have ill defined infiltrative border).
  - Relation of tumour in superficial lobe with facial nerve.

  - Differentiation between deep lobe tumours and para-pharyngeal space tumours.
  - Evaluation of bone involvement by tumour.

- Open surgical incisional biopsy is absolutely contraindicated. Open biopsy is indicated if there is skin infiltration or ulceration of over-lying skin. For tumours of minor salivary gland especially on palate open incisional biopsy is indicated as at these sites there are very high chances of malignancy and biopsy can be obtained without opening other tissue planes.

- Fine Needle aspiration cytology (FNAC) is a safe alternative to open biopsy for major salivary gland. There is no risk of needle seedling if the needle used is 18 gauge or more. FNAC is better in predicting benign than malignant lesions. Advantages of getting FNAC are:

  - Additional information may be provided to the patient which helps them in decision making regarding their treatment.
  - To identify certain subgroup of patients in whom surgery can be avoided
    - Non-neoplastic disease: Sjögren's syndrome, granulomatous disease
    - Poor surgical risk in whom alternative treatment can be planned if found malignant

- If there is suspicion of metastatic cancer or lymphoma
- In poor surgical risk patients with Warthin's tumour as they rarely become malignant so surgery can be avoided.
- To prepare the patient and surgeon for more extensive surgery if FNAC reveals high grade malignancy.

What is the treatment of pleomorphic adenoma?

Surgery is the treatment of choice. Various surgical options are:

a. *Extracapsular excision*: This comprises removal of tumour including wide margin of normal parotid tissue around the margins of mixed tumour. This is indicated for small tumour which are superficially located and less than 2 cm. Every effort should be made to preserve any branch of facial nerve in relation to tumour.

b. Enucleation and postoperative radiotherapy is just mentioned to condemn it as there are high chances of recurrence and radiotherapy may accelerate malignant transformation of pleomorphic adenoma.

c. Superficial parotidectomy with preservation of facial nerve is the operation of choice. It is indicated for big tumour in the superficial lobe of the parotid gland.

d. *Total conservative parotidectomy*: It is the removal of both superficial and deep parts of the gland with preservation of the facial nerve. It is indicated for tumour deep to the facial nerve and in recurrent tumour.

What is the treatment of malignant tumour of the parotid gland?

Total radical parotidectomy and block dissection of the neck is the treatment of choice. Postoperative radiotherapy appears to improve the cure rate and prevents the uncontrollable local recurrence.

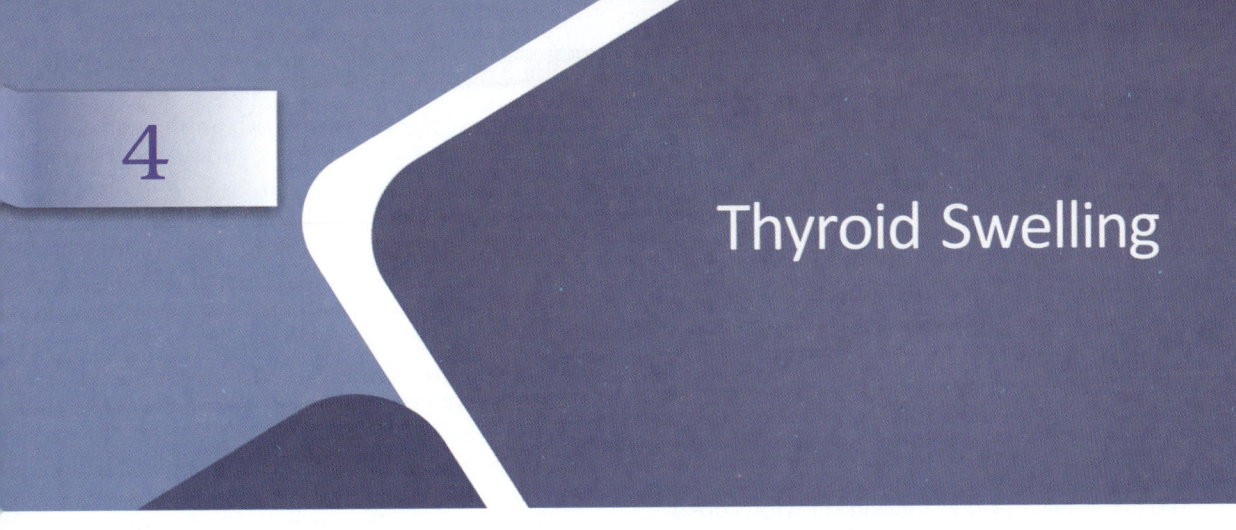

Thyroid Swelling

What is goitre?

The term Goitre means enlarged and palpable thyroid gland (Fig. 4.1). The normal weight of the thyroid gland is 18 gm in females and 25 gm in males. The thyroid gland becomes palpable when the volume of the gland is more than double of normal and the thyroid gland is visible when the volume becomes more than three times of normal.

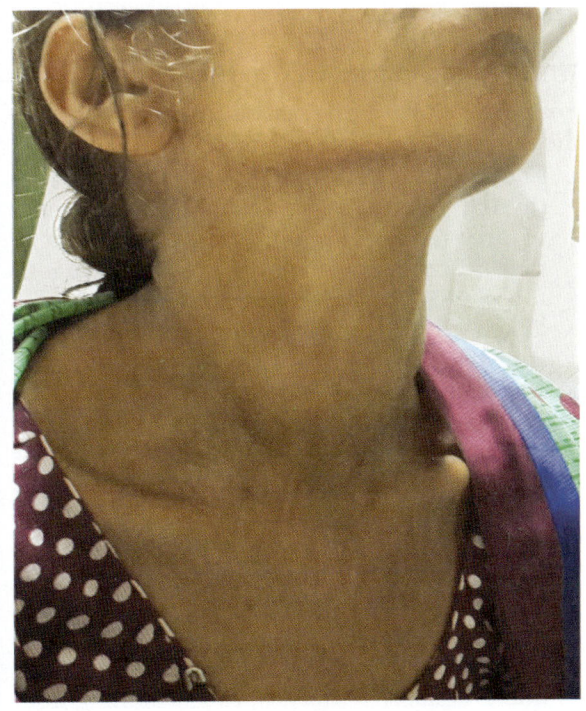

Fig. 4.1: Clinical picture of goitre

What is WHO classification of goitre?

This classification is used mainly for survey of endemic goitre in community.

Goitre can be classified as per WHO classification

- *Grade 0:* No goitre is found (the thyroid impalpable and invisible)
- *Grade 1:* Neck thickening is present as a result of enlarged thyroid, palpable, however, not visible in normal position of the neck; the thickened mass moves upwards during swallowing. Grade 1 also includes nodular goitre if thyroid enlargement remains invisible.
- *Grade 2:* Neck swelling, visible when the neck is in normal position, corresponding to enlarged thyroid—found on palpation.

Is the normal thyroid gland visible?

The normal thyroid gland is not visible except in young thin women when the isthmus may be visible.

Discuss examination of a thyroid case.

General Physical Examination

General inspection

Does the patient look ill, tense, agitated, irritable or sluggish?

Appearance of patient: Puffiness of face in hypo-thyroidism or anxious look in hyperthyroid.

Is the patient excessively sweating or feeling cold? Is he or she appropriately dressed for weather?

Pre-tibial myxoedema/generalised oedema (non-pitting)

Listen for a stridor, presence of which is suggestive of tracheal compression.

Dyspnoea

Hoarse voice, slow speech

Point to be noted in hands and arms in a thyroid case

Hypothyroid	Hyperthyroid
Bradycardia	Tachycardia—rapid/bounding pulse
Cool	Atrial fibrillation
Dry skin	Hot, sweaty
Carpal tunnel	Clubbing (Graves')
Raynaud	Onycholysis
	Fine tremor
	Systolic hypertension

Points to be noted in face in a thyroid case

Look for signs of anaemia, central cyanosis, dyspnoea as well as:

Hypothyroid	Hyperthyroid
Loss of outer eyebrow	Exophthalmos +/– ophthalmo-plegia (paralysis of one or more of extra occular muscles)
Thinning hair (women!)	Graves'
Xanthelasma	Lid lag
Corneal arcus/arcus senilis	Lid retraction
Pale, puffy face 'Toad-like'	Corneal ulceration

Inspection of the Neck

Inspection begins by looking for any scar, asymmetry, or masses. The inspection is best done from side of the neck and from the front. A scar of previous thyroid surgery points to the potential thyroid disease in patients with non-specific symptoms. The redness or erythematic skin overlying a tender swelling is seen in acute suppurative thyroiditis.

Pizillo's technique: This technique is used to make the thyroid more prominent in cases of short necked or obese persons. The patient is asked to put the hands behind the occipital region and push the head backwards against the clasped hands behind the head.

Signs of Thyroid Enlargement on Inspection

Assess the fullness on either side of the trachea below level of cricoid cartilage. To identify the thyroid gland, find the laryngeal prominence of the thyroid cartilage which is the most conspicuous prominence in the neck. Next, locate the cricoid cartilage. The isthmus of the thyroid lies just below the cricoid cartilage. Next, ask the patient to extend their neck. This will lift the trachea and stretch the skin against the thyroid, allowing for better visualization. Then, inspect the patient's neck from the side. You should see a straight line from the cricoid cartilage to the sternal notch. If there is an anterior bowing of this line, this suggests a goitre is present.

During inspection look for any tracheal deviation if it is obvious, otherwise deviation of trachea is confirmed on palpation. Inspect the swelling when the patient is swallowing water. Normally during swallowing the trachea and thyroid moves upwards from 1.5 to 3.5 cm and then hesitates momentarily before coming back to normal position. A neck swelling is likely not to be thyroid if it does not move with swallowing, or does not hesitate with trachea before coming down to original position or move in an asynchronous manner in relation to thyroid or trachea.

When will thyroid not move with swallowing?

a. When the thyroid is too big and has occupied the extensive space in the neck.
b. If there is fixation to surrounding structures as in:
   - Invasive carcinoma
   - Riedel's thyroiditis
   - Lymphoma.

Why does thyroid move with swallowing?

Following anatomical reasons are responsible for movement of thyroid with deglutination:
1. The pre-tracheal fascia splits to enclose the thyroid gland. The upper limit of attachment of pre-tracheal fascia is on oblique line of thyroid cartilage where the thyropharyngeus muscle (a part of inferior constrictor) is also attached. Thyropharyngeus muscle pulls the thyroid cartilage upwards along with the structures attached to it.
2. The pre-tracheal fascia gets thickened to form ligament of Berry. The ligament of Berry fixes the thyroid to trachea. The trachea moves upwards during second phase of deglutition.

What are the causes of breathlessness in relation to thyroid swelling?

a. Retrosternal goitre
b. Compression of trachea in long standing MNG due to collapse of tracheal rings resulting from pressure atrophy

c. Bilateral recurrent laryngeal nerve involvement due to malignancy or after surgery.

d. Erosion of trachea in malignancy

e. Congestive heart failure in thyrotoxicosis

What is pseudo goitre?

This refers to apparent thyroid enlargement when no true goitre is present. This pseudo goitre can be seen in the following situations:

a. In thin patients, thyroid lying high in the neck over thyroid cartilage may appear enlarged when actually there is no enlargement. These glands are actually of normal size on palpation. This situation commonly arises when the thyroid gland is placed more than 10 cm above the suprasternal notch.

b. Presence of other cervical masses like adipose tissue (diffuse or localised), cervical lymphadenopathy, brachial cleft cyst, or pharyngeal diverticulum that may simulate the appearance of goitre.

c. Modigliani syndrome is defined as a thyroid that appears enlarged when the person actually has an exaggerated cervical lordosis. This is named after the painter whose subjects demonstrated similar neck anatomy.

In which subgroup of patients palpation of thyroid is difficult?

Presence of kyphosis and emphysema in elderly may pose difficulties in palpation of thyroid as the cricoid bone is often displaced behind the sternum in these patients.

What is the normal size of each normal lobe?

Each normal lobe is estimated to the size of the distal phalanx of the individual thumb.

What are the different methods of palpation of thyroid gland?

A. The classical method of palpation of thyroid gland is to palpate from behind (Fig. 4.2). The clinician stands behind the patient and palpates with both hands on front. The first step is to identify the cricoid cartilage and palpate the

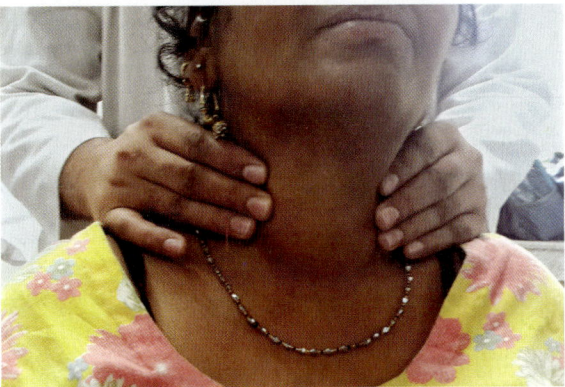

Fig. 4.2: Palpation of goitre from behind

isthmus of thyroid gland which lies horizontally just below cricoid cartilage. The isthmus can be palpated by thumb then the both lateral lobes are palpated together. Ask the patient to flex the neck slightly forward to relax the sternocleidomastoid muscles and place the three fingers of both hands on the patient's neck so that your index fingers are just below the cricoid cartilage, then ask the patient to sip and swallow water as before. Feel for thyroid isthmus rising up under the finger pads.

B. *Lahey's method:* The examiner stands in front of the patient. To palpate left lobe, the thyroid is pushed to the left from side by left hand so that left lobe becomes prominent. The left lobe is palpated by right hand and vice versa.

C. *Crile method of palpation:* Thyroid examination is done while patient is swallowing water. For palpating left lobe clinician stands on the right side. The left thumb is used to palpate the left lobe of thyroid. For palpating right lobe two fingers of right hand or the right thumb can be used.

What are the signs and symptoms of tracheal obstruction?

a. In a partially obstructed trachea a harsh noise is heard (stridor) as the patient breathes. If the obstruction is mild, one has to listen in a quiet room.

b. Later on as the obstruction becomes more obvious breathlessness cyanosis and restlessness become obvious.

c. The Kocher's test is used to detect tracheo-malacia or tracheal obstruction. The slight push on lateral lobes will produce stridor. However, this test is mentioned to condemn as it can cause acute respiratory distress due to collapse of tracheal rings by pressure of examiners finger.

What thyroid conditions give rise to tracheal obstruction?

a. Thyroid malignancy directly infiltrating into the lumen of trachea especially anaplastic carcinoma.
b. Retrosternal goitre
c. Long standing multi-nodular goitre giving rise to atrophy of tracheal rings
d. Riedel's thyroiditis

What is the consistency of normally thyroid gland and in various other conditions?

The consistency of normal thyroid gland is described as rubbery. In patients with Graves' disease thyroid gland feels softer than normal and is typically described as spongy and malleable. In Riedel's thyroiditis there is woody consistency. In malignancy and lymphoma the consistency is stony hard. Hard consistency can also be seen in calcification of nodule and haemorrhage into a nodule. Hashimoto's glands are firmer in consistency due to extensive fibrosis.

What is the accuracy of clinical examination in palpating nodules?

Only 6% of nodules less than 0.5 cm are palpable and about 50% of nodules more than 2 cm diameter are reliably detected by experienced examiner.

What are the signs of toxicity of goitre on clinical examination? (Rule of T)

Signs of toxicity in a goitre are following:
a. Tachycardia especially increased sleeping pulse rate
b. Tremors in the hands or tongue. These are fine tremors.
c. Thrill (bruit) over the goitre.
d. Toxic eye signs

What is Delphian node?

The Delphian node drains the thyroid gland and larynx. It lies anterior to the cricothyroid ligament just above the isthmus. The word Delphian refers to the ancient Greek "Delphi". Delphi was the site of the Delphic oracle, the most important oracle in the classical Greek world, and it was a major site for the worship of the God Apollo. The node is called "Delphian" because it is the first lymph node of the anterior neck structures exposed in surgery. It often heralds thyroid carcinoma, just as the oracle at Delphi in ancient Greek mythology foretold the future. Involvement of this node is the earliest sign of metastatic papillary carcinoma. It may also be enlarged in laryngeal cancer, subacute granulomatous thyroiditis, Graves' disease and rarely in Hashimotos's thyroiditis.

What are different methods to ascertain the possibility of retrosternal extension?

The retrosternal extension on clinical examination can be ascertained by following methods:
a. Inability to feel the lower border of thyroid or lower border only palpable at the peak of deglutition.
b. Dullness on percussion of manubrium sterni.
c. Positive Pemberton sign: The sign named after Hugh Spear Pemberton, an English physician (1890–1956) was described in a brief communication in the Lancet in 1946. Pemberton's sign is defined as the development of facial plethora, cyanosis, and distension of neck veins while raising both arms simultaneously. A positive test indicates thoracic inlet obstruction. This sign was originally described in patients with retrosternal goitre, but may also be seen in lung carcinoma, lymphomas, thymomas, dermoid cysts, or aortic aneurysms.
d. *How to perform Pemberton's test*: Have your patient hold his arms above his head, with elbows touching his ears. A negative Pemberton's sign occurs when nothing happens for three minutes. A positive sign is a sensation of stuffiness, dizziness, congestion, or a "funny feeling" in the head. The face can become dusky as well. When the arms rise anteroposterior diameter of thoracic inlet decreases as the thoracic inlet get raised by bilateral contraction of sternal heads of sternocleidomastoid muscles, and, if a retrosternal goitre or other similar enlargement is present, obstruction can occur.

What are the signs of malignancy on clinical examination of thyroid?

a. History of rapid increase in size of goitre.

b. History of radiation to the head and neck or thorax.

c. Presence of hard nodules

d. If the goitre is not moving with deglutition.

e. Involvement of recurrent laryngeal nerve leading to difficulty in breathing or hoarseness of voice.

f. Palpable cervical lymph nodes along with goitre.

g. *Berry's sign positive:* The positive Berry's sign means that the carotid pulsation are not palpable on the side of goitre as the malignant goitre engulfs the carotid sheath and the structures in it. On the other hand, benign enlargement of thyroid pushes the carotid pulsation laterally.

What questions one should be able to answer at the end of clinical examination of thyroid case?

a. The type of goitre, i.e. diffuse, multi-nodular, solitary nodular.

b. Functional status of thyroid gland, i.e. hyper-functioning, hypo-functioning or euthyroid on the basis of clinical examination.

c. Any feature of malignancy as discussed above.

d. Is there any feature of retrosternal extension as discussed above?

What is the pathology of eye signs in Graves' disease? (Adapted from institute of ophthalmology, RUMS)

In patients with Graves' disease, eye signs may precede, coincide with or follow the hyper-thyroidism.

Activated T cells infiltrate orbital contents and stimulate fibroblasts, leading to:

1. Enlargement of extra ocular muscles

2. Cellular infiltration of interstitial tissues

3. Proliferation of orbital fat and connective tissue

Enlargement of extra ocular muscles occurs by following mechanism:

    a. The stimulated fibroblasts produce glycosaminoglycans (GAGs) which cause the muscle to swell

    b. Muscle size may increase by up to 8 times

c. The swollen muscles occupy orbital space and can compress the optic nerve

d. These swollen muscles can cause a forward propulsion of the globe (proptosis) so that the eyelids do not cover well and eyes dry out, causing exposure keratopathy

Five Main Clinical Manifestations

1. Soft tissue involvement
2. Eyelid retraction
3. Proptosis
4. Optic neuropathy/exposure keratopathy
5. Fibrosed muscles

Soft Tissue Involvement

Symptoms

a. Variable grittiness

b. Photophobia

c. Lacrimation

Signs

a. Periorbital and lid swelling

b. Conjunctiva hyperemia—sensitive sign of disease activity

c. Chemosis (oedema of the conjunctiva)

d. Severe cases: Conjunctiva prolapses over lower eyelid—watery eyes

Eyelid Retraction

1. Retraction of both upper and lower eyelids occur in 50% of patients

2. Normally, upper eyelid rests about 2 mm below the limbus, with lower eyelid resting at the inferior limbus

3. When retraction occurs, the sclera (white) can be seen. Causes cosmetic problems

4. Pathogenesis not clear

5. May be due to contraction of the levator muscle by fibrosis, or be chemically induced by high thyroid hormone levels

6. If persists when disease is inactive, can be helped by eyelid surgery

Eyelid Retraction

Clinical Features

Clinical signs:

A. Lid retraction in 1° (front) gaze

B. Lid lag, i.e. delayed descent of upper lid in downgaze

C. Staring appearance of the eyes

Proptosis is axial

- Thyroid eye disease is the most common cause of both bilateral and unilateral proptosis in adults
- Proptosis is uninfluenced by Rx of hyper-thyroidism and is permanent in 70% of cases
- Severe proptosis prevents adequate lid closure, and may lead to severe exposure keratopathy and corneal ulceration.

Optic Neuropathy

- Serious complication affecting about 5% of patients
- Caused mainly through direct compression of the optic nerve or its blood supply by enlarged and congested rectus muscles at the orbital apex
- May occur in the absence of proptosis
- Can cause severe but preventable visual impairment
- An early sign is decreased colour vision
- Slow progressive impairment of visual acuity
- Visual defects, especially central scotomas
- Optic atrophy in chronic advanced cases

What are causes of thyroid nodules?

Causes of thyroid nodules

Benign aetiology
- Multinodular (sporadic) goitre ("colloid adenoma")
- Hashimoto's (chronic lymphocytic) thyroiditis
- *Cysts:* Colloid, simple, or haemorrhagic
- Follicular adenomas
  - Macrofollicular adenomas
  - Microfollicular or cellular adenomas
  - Hurthle-cell (oxyphil-cell) adenomas

Malignant Aetiology

- Papillary carcinoma
- Follicular carcinoma
- Minimally or widely invasive oxyphilic (Hurthle-cell) type
- Medullary carcinoma
- Anaplastic carcinoma
- Primary thyroid lymphoma
- Metastatic carcinoma

What are different types of goitre?

The goitre can be diffuse, multinodular goitre (MNG) or solitary nodular goitre (SNG).

The diffuse goitre means both lobes of thyroid are enlarged and smooth surfaced.

The multi-nodular goitre means more than one nodule is palpable on the surface of thyroid gland.

The solitary nodular goitre means except one nodule nothing else is palpable in the region of thyroid.

The goitre can be hyper-functioning, hypo-functioning or euthyroid.

Causes of Multinodular Goitre

- *Endemic or sporadic:* Endemic goitre is one when more than 10% of population is suffering from goitre.
- Iodine deficiency
- Environmental goitrogens
- *Dietary goitrogens:* Vegetables with goitrogenic effect contain thioglycosides or cyanogenic glycosides. In this context cigarette smoking is thought to be a cofactor for goitrogenesis, since it increases serum thiocyanate concentration.
- Genetic defects of thyroid hormone action like T4 receptor defects
- Genetic defects of thyroid hormone synthesis
- *Goitrogenic drugs:* Lithium, carbutamide, aminoglutehiemide and fluoride
- *Thyroiditis syndrome:* They give rise to acute development of goitre. This inflammatory thyroid disease may be painful as in acute thyroiditis or sub-acute thyroiditis of de Quervain. Pain in acute MNG gives rise to suspicion of granulomatous thyroiditis such as sarcoidosis or tuberculosis.
- TSH producing pituitary adenoma

Clinical Symptoms of Multinodular Goitre

- Feeling of tightness or feeling of foreign body are non-specific and are independent of actual thyroid volume or nodules.
- Dysphagia and urge to cough are usually caused by retrotracheal thyroid tissue and usually detected during surgery.
- Hoarseness is due to functional impairment of recurrent laryngeal nerve resulting from pressure.
- Dyspnaea and stridor are usually due to tracheal compression or by dislocation of trachea by episternal or intra-thoracic goitre
- Venous obstruction

What is the rate of enlargement of benign non-toxic MNG?

There is linear relationship between age, thyroid volume and nodularity with an average yearly increase of 4.5% of thyroid volume.

Enumerate different causes of solitary nodular goitre (SNG)?

Causes of SNG are

a. *Dominant nodule:* In this condition only one nodule is palpable and other nodules are small not clinically palpable. Dominant nodule is the cause of SNG in more than 50% of cases.
b. Papillary carcinoma
c. Follicular carcinoma
d. Anaplastic carcinoma
e. Follicular adenoma
f. Haemorrhage in one of the necrotic nodule of MNG and become large
g. If only one lobe is enlarged in Hashimoto's thyroiditis

How much is the prevalence of cancer in thyroid nodules?

Clinical importance of thyroid nodules lies in excluding thyroid cancer, which accounts for 4.0 to 6.5% of all thyroid nodules in non-surgical series. Non-palpable nodules have the same risk of malignancy as palpable nodules.

In which subgroup of patient the prevalence of cancer is high in thyroid nodules?

The prevalence of cancer is higher in several groups:

- Children
- Adults less than 30 years or over 60 years old
- Patients with a history of head and neck irradiation
- Patients with a family history of thyroid cancer
- Serum TSH is an independent risk factor for predicting malignancy in a thyroid nodule. The prevalence of malignancy is around 29.7% for patients with serum TSH >5.5 mU/L. When cancer is diagnosed, a higher TSH is associated with a more advanced stage of cancer.

On the other hand, the prevalence of cancer is lower in nodules in multi-nodular goiters. All autonomously hyper-functioning ("hot") nodules are practically benign.

What investigations should be performed in a case of goitre?

Serum TSH: Thyroid function should be assessed in all patients with thyroid nodules. If the serum TSH concentration is low, it indicates overt or subclinical hyperthyroidism, the thyroid scintigraphy should be performed next.

If the serum TSH concentration is normal or elevated, then fine needle aspiration biopsy is indicated. The patients with a high serum TSH concentration also require an evaluation for hypothyroidism.

Thyroid Ultrasonography

It should be performed in all patients with thyroid nodules. The nodularity in goitre can be due to varied aetiology like from Hashimoto's thyroiditis resulting from focal enlargement from lymphocytic infiltrates, TSH-induced hyperplasia of follicular tissue, or a thyroid tumour.

Ultrasonography may also help to distinguish among these possibilities.

It gives following information:

- Gives information regarding size and anatomy of gland and adjacent structures
- It provides much more information than physical examination and thyroid scan
- Ultrasound findings can be used to select nodules for FNA biopsy
- Ultrasound can identify nodules on posterior aspect of thyroid or predominantly cystic nodules
- Thyroid volume can be calculated by USG using formula of ellipsoid with empirical correction factor of 0.479. Thickness, width and length of both thyroid lobes is measured and thyroid volume is corrected by following formula:

  axbxcx0.479

  a, b, c represent maximum length, maximum width and maximum thickness.

Thyroid Scintigraphy

Thyroid scintigraphy determines the functional status of a nodule. A low serum TSH, indicating overt or subclinical hyperthyroidism, increases the possibility that a thyroid nodule is hyperfunctioning. Thus, thyroid scintigraphy should be performed in patients with a low serum TSH concentration.

Thyroid scintigraphy can be used to select nodules for FNA. Scintigraphy is done by using one of the radioisotopes of iodine (usually ^{123}I) or technetium-99m pertechnetate, however, radio-iodine scanning is preferred as 5% of thyroid cancers concentrate pertechnetate, but not radio-iodine These nodules may appear hot or indeterminate ("warm") on pertechnetate scans and cold on radioiodine scans. The nodule may appear cold (non-functioning), warm or hot on scintiscan.

Fine Needle Aspiration Cytology (FNAC)

The American Thyroid Association recommends FNA biopsy as the procedure of choice for evaluating thyroid nodules and selecting candidates for surgery. FNA biopsy has resulted in improved diagnostic accuracy, a higher malignancy yield at the time of surgery, and significant cost reductions.

FNA

a. A simple and safe office procedure

b. In this procedure tissue samples are obtained for cytological examination using 23 to 27 gauge (commonly 25 gauge) needles with or without ultrasound guidance.

c. The adequate samples can be obtained in 90 to 97% of aspirations of solid nodules.

Recommendations for FNA in Thyroid Nodules

a. Solid hypo-echoic nodules (palpable or non-palpable) measuring >1 cm in the absence of risk factors

b. Solid nodules that are iso-echoic or hyper-echoic, if they are $\geq$1.0 to 1.5 cm

c. Mixed cystic-solid nodules without suspicious features on ultrasound, if they are $\geq$ 2.0 cm

d. Spongiform nodules, defined as an aggregation of multiple micro-cystic components in more than 50% of the nodule volume, may not require FNA regardless of size, although it may be prudent to biopsy spongiform nodules >2.0 cm.

e. In presence of abnormal cervical lymph nodes all nodes should be biopsied

f. Solid nodules with micro-calcification nodules more than 1 cm should be biopsied

In High-risk History all Nodules should be Biopsied

a. History of thyroid cancer in one or more first degree relatives;

b. History of external beam radiation as a child;

c. Exposure to ionising radiation in childhood or adolescence;

d. Prior hemi-thyroidectomy with discovery of thyroid cancer;

e. 18FDG avidity on PET scanning;

f. MEN2/FMTC-associated RET proto-oncogene mutation;

g. Calcitonin >100 pg/mL

When cytologic results show follicular lesion/atypia or follicular neoplasm, the results are often called indeterminate. The risk of malignancy with these cytologic classifications ranges from 5 to 32% and the majority of these patients undergo thyroid surgery.

However, in most of these patients who undergo surgery the pathology is found to be benign. There are two approaches to the molecular characterisation of FNA aspirates that are commercially available: Identification of particular molecular markers of malignancy, such as BRAF and RAS mutational status, and use of high density genomic data for molecular classification (an FNA-trained mRNA classifier). The mRNA classifier measures the activity level of 167 genes within the nodule (using the FNA aspirate).

What are the different approaches regarding treatment of goitre?

a. *Observation:* Patients with an asymptomatic non-toxic MNG can be safely observed without specific treatment. Growth preventing intervention is usually unnecessary, as benign nodules usually grow quite slowly.

b. *Iodine supplementation:* Iodine supplementation is usually effective in reducing thyroid size in children and adolescents living in iodine deficient areas.

c. *Thyroxine suppression:* Recent trials have shown a beneficial effect of thyroxine treatment for both diffuse goitres and thyroid nodules. A goitre reduction of 20–40% can be achieved, but results are variable. The suppression of the serum TSH level should be between 0.5 and 0.1 mIU/L without going below this limit. Thyroid nodule reduction has been achieved with TSH being kept in the lower part of the normal range to minimize potential side effect.

d. *Radioactive iodine therapy:* Radioiodine therapy of non-toxic goitres is commonly performed in Europe as it is a reasonable therapeutic option, especially in patients who are older or have a contraindication to surgery. Careful studies have shown a reduction in thyroid volume in nearly all patients after a single dose of therapy. Of patients with non-toxic diffuse goitre treated with radioactive iodine, 90% have an average of 50–60% reduction in goitre volume after 12–18 months, with a reduction in compressive symptoms. The decrease in goitre size has positively correlated with the dose of iodine-131. Reduction in goitre size is greater in younger patients and in individuals who have only a short history of goitre or who have a small goitre. Baseline TSH is not a predictor of response to radioactive iodine. Obstructive symptoms improved in most patients who received radioactive iodine. Adverse effects, including thyroiditis occurred, but no patient reported worsening of compressive symptoms requiring treatment. No long-term follow-up reports on patients treated with radioactive iodine exist. Patients should always be monitored clinically after ^{131}I therapy, for evidence of goitre re-growth.

Transient hyperthyroidism is rare and typically occurs in the first 2 weeks after treatment. Only a small percentage (~20%) of patients with non-toxic goitre develop hypothyroidism after radioactive iodine treatment. Recombinant human TSH (rhTSH) may have a role in radioactive iodine treatment for nontoxic goitre. Pretreatment with rhTSH 24 hours prior to therapy can reduce the amount of radioiodine needed to shrink the goitre (up to a 50% reduction).

Surgery

Indications of Surgery for Nontoxic MNG

a. Cosmetic reasons
b. Compressive symptoms (tracheal or esophageal)
c. Retro-sternal goitre
d. Suspicious nodules

Type of Surgery

Subtotal thyroidectomy is performed leaving normal amount of thyroid tissue on each side (8 gm). Care is taken to remove all visible nodules.

Another option is Dunhill procedure in which total lobectomy is performed on the side which is mainly involved in the pathology and on less involved side partial lobectomy is done.

After bilateral subtotal thyroidectomy, all patients require thyroid hormone replacement therapy. The full replacement therapy should start immediately after surgery, with TSH levels checked 3–4 weeks postoperatively. Adjust thyroid hormone therapy, such as T4, to maintain a TSH level in the reference range. Some evidence exists that thyroid hormone replacement therapy prevents recurrence of non-toxic goitre after surgical removal.

What is toxic nodular goitre?

A toxic nodular goitre (TNG) contains autonomously functioning thyroid nodules, with resulting hyperthyroidism. TNG, also known as Plummer's disease, was first described by Henry Plummer in 1913. It is the second most common cause of hyperthyroidism after Graves' disease. In areas of endemic iodine deficiency, it is the most common cause of hyperthyroidism especially in elderly persons.

What is the pathophysiology of TNG?

- There are single or multiple nodules in MNG which are autonomour and hyper-functioning.
- The single hyper-functioning nodule is known as toxic adenoma.
- The nodules become autonomous due to somatic mutation in the thyrotropin or TSH receptor.
- Autonomous nodules become toxic in 10% of patients particularly if the nodule is more than 2.5 cm in diameter.

Treatment of Toxic Nodular Goitre?

As TNG is not an autoimmune disease so it rarely remits. All patients who have autonomously functioning nodules should be treated definitely with radioactive iodine or surgery.

Radioactive ^{131}I treatment (RAI): In the Western countries radioactive iodine is considered the treatment of choice for TNG. Except for pregnancy, there are no absolute contraindications to radio-iodine therapy.

A fixed dose of using 370 megabecquerels is used. A single dose of radioiodine therapy has a success rate of 85–100% in patients. Radioiodine therapy may reduce the size of the goitre by up to 40%.

- Failure of initial treatment with radioactive iodine has been associated with increased goitre size and higher T3 and free T4 levels and suggests a need for higher doses of radioactive [131]I.
- A positive correlation exists between radiation dose uptake by the thyroid and decrease in thyroid volume. In patients with uptake of less than 20%, pretreatment with lithium, PTU, or recombinant TSH can increase the effectiveness of iodine uptake and treatment. This treatment may be valuable in elderly patients in whom surgery is considered high risk.

Complications RAI

- Hypothyroidism occurs in 10–20% of patients.
- Tracheal compression due to thyroid swelling after radiation therapy is no longer considered to be a risk.
- In about 4% of patients clinically significant radiation-induced thyroiditis develop with features of mild hyperthyroidism. These patients should be treated symptomatically with beta blockers.
- Elderly patients may have exacerbation of congestive heart failure.
- Thyroid storm is a rare complication which can develop in patients with rapidly enlarging goitres or high total T3 levels. Patients with these conditions should receive pretreatment with anti-thyroid drugs.

Pharmacotherapy

Anti-thyroid drugs and beta blockers are used for short courses in the treatment of TNG; to make patients euthyroid in preparation surgery and in treating hyperthyroidism while awaiting full clinical response to radioiodine. Patients with subclinical disease at high risk of complications (e.g. atrial fibrillation, osteopenia) may be given a trial of low dose methimazole (5–15 mg/d) or beta blockers and should be monitored for a change in symptoms or for disease progression that requires definitive treatment.

Surgical therapy

Surgical therapy is usually reserved for
- Young individuals
- Patients with 1 or more large nodules
- Patients with obstructive symptoms,
- In patients with dominant nonfunctioning or suspicious nodules,
- In patients who are pregnant,
- In patients in whom radioiodine therapy has failed.
- In patients who require a rapid resolution of the thyrotoxic state.
  - Subtotal thyroidectomy results in cure of hyperthyroidism in 90% of patients and allows for rapid relief of compressive symptoms.
  - Restoring euthyroidism prior to surgery is mandatory
  - Complications of surgery include the following:
    - In patients who are treated surgically, the frequency of hypothyroidism is similar to that found in patients treated with radioiodine (15–25%).
    - Complications include permanent vocal cord paralysis (2.3%), permanent hypoparathyroidism (0.5%), temporary hypoparathyroidism (2.5%), and significant postoperative bleeding (1.4%).
    - Other postoperative complications include tracheostomy, wound infection, wound hematoma, myocardial infarction, atrial fibrillation, and stroke.
    - The mortality rate is almost zero.

How are tumours of the thyroid classified?

As per WHO 2010 the thyroid tumours can be classified as (Fig. 4.3):
- Primary
  - Epithelial
    - Follicular origin
      □ Benign
        ▫ Follicular adenoma (conventional type)
        ▫ Follicular adenoma (oncocytic type)
      □ Uncertain malignant potential
        ▫ Hyalinizing trabecular tumour
      □ Malignant
        ▫ Papillary carcinoma

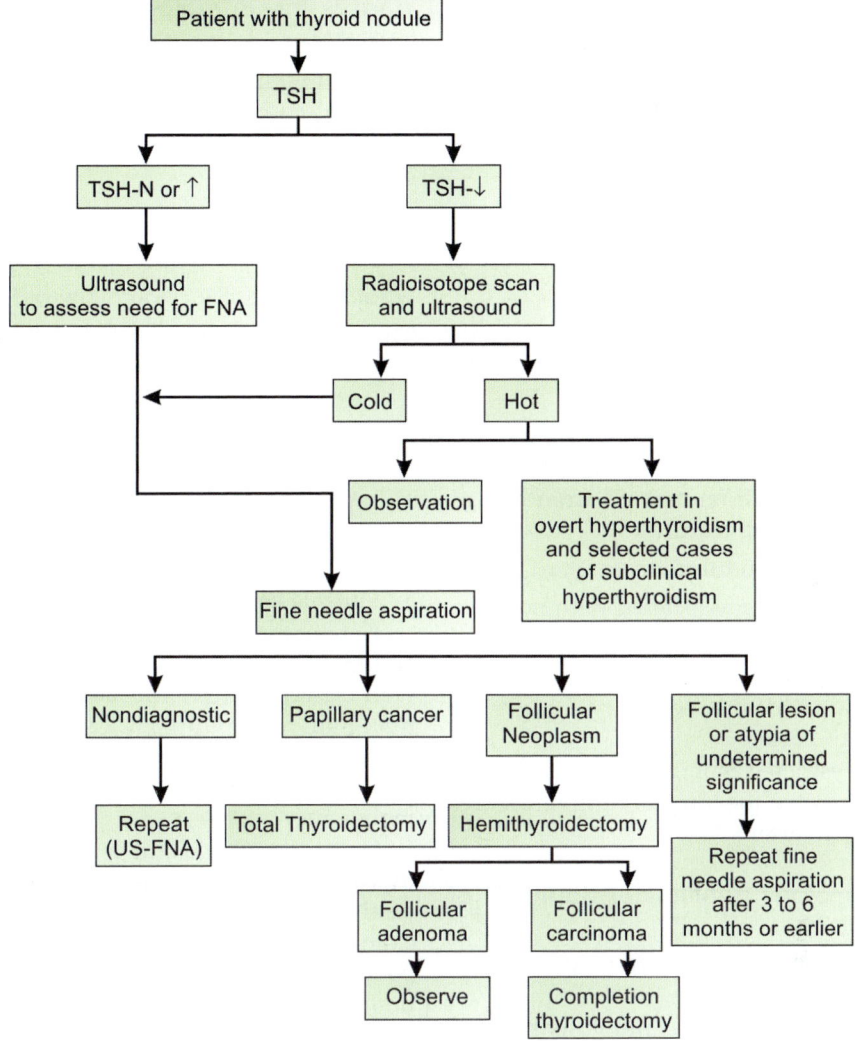

Fig. 4.3: Algorithm showing management of thyroid nodule

- Follicular carcinoma
  - ✧ Conventional type
  - ✧ Oncocytic type
- Poorly differentiated carcinoma
- Anaplastic (undifferentiated) carcinoma
- C-cell origin
  - Medullary carcinoma
- Mixed follicular and C-cell origin
  - Mixed medullary and follicular carcinoma
  - Mixed medullary and papillary carcinoma

- Epithelial tumours of different or uncertain cell origin
  - Mucoepidermoid carcinoma
  - Sclerosingmucoepidermoid carcinoma with eosinophilia
  - Squamous cell carcinoma
  - Mucinous carcinoma
  - Spindle cell tumour with thymus-like differentiation (SETTLE)
  - Carcinoma showing thymus-like differentiation (CASTLE)
  - Ectopic thymoma
- Nonepithelial

– Primary lymphoma and plasmacytoma
– Angiosarcoma
– Teratoma
– Smooth muscle tumours
– Peripheral nerve sheath tumours
– Paraganglioma
– Solitary fibrous tumour
– Follicular dendritic cell tumour
– Langerhans cell histiocytosis
– Rosai-Dorfman disease
– Granular cell tumour
• Secondary (metastatic)

What are the characteristics of thyroid tumours?

Thyroid tumours are differentiated from benign lesions by the following features:

1. The new nodule is in tumours are hard
2. Thyroid tumours are associated with nodes in the neck
3. They grow rapidly
4. They are associated with secondary changes like hoarseness of voice
5. They have restricted mobility
6. They may involve the surrounding structures like the carotid artery

What is the etiology behind development of thyroid tumours?

The risk factors for development of thyroid carcinoma include:

• *Ionizing radiation*: Thyroid gland is sensitive to medical or accidental exposure to ionizing radiation. Latency period after medical radiation exposure for treatment of various conditions is about 30 years or more. Papillary carcinoma is common in such situations.
• Genetic syndromes like Gardner's syndrome, familial adenomatous polyposis and Cowden's disease may be associated with papillary carcinoma. MEN syndrome is associated with medullary carcinoma where the tumour is bilateral and multicentric.
• In patients of long standing goitre follicular carcinoma may develop due to overstimulation by TSH or prolonged stimulation.
• Thyroid may be involved in lymphomas or lymphoma may arise de novo in cases of Hashimoto's or autoimmune thyroiditis.

What is the common differential of thyroid tumours?

The common differential diagnosis includes:
1. Calcified nodular goitre
2. Thyroid carcinoma
3. Thyroiditis
4. Neurofibroma
5. Malignant involvement of lymph nodes

What is the classification of thyroid malignancy?

Thyroid malignancy may be divided into the following types:
• Papillary carcinoma of thyroid
• Medullary carcinoma of thyroid
• Follicular carcinoma of thyroid
• Lymphoma
• Secondary metastases to thyroid
• Anaplastic carcinoma
• Hurthle cell variant

Carcinoma of the thyroid is the most common endocrine malignancy. Most of these tumours are well differentiated. The most common thyroid malignancy is papillary carcinoma thyroid. It accounts for more than 50% of all thyroid cancers. Follicular carcinoma is the next most common malignancy.

Hurthle cell variant is a form of follicular thyroid cancer that arises from the oxyphyllic cells of the thyroid which secrete thyroglobulin. Compared to the follicular carcinoma only a small percentage of these tumours (15–20%) are malignant but they have a propensity to be multifocal, bilateral and associated with positive lymph nodes. This tumour does not take up radio-iodine but is detected using sestamibi scan.

Papillary, follicular and Hurthle cell variant are classified together as differentiated thyroid cancers.

Describe the TNM Staging of thyroid tumours.

TX   Primary tumour cannot be assessed

T0   No evidence of primary tumour is found

T1   Tumour size ≤2 cm in greatest dimension and is limited to the thyroid

T1a   Tumour ≤1 cm, limited to the thyroid

T1b   Tumour >1 cm but ≤2 cm in greatest dimension, limited to the thyroid

T2   Tumour size >2 cm but ≤4 cm, limited to the thyroid

T3   Tumour size >4 cm, limited to the thyroid or any tumour with minimal extrathyroidal extension (e.g. extension to sternothyroid muscle or perithyroid soft tissues)

T4a   Moderately advanced disease; tumour of any size extending beyond the thyroid capsule to invade subcutaneous soft tissues, larynx, trachea, esophagus, or recurrent laryngeal nerve

T4b   Very advanced disease; tumour invades prevertebral fascia or encases carotid artery or mediastinal vessel

All anaplastic carcinomas are considered as stage IV:

T4a   Intrathyroidal anaplastic carcinoma

T4b   Anaplastic carcinoma with gross extrathyroid extension

Regional Lymph Nodes (N)

Regional lymph nodes are the central compartment, lateral cervical, and upper mediastinal lymph nodes:

NX   Regional nodes cannot be assessed

N0   No regional lymph node metastasis

N1   Regional lymph node metastasis

N1a   Metastases to level VI (pretracheal, paratracheal, and prelaryngeal/Delphian lymph nodes)

N1b   Metastases to unilateral, bilateral, or contralateral cervical (levels I, II, III, IV, or V) or retropharyngeal or superior mediastinal lymph nodes (level VII)

Distant metastasis (M)

M0   No distant metastasis is found

M1   Distant metastasis is present

What is the difference between follicular and papillary thyroid carcinoma?

- Papillary carcinoma is the most common thyroid malignancy accounting for 60% of the cases of thyroid carcinoma that spreads mainly by lymphatics. Follicular carcinoma spreads by blood-borne route, therefore involvement of lymph nodes is a rare.
- Papillary carcinoma does not invade the capsule or vessels, whereas follicular carcinoma commonly involves both
- Papillary carcinoma has a good prognosis compared to follicular carcinoma of the thyroid
- Histopathological examination reveals presence of orphan Annie eyed nuclei and papillary

distribution of cells along with psammoma body in more than half of the cases.

How is a case of suspected thyroid carcinoma worked up?

Fine needle aspiration cytology can be used to confirm the diagnosis of thyroid carcinoma. However, this test cannot differentiate between follicular carcinoma and follicular adenoma. The only reliable way of differentiating these two lesions is by demonstration of capsular invasion or vascular invasion.

In papillary carcinoma of thyroid orphan Annie eyed nuclei will be seen. The nuclear membrane is irregular and there is grooving around the cells. There may be inclusions within the nucleus or cytoplasm.

An ultrasound scan is also needed as that can tell about the number of foci, status of surrounding structures and assessment of lymph nodes. In all cases a thyroid profile must also be done which includes T3, T4 and TSH.

On the radioiodine scanning these lesions appear cold as there is no update due to loss of function in most cases. Technetium-99m sestamibi scan may be helpful in cases of suspected Hurthle cell cancer. These investigations are not routinely required.

An indirect laryngoscopy should also be done to assess the vocal cords prior to surgery. In a number of cases the vocal cord may be affected without change in the voice. Also in about 1% of patients there may be congenital paresis of the vocal cord.

What is lateral aberrant thyroid?

In a papillary carcinoma of the thyroid the primary tumour may not be palpable, instead of lymph node may be palpable. This represents metastasis from the occult primate tumours and is often wrongly called lateral aberrant thyroid.

Papillary microcarcinoma was initially regarded as an occult thyroid carcinoma presenting as lateral aberrant thyroid. It is now classified separately as any papillary tumour ≤1 cm in size.

What are the prognostic markers for thyroid carcinoma?

As per AGES criteria the favorable prognostic factors are:

- *A*: Age <40 years in female and <50 in males

- *Grade of tumour*: Well differentiated tumour
- *Extent*: Intrathyroidal
- *Size*: <1cm for papillary and <4 cm for follicular

Other prognostic systems that have been used include:

- *AMES system*: Includes age, metastases, extent of spread and size of tumour
- *MACIS system*: Includes metastases, age, completeness of resection, invasion of surrounding structures and size of tumour
- *Sloan kettering system*:
  - *High risk*: Age >45 years, size >4 cm, Presence of unfavorable factors
  - *Intermediate risk*: High risk patients with low risk tumours or vice versa
  - *Low risk*: Age <45 years, size <4 cm, presence of favorable factors.

What are the indications of performing Tru-cut biopsy of the thyroid?

Tru-cut biopsy is a method to obtain tissue for histopathology and can more precisely define the type of tumour. It is indicated when one is suspecting lymphoma (in presence of organomegaly or multiple lymph nodes), anaplastic tumour (history of rapid growth) or other lesions like tuberculosis. It is not preferred over FNAC because it is associated with complications like pain, hematoma formation and injury to surrounding structures like trachea, or the nerves.

What is the management of papillary and follicular carcinoma of the thyroid?

Differentiated thyroid cancers which include papillary and follicular carcinoma of the thyroid are best managed by total or near total thyroidectomy. Total thyroidectomy includes removal of all of the thyroid tissue eliminating any chance of residual thyroid cancer in any of the lobes. In near total thyroidectomy a small amount of thyroid tissue (≈1–2 grams on either side) that lies within the trachea-esophageal groove is removed. This preserves the parathyroids and their vascular supply and lessens chances of damage to the recurrent laryngeal nerve. In the event that vascular supply (superior and inferior parathyroid artery) to parathyroid glands are accidentally damaged, parathyroid glands can be divided into small fragments and implanted over the sternocleidomastoid muscle or the forearm muscles.

What is the difference in management of Hurthle cell tumour and differentiated thyroid cancers?

Hurthle cell tumours have fewer propensities to be malignant. If they are limited to one lobe only, hemithyroidectomy can be performed and subjected to frozen section analysis. Only if carcinoma is present that a completion thyroidectomy with removal of lymph nodes (central neck dissection) is indicated. If a pre-operative diagnosis of Hurthle cell carcinoma has been made already by core biopsy, then one may proceed straightaway to surgery. If lymph nodes are palpable, modified radical neck dissection is also needed.

How are lymphnodes managed in patients with differentiated thyroid cancers?

Modified radical neck dissection is performed when lymph nodes are involved. Alternatively functional neck dissection can also be performed. In this procedure structures like the internal jugular vein, spinal accessory nerve and sternocleidomastoid are preserved.

When lymph nodes are not involved but tumour is T3 or T4 central compartment, dissection can be done which involves removal of thymus, paratracheal, pretracheal and prelaryngeal nodes along with tracheoesophageal nodes and thyroid gland. The boundaries of dissection include hyoid bone superiorly, innominate artery inferiorly and carotid arteries laterally on each side. However, majority of surgeons do not remove thymus gland.

Up to 50% of the patients with thyroid cancers may have positive nodes in the central compartment which may be difficult to manage later on and lead to recurrence and difficulties in follow up.

What is Radio remnant ablation and when is it indicated?

Radio remnant ablation is administered when any remnant tumour is detected on radioiodine scan. In this Iodine 131 is administered which is taken up by the remnant tissue and destroys it. Usual dose is 30 mCi. RRA is indicated in tumours >4 cm, gross extension of tumour beyond thyroid capsule, involvement of lymph nodes and distant metastasis. If there is evidence of distant metastasis a higher dose of 100–200 mCi radioiodine can be given. For ablation of skeletal metastasis an even higher dosage of 300 mCi is administered.

How are patients followed up after thyroidectomy?

Patients are followed up after thyroidectomy by radionuclide whole body scan (I131 in a dose of 3mCi) to look for any evidence of residual disease usually one week after surgery. The patient is given suppressive doses of L-thyroxine. Alongside, serum thyroglobulin is also used as a marker for metastatic, residual or recurrent disease. Its levels should ideally be undetectable after total thyroidectomy and suppressive therapy but level <2 ng/mL is considered normal.

Whole body radioiodine scanning can be repeated after 6 months to one year along with yearly thyroglobulin for follow up.

What are the clinical features of anaplastic carcinoma of the thyroid?

Anaplastic carcinoma thyroid is an aggressive form of thyroid cancer with a dismal outcome. It can be clinically differentiated from other thyroid tumours by presence of:

- Rapidly growing swelling in the neck
- Hard and irregular swelling that appears to be fixed to underlying structures and often engulfs surrounding structures
- Associated with compressive symptoms arising from involvement of the nearby structures like difficulty in breathing, stridor and hoarseness of voice and difficulty in swallowing.
- Usually involves the elderly patients. F>M

How is anaplastic thyroid cancer managed?

When detected at an early stage by FNAC, anaplastic thyroid cancer can be managed by total thyroidectomy along with radical lymph node dissection. Adjuvant chemotherapy can be given after surgery. However, most patients present in the advanced stage and management is essentially palliative. Radiotherapy and chemotherapy may be given and to relieve pressure on the trachea an isthumusectomy can be performed.

What are the systemic agents used in management of anaplastic carcinoma of thyroid?

The various systemic chemotherapy agents used are:
- Paclitaxel or carboplatin
- Cisplatin
- Doxorubicin

What are the common syndromes associated with thyroid carcinoma?

Although a number of syndromes are associated with thyroid carcinoma, Cowden syndrome and Multiple Endocrine Neoplasia Syndrome (MEN) are frequently associated with thyroid cancer.

Cowden syndrome: Cowden syndrome or disease is an autosomal dominant condition caused by mutation in the PTEN gene. This gene is located on the long arm of chromosome 10. This syndrome is also well known by the name of multiple hamartoma syndrome as it is associated with hamartomatous lesions on the mucosa, bones, eyes, gastrointestinal and genitourinary tract. This syndrome involves the thyroid in 60–70% of the cases. There is increased incidence of differentiated thyroid cancers in this syndrome along with breast cancer. Colon cancer and renal cancer may also be associated.

MEN syndrome: MEN syndrome has been summarized in the table below.

Familial medullary thyroid cancer is another type of MEN2 syndrome where medullary thyroid cancer may present in isolation.

What are the different forms of medullary thyroid carcinoma?

Medullary carcinoma of the thyroid can occur as a sporadic tumour which usually represents as a solitary nodule in the elderly patient. Most cases of MTC are sporadic (up to 75%).

Up to 20% of the tumours are familial and such tumours are bilateral, multifocal and aggressive in nature. There tumours are poorly responsive to radiotherapy and associated with higher rate of recurrence and mortality. They occur at a younger age usually in the 2nd or 3rd decade. History of other family members having such tumours, presence of diarrhea, abdominal pain and hypertension should be taken in suspected cases.

What is the role of genetic screening and screening of family members?

When a diagnosis of medullary thyroid cancer is made, genetic screening is advocated for the RET proto-oncogene. All family members must be screened if the patient is positive for RET. Screening tests should include ultrasound of the neck, serum calcitonin, calcium and parathormone assay. Stimulated calcitonin test may uncover the defect when basal calcitonin levels are normal. For this test pentagastrin injection is given sub-cutaneously in a dose of 5 microgram/kg and a rise in serum calcitonin is noted.

Prophylactic thyroidectomy should be considered in family members as early as 1 year of age.

What are the additional tests required when medullary thyroid cancer is suspected?

Medullary thyroid cancer is associated with many other clinical disorders. Screening should be done additionally for:

- Ultrasound abdomen is required to screen for pheochromocytoma
- CEA may be raised up to 50% of the cases
- 24 hours urinary metanephrines
- Calcitonin levels unstimulated and stimulated.

What are the special precautions and prognostic factors in medullary carcinoma of the thyroid?

Medullary thyroid cancers are managed with total thyroidectomy and central node dissection even in the absence of palpable nodes. If nodes are present modified radical neck dissection along with central neck dissection should be performed.

Prognostic factors that must be looked to include:

- Calcitonin level
- CEA level
- DNA ploidy
- Stage
- Type of MEN associated (MEN 2A is most favorable).

	Men 1	Men 2A	Men 2B
Name	Werner syndrome	Sipple syndrome	Mucosal neuronal syndrome
Associated tumours	Pituitary adenoma, pancreatic tumours (M/C gastrinoma, followed by insulinoma, VIPoma, glucagonoma) and parathyroid hyperplasia	Parathyroid hyperplasia, pheochromocytoma and medullary thyroid carcinoma (occurs in up to 100% patients)	Medullary carcinoma of thyroid, pheochromocytomas, multiple mucosal neuromas in a patient with marfanoid habitus

5

Common Neck Swelling

What is thyroglossal duct cysts (Fig. 5.1)?

- Anterior midline neck masses seen in 1st year of life arising from thyroglossal duct remnant.
- Incidence is >25% before 5 years, 40% by 10 years and 10% per decade thereafter.

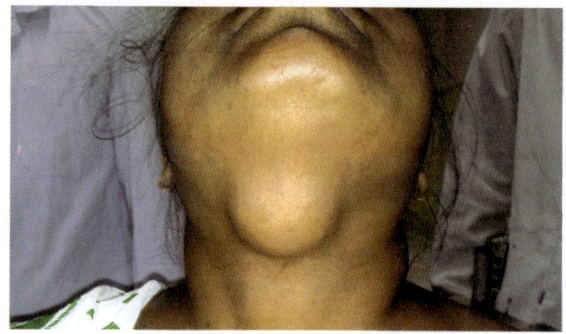

Fig. 5.1: Clinical picture of thyroglossal cyst

Describe the embryology of thyroglossal duct cyst.

Tuberculum impar arises from the anterior pharyngeal wall

↓

Thickening appears in the 3rd week Median Thyroid Anlage

↓

Rostral growth of embryo leads to caudal displacement of median thyroid anlage

↓

Thyroglossal duct formed by canalization of median stalk till the tuberculum impar courses ventral to the hyoid anlage but may go through/dorsal to it

↓

Degenerates by 5th week of gestation (Thyroglossal duct cyst formed by the secretions of the epithelial lined duct remnants by an unknown stimulus)

Describe the course of thyroglossal duct.

From foramen caecum it passes down exactly in the midline through the genioglossi muscles, geniohyoid muscle and myelohyoid muscle and then lies in close contact with central part of body of hyoid bone. It can lie in front of hyoid or traverse through hyoid bone or hook behind the hyoid. From hyoid bone it comes down to upper border of thyroid cartilage where it diverges slightly to one side of the midline. It continues down to the pyramidal lobe or isthmus. Thyroid follicles are seen in one-third of specimens of thyroglossal duct remnant.

Describe clinical features.

- Sudden appearance of a neck mass which may or may not be inflamed.
- Usually within 2 cm of the midline over the hyoid bone.
- Smooth mobile, without communication with overlying skin.
- Spontaneous drainage of an infected cyst or incision and drainage can lead to a sinus tract.
- Rises in the neck with swallowing and protrusion of the tongue.

Sites of thyroglossal cyst:

1. Subhyoid
2. Supra hyoid
3. Region of thyroid cartilage
4. At cricoid cartilage
5. Floor of mouth

Differentials

- Dermoid cyst
- Lymphadenitis

- Enlargement of pyramidal lobe of thyroid
- Neoplasia
- Thyroglossal duct carcinoma (<1%)—all types except medullary type can be seen.

Investigations needed

- USG
- Thyroid scintigraphy as sometimes it may contains functioning thyroid tissue.
- CECT/MRI/FNAC—may be considered if there is:
  - Suspicious lymphadenopathy
  - Compression of neighbouring structures
  - Multiple recurrences

What are the surgical techniques used in treatment?

- *Sistrunk procedure*
  - Resection of the tract of the thyroglossal duct with the central portion of the hyoid bone along with the cyst. Tract is removed right up to the base of the tongue.
  - It decreases the rate of recurrence to <5%.

Complications

- Postoperative wound haemorrhage leading to airway compromise
- Surgical site infection
- Recurrence.

What is cystic hygroma (Fig. 5.2)?

Basic defect is failure of lymphatic structures to anastomose with the venous system resulting in collection of lymphatic sacs with clear, colourless lymph

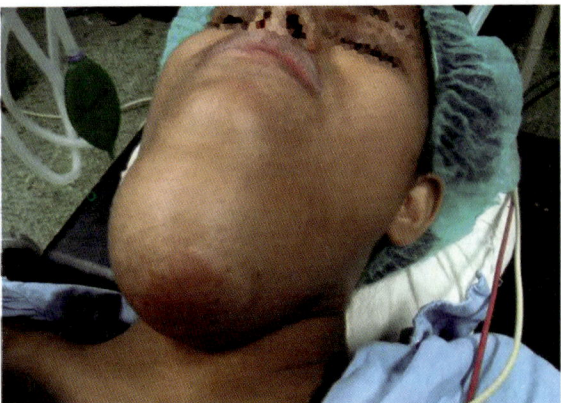

Fig. 5.2: Clinical picture showing cystic hygroma in submandibular reason

What is the common location?

- 75%: From the jugular lymphatic network → posterior triangle of neck
- 20%: Axilla
- 5%: Retroperitoneum/mediastinum/inguinal region/pelvis
- It does not have any communication with normal lymphatic channels.

Describe embryology.

- *Centrifugal spread*: Venous origin and lymphatic channels sprout from a single central vein
- *Centripetal spread*: Mesenchymal origin. Lymphatics arise from mesenchymal space
- Combination

Describe pathology of cystic hygroma.

- It is multiloculated, multicystic, thin-walled masses in subcutaneous tissues.
- Classically have soap bubble appearance.
- Large cysts lie superficially and smaller cysts are in deeper planes.
- Various cysts communicate with each other.
- Cysts are lined by single layer of flattened epithelium.
- Four types:
  a. Cavernous lymphangioma
  b. Lymphangioma
  c. Cystic hygroma
  d. Hemangio-lymphangioma

What are common presentation?

- *At birth* it can present with airway obstruction if large
  - Prenatal EXIT procedure (*exutero*, intrapartum) may be helpful to deliver the child safely
- *After birth*
  - Disfigurement
  - Pressure on oesophagus trachea, neck vessels resulting in interference with speech or swallowing.
  - Traumatic haemorrhage
  - Acutely infection/inflammation
(There may be sudden increase in size leading to respiratory distress)

Clinical signs

- Present as cystic fluctuant swelling

- Brilliant transilluminescence/Chinese lantern appearance (clear cyst contents)
- Swelling partially compressible
- Overlying skin is free from swelling

Investigations

- X-ray neck and chest
- Contrast enhanced computed tomography (CECT) for extension into thorax
- *Findings*: Multiloculated cystic structures with well-defined boundaries with or without associated vascular malformations

Describe management.

- Small/uncomplicated swelling—observation and expectant management
- *Intralesional sclerosant*: Repeated aspiration of macrocystic lesions and injection of sclerosing agents such as sodium tetradecyl sulphate and OK-432 (Picibanil, a streptococcal product)
- Surgical excision in case of a large swelling causing obstructive symptoms and compression of vital structures.

BRANCHIAL SINUS OR FISTULA (Fig. 5.3)

Describe embryology of branchial sinus.

- *Development of pharyngeal apparatus*
  - Pharyngeal arches
  - Pharyngeal pouches
  - Pharyngeal grooves/clefts
  - Pharyngeal membranes

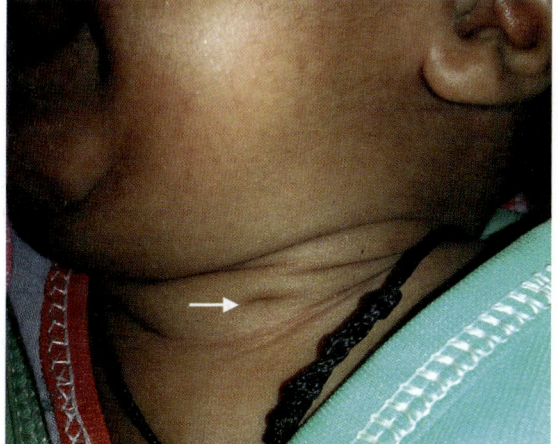

Fig. 5.3: Clinical picture showing left branchial sinus

- *Formation of the cervical sinus*
  - Proliferation of the mesenchyme of the second arch which grows into the mesenchyme → grows caudally → overlaps the 3rd and 4th arches and merges with the epicardial arches → cervical sinus of His
- *External branchial sinus*
  - Failure of cervical sinus to obliterate
  - Extends along anterior border of sternocleidomastoid (SCM) in lower third of neck
- *Internal branchial sinus*
  - Persistence of proximal part of second pharyngeal pouch
  - Opens into pharynx in tonsillar sinus

What is branchial fistula?

- Internal opening is located tonsillar sinus
- External opening is at anterior border of SCM usually at lower one-third
- *Course of tract*: Courses upwards and backwards → pierces deep fascia near the upper border of thyroid cartilage → passes between external carotid and internal carotid artery → tract remains superficial to 9th and 10th cranial nerve → hypoglossal nerve crosses the tract
- Usually congenital but can be acquired nature if the incision drainage of infected branchial cyst is carried out.

What is the aetiology?

- 90% cases due to failure of fusion of second branchial arch with fifth branchial arch. Origin from the 1st, 3rd and 4th pouches—less common.
- *Epithelial lining*: Usually respiratory or squamous.
- *Wall of the fistula*: Muscle fibres or lymphoid tissue.

Describe clinical features.

- It is bilateral in 10–20% of cases
- Presentation may range from complete lack of symptoms, intermittent clear mucus discharge from an opening in the mid-neck along the anterior border of the SCM or even an abscess.

How will you investigate?

- Fistulogram is done to know the extent of fistula and to find out if the internal opening is present or absent.

Describe treatment.

- If asymptomatic no treatment is needed.
- Excision of whole of the tract is indicated in symptomatic or for cosmetic reasons.

BRANCHIAL CYST (Fig. 5.4)

What is the embryology?

- It occurs due to persistence of part or whole of ectoderm lined cervical sinus.
- It can also occur due to epithelial inclusion within the lymph node.

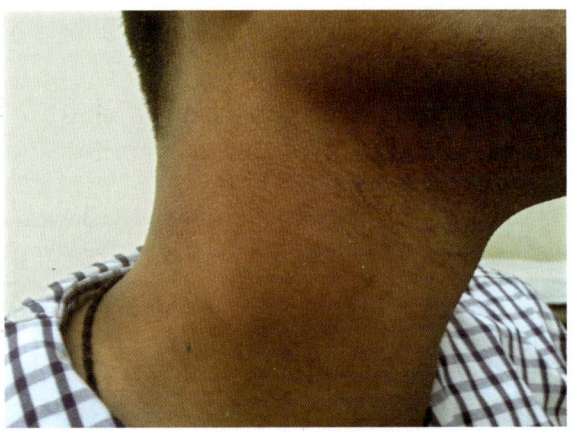

Fig. 5.4: Clinical picture showing right branchial cyst

What is the common location?

- Branchial cyst usually lies at the anterior border of the sternocleidomastoid at the junction of upper 1/3rd and lower 2/3rd—a palpable neck mass at the level of the carotid bifurcation
- Location in the neck is higher than that of sinuses/fistulae.

Describe clinical features.

- Usually after the first decade of life and detected in 3rd decade of life
- 60% of patients are males
- In 60%, it lies on left side
- In 2%, it can be bilateral

What is the differential diagnosis?

- Branchial cyst must be differentiated from cold abscess.

Describe anatomical relations.

- Branchial cyst lies deep to lesser cornu of hyoid bone, stylohyoid ligament, facial nerve and external carotid artery.
- It lies superficial to internal carotid artery, 9th cranial nerve and stylopharyngeus muscle.

What is the treatment?

- Surgical excision.

6

Generalised Lymphadenopathy

Generalised lymphadenopathy is defined as enlargement of lymph nodes of two or more noncontiguous areas. Of all the patients presenting with nodal enlargement, 25% patients have generalised lymphadenopathy. Rest of the 75% patients present with localised lymphadenopathy. Most commonly involved groups of lymph nodes are those in the head and neck which account for 55% of the total presentations. Inguinal group of nodes are next most commonly involved group accounting for 14% of the presentations. Axillary nodes are involved in 5% of the cases and supraclavicular nodes may be present in 1% of the presentations. Overall there are more than 600 nodes in the body (Fig. 6.1).

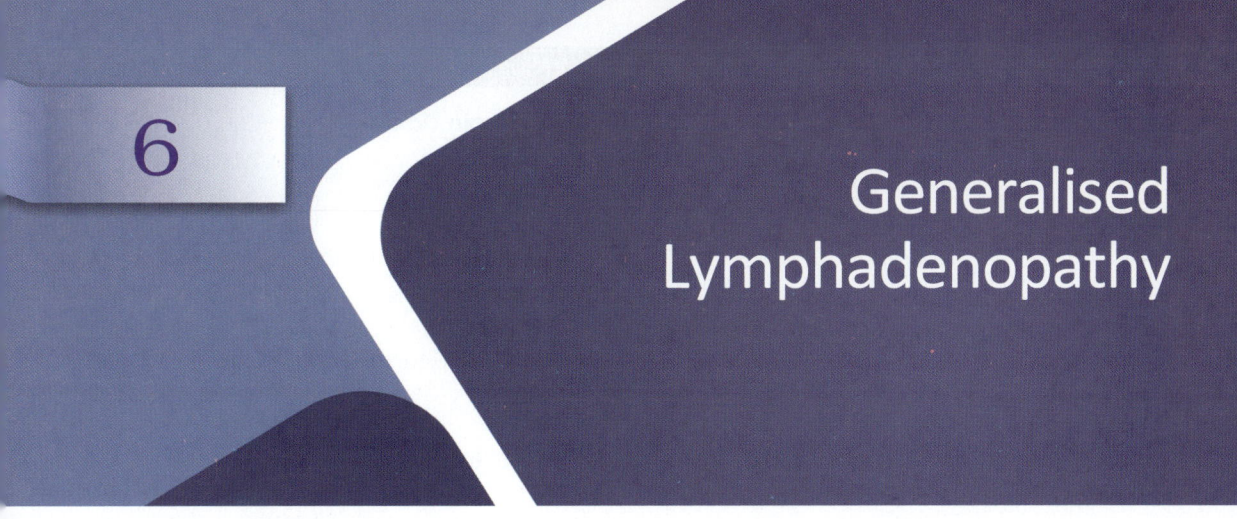

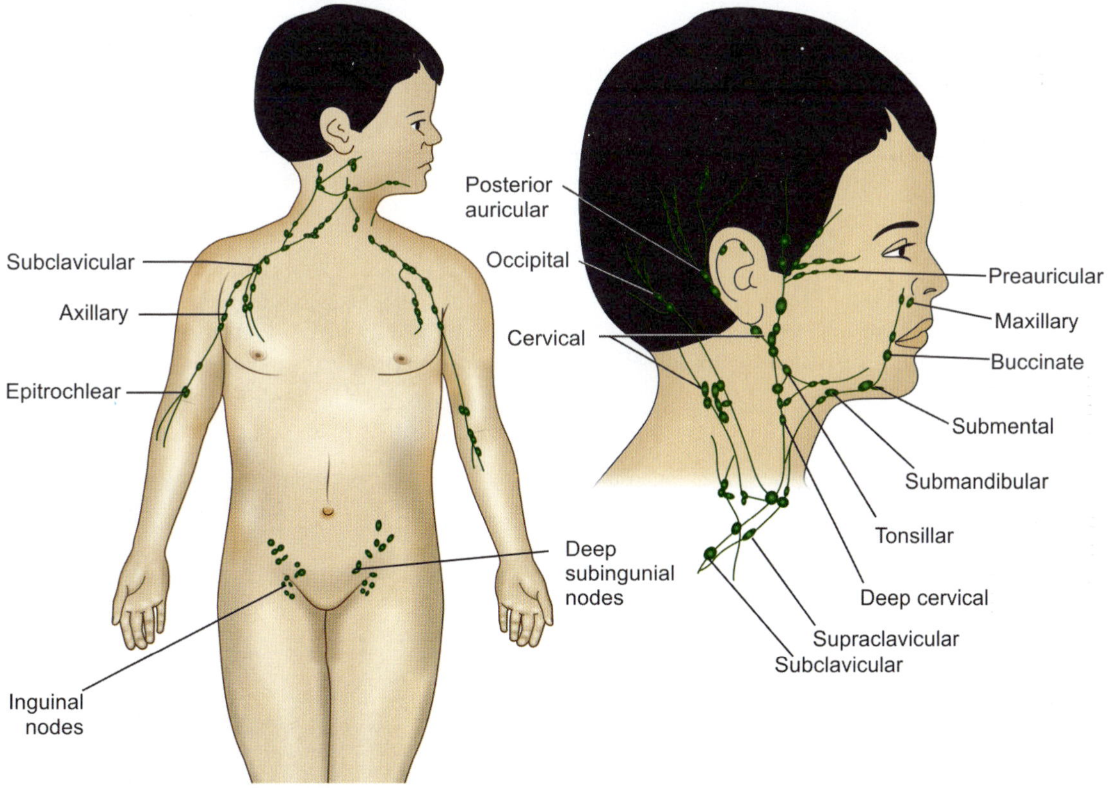

Fig. 6.1: Distribution of superficial lymph nodes in the body

Various groups of lymph nodes and the regions that they drain (Table 6.1)

Table 6.1: Drainage area of different lymph nodes			
Lymph nodes enlarged	*Drainage area*	*Infections*	*Malignancy*
Pre-auricular	Scalp, skin	Scalp infection, mycobacterial infections	Skin neoplasms, lymphomas, head and neck squamous cell carcinomas
Posterior cervical	Scalp, neck, upper thoracic skin	Scalp infection, mycobacterial infections	Skin neoplasms, lymphomas, head and neck squamous cell carcinomas
Supraclavicular	Gastrointestinal tract, genito-urinary tract, respiratory system	Mycobacterial/fungal infections	Abdominal/thoracic neo-plasms, thyroid/laryngeal diseases
Submandibular	Oral cavity	Mononucleosis, upper respiratory bacterial/viral infections, mycobacterial infections, toxoplasma, cytomegalovirus, dental disease, rubella	Squamous cell carcinoma of head and neck, lymphomas, leukaemias
Anterior cervical	Larynx, tongue, oropharynx, anterior neck	Mononucleosis, upper respira-tory bacterial/viral infections, mycobacterial infections, toxo-plasma, cytomegalovirus, dental disease, rubella	Squamous cell carcinoma of head and neck, lymphomas, leukaemias
Infra-clavicular			Highly suspicious for non-Hodgkin's lymphoma
Axillary	Breast, upper extremity and thoracic wall	Skin infection, trauma, cat-scratch disease, sarcoidosis, syphilis, leprosy, brucellosis, leishmaniasis	Breast adenocarcinoma, skin neoplasms, lymphomas, leukaemias, soft tissue
Epitrochlear	Ulnar forearm, hand	Skin infections	Lymphoma, skin malignancies
Horizontal node group	Lower abdomen, external genitalia (skin), anal canal, lower half of vagina, lower extremity	Benign reactive lymphadeno-pathy, sexually transmitted diseases, skin infections	Lymphomas, squamous cell carcinoma of the penis, vulva and anus, skin neoplasms, soft tissue/Kaposi's sarcoma

Axillary lymph nodes and the structures that they drain (Fig. 6.2)

- Most of cases are nonspecific or reactive.

- Persistent lymphadenopathy is less common.

- Breast adenocarcinoma often metastasizes initially to axillary nodes.

- Ante-cubital or epitrochlear lymphadenopathy can suggest lymphoma or melanoma of the extremity.

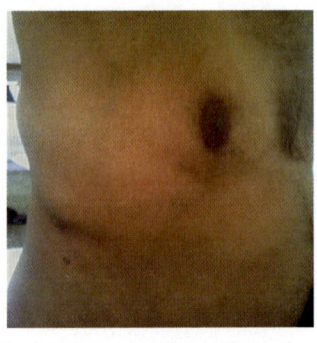

Fig. 6.2: Clinical picture showing enlarged axillary nodes

Inguinal lymph nodes and the structures that they drain

It is common, with nodes enlarged up to 1 to 2 cm in diameter in many healthy adults, but it is of low suspicion of malignancy.

Benign reactive lymphadenopathy and infection are the most common aetiologies.

Although some tumours, such as Hodgkin's lymphomas, penile/vulvar SCC, melanoma in this area, may present with inguinal lymphadenopathy but it is not a typical presenting finding in neither case.

What are the common causes of generalised lymphadenopathy?

The common causes of lymphadenopathy can be categorised into infectious, inflammatory and neoplastic causes. These include:

- *Infectious*
  - Tuberculosis
  - Human immunodeficiency virus infection
  - Chronic pyogenic lymphadenitis
  - Measles
  - Varicella
  - Brucellosis
  - Mononucleosis and Epstein-Barr virus infection
  - Coccidioidomycosis
  - Histoplasmosis
  - Taenia
  - Pediculosis
  - Plague
  - Rubella
  - Toxoplasmosis
  - Syphilis
- *Inflammatory and autoimmune*
  - Cystic fibrosis
  - Histiocytosis
  - Juvenile rheumatoid arthritis
  - Kawasaki disease
  - Systemic lupus erythematosus
  - Sarcoidosis
  - Diaper dermatitis
  - Serum sickness
  - Graft-versus-host disease
  - Primary biliary cirrhosis
  - Dermatopathic lymphadenitis
  - Castleman's disease
  - Inflammatory pseudotumour
  - Familial mediterranean fever

- *Neoplastic lesions*
  - Hodgkin disease
  - Non-Hodgkin lymphoma
  - Acute lymphoblastic leukaemia
  - Acute myelocytic leukaemia
  - Rhabdomyosarcoma
  - Neuroblastoma
- *Metabolic*
  - Gaucher disease
  - Niemann-Pick disease
  - Hyperthyroidism
  - Other lipidosis
  - Hypertriglyceridemia

How is case of generalised lymphadenopathy evaluated?

Painless lymphadenopathy is usually the most common chief complaint. Associated systemic symptoms include fever, night sweats, weight loss, fatigue, pruritus (NS type of HL), Pel-Ebstein fever, alcohol induced pain (pathognomic of HL) abdominal pain (splenomegaly, bowel dysfunction, hydronephrosis, bone pain (bone destruction/marrow infiltration), neurogenic pain (cord/nerve root compression, nerve root infiltration, plexopathy, meningeal involvement, complicating varicella zoster) and back pain (retroperitoneal involvement, psoas invasion).

Travel history, occupational history, recent blood transfusion, dietary history (ingestion of undercooked meat), intravenous drug abuse and sexual history are especially relevant to this case. It must be kept in mind that certain drugs like allopurinol, atenolol, captopril, carbamazepine, cephalosporins, gold, hydralazine, penicillin, phenytoin, primidone, pyrimethamine, quinidine, sulfonamides, sulindac, etc. may also cause enlargement of the lymph nodes which may even be painful.

Examination

First and foremost the size of lymph nodes should be ascertained. Since many lymph nodes lie deep to the fascia, it is useful to relax the nearby joints and muscles to be able to palpate the nodes easily. Look for associated tenderness, consistency, location, mobility, matting and signs of lymphangitis apart from thorough examination of the draining

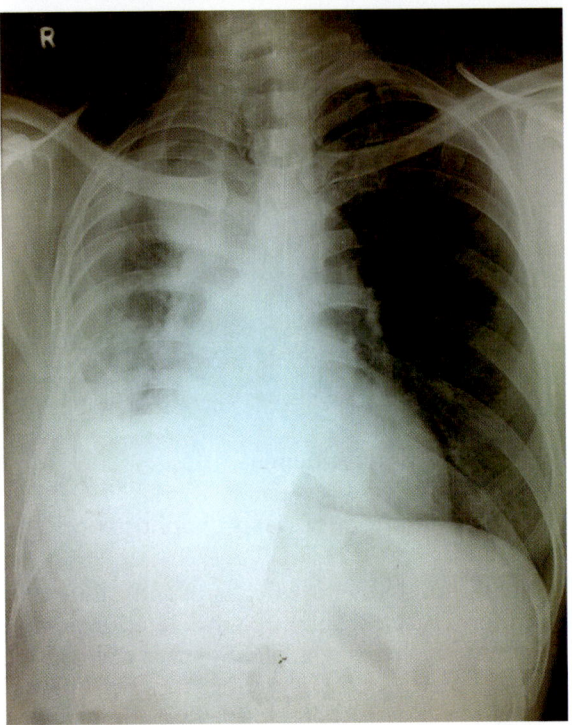

Fig. 6.3: Chest X-ray showing pleural effusion resulting from metastatic spread of non-Hodgkin's lymphoma

area. Associated features of lymphoma like hepatosplenomegaly, pleural effusion (Fig. 6.3), neuropathy and other obstructive signs like edema, SVC syndrome, and spinal cord compression should be looked for actively.

Also perform examination of other lymph node chains, tonsils and oropharynx, pharyngeal infections, ear infections, sexually transmitted infections, underlying malignancies like those of lung, gastrointestinal, retroperitoneal and testicular may lead to enlargement of lymph nodes unrelated to the site of origin.

What are the necessary investigations that must be done in patients with generalised lymphadenopathy?

Routine blood examination that includes haemoglobin, differential and total leukocyte counts, total RBC count, platelet count and absolute eosinophil count along with peripheral blood smear and ESR can be informative in most cases. Additional tests like blood sugar, lipid profile, kidney function tests, liver function tests and cultures from draining areas may be useful. Liver function tests

may show increase in alkaline phosphatase and cholestasis in para neoplastic syndromes associated with malignancies. Hyperuricemia results from a high cell turn over, sometimes in HL. Deranged kidney function may suggest urinary obstruction due to mass effect or direct renal involvement. Hypercalcemia may be present secondary to PTHrP secreted by tumour cells. LDH level reflects tumour bulk and turn over and is raised in malignancies, tuberculosis, toxoplasmosis, bacterial pneumonitis and many other inflammatory and infectious diseases. Immunoglobulin levels reflect polyclonal hypergammaglobulinemia in Hodgkin's and non-Hodgkin's lymphoma and hypogammaglobulinemia in NHL variants.

Other specialised tests must be directed at the likely diagnosis. If tuberculosis is suspected, a Mendel-Mantoux test, chest X-ray, sputum examination for AFB (2 samples) and occasionally immunoglobulin levels and PCR assay may be required. For suspected malignancies bone marrow aspirate or biopsy may be required. Fine needle aspiration cytology from the enlarged lymph nodes often solves the mystery in a large number of cases. Microbial culture of swabs from throat, sputum and other secretions and fluids may be needed when diagnosis cannot be ascertained.

Excisional biopsy of the lymph node is another useful alternative that provides enough tissue to run a battery of pathological tests and study the structure of the lymph nodes. It must be remembered that for suspected lymphomas, biopsy is not placed in a fixative but directly handed to the pathologist. Touch preparations/imprints are used for immunological phenotyping. Tissue may also be used for culture of fastidious organisms.

Routine CSF examination is required in Burkitt/ lymphoblastic lymphoma and intermediate/high grade lymphoma involving testis, paranasal sinuses or bone marrow.

PET scan has high sensitivity (up to 95%) in detecting metastasis in lymphoma while a Gallium scan (Ga67) can be useful in detecting residual mediastinal/retroperitoneal and abdominal infections. Other routine imaging investigations include CT scan and MRI.

Immunological phenotyping for non-Hodgkin's lymphoma includes CD2/3, CD5, CD19, CD20 and CD23, while Hodgkin's lymphomas demonstrate

CD15 and CD30 positivity. Special handling in the form of cytogenetics and molecular genetic analysis may also be required.

What are the typical characteristics of tubercular lymphadenopathy?

Tubercular nodes pass through five different stages of disease as described first by Jones and Campbell.

Stage I: The bacteria are brought by macrophages to the nodes and there is inflammation and enlargement of the nodes along with tenderness.

Stage II: Inflammation spreads to the surrounding tissues leading to periadenitis.

Stage III: Caseous necrosis leads to central liquefaction and pus formation with breach in the continuity of the node.

Stage IV: Pus breaches through the deep fascia that is containing it and forms a typical collar stud abscess (dumbbell abscess) with a part of it lying outside the deep fascia and communicating with the underlying abscess deep to the fascia (Fig. 6.4).

Stage V: Pus extrudes through the skin forming a visible abscess and subsequently a sinus.

Typically the tubercular nodes are firm, painless and matted or fixed to each other due to resulting periadenitis. They may present as small abscesses which keep discharging even when drained because of the deeper communication that has not been dealt with.

How is tuberculosis diagnosed and managed?

Histopathological demonstration of tubercular changes in the form of epithelioid granuloma formation, demonstration of Langerhans type giant cells (Fig. 6.5), and evidence of caseous necrosis can

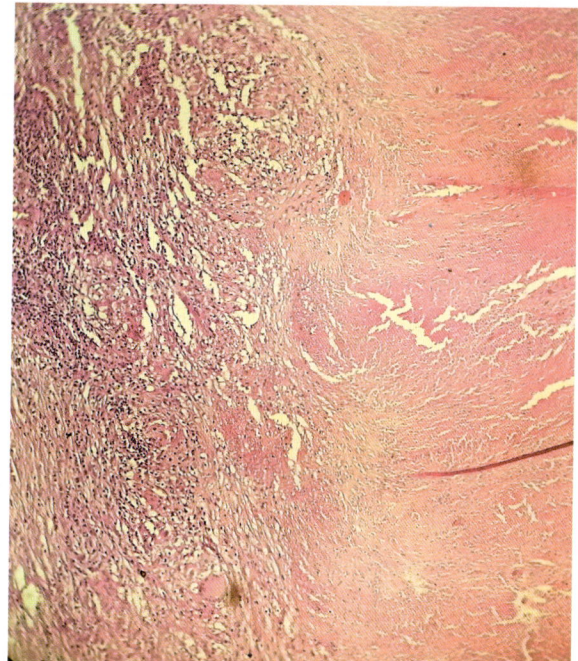

Fig. 6.5: Microscopic section showing Langerhans type of giant cells

guide the surgeon to start anti-tubercular therapy. Two sputum samples are taken to look for AFB and rule out associated pulmonary tuberculosis.

New patients with pulmonary or extrapulmonary disease are managed as category I and III patients using 2 months initial therapy with HRZE followed by 4 months continuous therapy with HR. Previously treated patients with relapse, failure or other reasons of resurgence are treated with initial therapy with HRZES for 2 months followed by HRZE for 1 month and then a continuation therapy with HRE for 5 months making it a total treatment of 8 months.

If sputum positive follow-up sputum examination is done at the end of intensive phase and two months after start of continuation phase and finally at the end of treatment. For new patients it is thus done at 0, 2, 4 and 6 months and for previously treated patients, it is done at 0, 3, 5, and 8 months.

What is MDR TB and when is it suspected?

Multidrug resistant tuberculosis is suspected when sputum culture is positive for mycobacterium tuberculosis with *in vitro* resistance to isoniazid and rifampicin with or without resistance to other

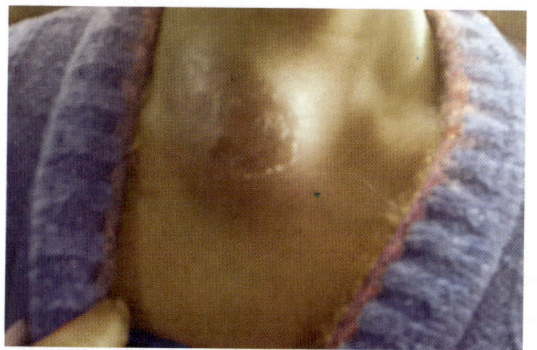

Fig. 6.4: Dumbbell shaped cold abscess in the neck

drugs from an RNTCP accredited laboratory. Multi-drug resistance levels of 3% have been found among new TB cases and 12–17% among previously treated patients of tuberculosis.

Multi-drug resistant tuberculosis should be suspected if the patient remains sputum positive even after 5 months of treatment (4 months if previously treated). Close contacts of MDRTB with pulmonary tuberculosis should also be considered with high suspicion. These patients are labeled as Category IV under the DOTS plus regime.

What is XDR tuberculosis and when is it suspected?

When the mycobacterium demonstrates *in vitro* resistance to isoniazid and rifampicin along with resistance to any second line injectable aminoglycoside and any fluoroquinolone, it is referred to as XDR tuberculosis. The criteria of suspicion are same as that of MDR TB and treatment is based on administration of a cocktail of culture sensitive antibiotics. These patients are labeled as Category V under the DOTS plus regime.

What are the commonly used second line drugs for tuberculosis?

The commonly used second line drugs include:
- Amikacin
- Capreomycin
- Ciprofloxacin
- Clofazimine
- Cycloserine
- Ethionamide
- Kanamycin
- Levofloxacin
- Ofloxacin
- Para-aminosalicylic acid

What are the risk factors for Hodgkin's lymphoma?

Hodkin's lymphoma affects patients with a bimodal age distribution and 85% patients are males. Risk increases with higher social class, small family size, advanced education, EBV and HIV association.

What are the various types of Hodgkin's lymphomas?

Hodgkin's lymphomas have been classified based on various systems. According to Rye's classification there are four types of Hodgkin's lymphoma:
1. Lymphocyte predominant
2. Nodular sclerosing
3. Mixed cellularity
4. Lymphocyte depleted

According to WHO classification

- *Nodular lymphocyte predominant (5%)*: This form is usually localised to peripheral nodes and bears an excellent prognosis. Contains L and H popcorn cells on histological examination.
- *Lymphocyte rich (5%)*: Affects older males usually leading to enlargement of peripheral nodes, excellent prognosis due to earlier detection. There are RS cells scattered in background of small lymphocytes, with absent eosinophils and neutrophils.
- *Nodular sclerosing (70%)*: Usually affects females and presents as mediastinal masses and peripheral nodes. Lacunar cells are found on histological examination. They have nodular growth pattern with collagen bands with numerous eosinophils and neutrophils.
- *Mixed cellularity (25%)*: These lymphomas frequently involve retroperitoneal nodes and present at an advanced stage of the disease. RS cells are more frequent in mixed inflammatory background without nodular sclerosing fibrosis.
- *Lymphocyte depleted (5%)*: This variant of Hodgkin's lymphoma bears an aggressive course with early involvement of liver and bone marrow.

Hodgkin's lymphomas have also be classified using REAL classification into classical and non-lymphocyte predominant disease.

What are Reed-Sternberg (RS) cells and their variants?

Reed-Sternberg cells are very large lymphoid clonal B-cells with abundant pale cytoplasm and two or more oval lobulated nuclei containing large nucleoli. Four types of cells have been described:
1. *Classical RS cell*: B cells that originate in the germinal centres, CD15+, CD45+, CD20+/–, CD45 (LCA)–
2. *Lacunar cell*: Usually plentiful in NS: CD30+
3. *L and H cell*: CD 20+, CD45+, CD79a+, CD19
4. *L and M cells*: CD20+, CD45+, 79a+, EMA+/–, found in nodular LPHL

RS-like cells are seen in infectious mononucleosis, lymphoid hyperplasia with phenytoin, and variants of immunoblastic lymphoma.

How does Hodgkin's lymphoma spread?

Hodgkin's lymphoma has a very predictable pattern of spread along the central axis with contagious involvement of nodes. Except for the nodular sclerosis variant, others may skip the mediastinum and no extra-nodal involvement is seen. Late haematogenous dissemination is usually seen with LD variant. The common sites of involvement of HL are most commonly the cervical and supraclavicular nodes. Axillary and inguinal are less common involved and an axial nodal distribution is seen. Epitrocheal and popliteal nodes are rarely involved. Anterior mediastinum is prime location for nodular sclerosing variant and SVC syndrome is uncommon in HL, compared to non-Hodgkin's lymphoma. Spleen, splenic hilum, and celiac nodes are involved in infra-diaphragmatic disease but mesenteric nodes rarely involved. Liver involvement is almost always associated with splenomegaly. Bone marrow involvement and retroperitoneal lymphadenopathy develop late and bone infiltration produces prostate like osteoblastic reaction which may form extradural masses and cause cord compression. Extra-nodal sites are rarely involved.

What is Cotswolds modification of Ann Arbor staging for Hodgkin's lymphoma?

I   Single lymph node group
II   2 or more lymph node regions on same side of diaphragm
III   Multiple lymph node groups on both sides of diaphragm
III1   Splenic hilar, celiac, portal
III2   Para-aortic, iliac, mesenteric
IV   Multiple extra-nodal sites or lymph nodes and extra-nodal disease
X   Nodal mass bulk >10 cm, mediastinal mass >1/3rd of maximum chest diameter
E   Extra-nodal extension or single, isolated site of extra-nodal disease
A   No symptoms
B   Symptoms: Unexplained weight loss >10%, fever, drenching night sweats.

What are the poor prognostic factors for Hodgkin's lymphoma?

The various factors signifying poor prognosis in patients with Hodgkin's lymphoma are:
- Higher stage III/IV
- Males
- Age >45 years
- Hb <10.5 g%
- WBC >15,000/µL
- Lymphocyte <600/µL or <8% of WBC
- Serum albumin <4 g%
- Eosinophilia
- RS atypia
- Bulky (X) disease
- ESR >50
- Four or more sites involved

What are the various treatment modalities used for the management of Hodgkin's lymphoma?

Surgery, radiotherapy and chemotherapy are all used in management of Hodgkin's lymphoma. Role of surgery is limited to diagnosis and occasionally laparotomy and laminectomy.

RT as a solitary therapy may be used at a dose of 30–44 Gy. Commonly employed fields for RT include: Mantle: Cervical, supraclavicular, infra-clavicular, hilar, mediastinal. Lung and heart are shielded by lead blocks. Inverted Y radiation is given to splenic pedicle, coeliac, iliac, inguinal and femoral nodes. Shielding is done over kidney, pelvic marrow and testis.

Various options for chemotherapy include:
- MOPP/COPP (28 days/21 days)
  MOPP is erpetogenic, myelosuppressive, with leucogenesis and infertility and COPP is better tolerated.
  (Nitrogen mustard) meclorethamine 6 mg/m^2 (day 1+8)/cyclophosphamide 400–650 mg/m^2
  Vincristine   1.4 mg/m^2
  Prednisone   40 mg/m^2
  Procarbazine   40 mg/m^2
- ABVD (28 days)
  Superior to MOPP as it causes less leukaemia and infertility
  Doxorubicin—cardiotoxic
  Bleomycin—pulmonary toxicity
  6–8 monthly cycles, 2 cycles minimum beyond maximum response
  Vinblastine 6 mg/m^2 (day 1 + 15)
  Daunorubicin 25 mg/m^2 (day 1 + 15)
  Bleomycin 10 mg/m^2 (day 1 + 15)
  Dacarbazine 375 mg/m^2 (day 1 + 15)
- MOPP + ABVD—alternating cycles. (3rd generation)
- MOPP/ABV hybrid

Dose intense regimens used for high grade HL include:
- BEACOPP (21 days)—higher risk for leukaemia
  Bleomycin   10 mg/m^2 (day 8)
  Etoposide   100 mg/m^2 (day 1–3)
  Adriamycin   25 mg/m^2 (day 1)

Cyclophosphamide   650 mg/m^2 (day 1)
Oncovin   1.4 mg/m^2 (day 8)
Prednisone   40 mg/m^2 (day 1–14)
Procarbazine   100 mg/m^2 (day 1–7)
(Escalated BEACOPP has higher doses of CEA)

- Stanford V
  (Similarly ABVD/MOPP)
  Methylchlorethamine   6 mg/m^2 (day 1 + 15)
  Vinblastine   6 mg/m^2 (day1 + 15)
  Doxorubicin   25 mg/m^2 (day 1 + 15)
  Etoposide   60 mg/m^2 (day 15)
  Vincristine   1.4 mg/m^2 (day 8, 22)
  Bleomycin   5 mg/m^2 (day 8, 22)
  Prednisone   40 mg/m^2 alternate day

Recommended treatment for Hodgkin's lymphoma stagewise is summarised as under:

Classical HL IA-IIA	ABVD × 4 cycles + IFRT 20–30 Gy (inv. Field RT) Stanford V × 2 cycles + IFRT
Lymphocyte predominant IA-IIA	IFRT alone
IB, IIB	Full course chemotherapy × 6 cycles
Bulky I–II	ABVD × 6/Stanford V × 3 + IFRT
III–IV	ABVD × 6–8 cycles BEACOPP + RT for residual
Multiple E/extensive E	Needs continued treatment

How are patients with HL restaged and followed up?

All complete remissions must be restaged using repeat biopsy and imaging. The following treatment and investigations are recommended:

Fluorouracil:
    2–4 months × 2 years
    3–6 months × 3–5 years

- CT scans every 6 months × 3 years
- Annual TSH if neck irradiated
- Annual mammogram after 40 or 5–8 years following treatment
- Routine PET is not recommended due to a high false positive rate

Salvage treatment should be offered when there is

- Failure to achieve complete remission—stem cell/bone marrow transplant

- Relapse after chemotherapy induced complete remission. In such cases initial combination can be used again if CR lasts more than 1 year
- Consider transplant if resistant to MOPP/ABVD
- Other options include:
  - *2nd and 3rd line chemotherapy:* Consider gemcitabine with vincristine or platinum
  - *Intensive chemoradiotherapy:* Myeloablative high dose chemotherapy with total body RT (conditioning regimen)
  - Autologous BM transplant/peripheral stem cell transplant
  - *Immunoconjugation:* Anti CD30 immuno-toxins
  - Radioimmunotherapy, rituximab.

What are the complications of therapy for Hodgkin's lymphoma?

The common complications of therapy include:

- Hypothyroidism: 10–20% with mantle therapy
- Sterility
- Radiation/bleomycin induced pneumonitis
- Cardiac damage
- Femoral head necrosis
- Decreased cell mediated immunity leading to listeria, toxoplasmosis, mycobacterium, pneumocystis, CMV, herpes zoster, OPSI
- *Secondary neoplasms*
  - Acute myelogenous leukaemia 2–10%
  - Non-Hodgkin's lymphoma—high grade B cell tumours
  - Epithelial tumours and sarcomas
- *Neurological complications*: Lhermitte/transverse myelopathy
- Retroperitoneal fibrosis
- *Synchronous neoplasms*: Kaposi sarcoma, leukaemia, NHL, myeloma
- Nephrotic syndrome
- Acute onset icthyosis

What is the role of laparotomy in patients with HL?

Laparotomy is indicated for more thorough staging of the patient but with advances in imaging its role has reduced. It is done only in cases where RT is planned as treatment. As a part of the procedure FNAC is taken from the liver along with wedge biopsy from both lobes. Splenectomy with lymph nodal examination of para-aortic, splenic, mesenteric, portal (as they may be found to have stage II/IV disease) nodes is done. Biopsy is taken from the iliac crest bone marrow.

How does non-Hodgkin's lymphoma differ from HL?

Table 6.2: Differences between Hodgkin's lymphoma and non-Hodgkin's lymphoma

Hodgkin's lymphoma	Non-Hodgkin's lymphoma
Contiguous predictable involvement	Non-contiguous involvement
Better prognosis	Worse prognosis
Malignancies are also found in the chest area	Malignancies mainly in abdomen
Systemic symptoms common	Systemic symptoms not so common
Extra-nodal spread uncommon (<5%)	Extra-nodal spread common
Bone marrow less commonly involved	Bone marrow involvement is more common
Cells of origin are usually the monocytes and macrophages	B cells are the common origin

What are the proposed aetiological factors for non-Hodgkin's lymphoma?

The proposed aetiological factors include HTLV-1, ATLL, chronic hepatitis C (indolent B cell lymphoma), EBV, chronic *H. pylori*, AIDS, agammaglobulinemia, Wiskott-Aldrich syndrome, Sjögren's syndrome, rheumatoid arthritis, LE, phenytoin and treatment related to HL.

What are the distinct clinical signs and symptoms of NHL?

Some of the distinct signs and symptoms of NHL are:
- Early bone marrow involvement, hematogenous and non-contiguous dissemination
- Extra-axial nodes including epitrochlear and mesenteric nodes
- Extra-nodal involvement: Waldeyer's ring, GI tract, skin, bone, CNS

How are NHL tumours classified?

NHL tumours are classified based on the WHO working classification:

Low grade
- A Small lymphocytic small round cleaved, low mitotic rate
- B Follicular, small cleaved
- C Follicular, mixed

Intermediate grade
- D Follicular, large cell
- E Diffuse, small cleaved
- F Diffuse, mixed
- G Diffuse, large cell

High grade
- H Immunoblastic (large cell)
- I Lymphoblastic
- J Small non-cleaved

What are the various immunological phenomenon seen in NHL?

Small lymphocytic lymphoma related
- Hypogammaglobulinemia
- Warm/cold antibody haemolytic anaemia
- Acquired vWF disease
- Angioedema

Lymphoplasmacytic lymphomas related
- Paraprotein spikes-IgM
- Polyclonal hypergammaglobulinemia

What are the important prognostic factors in patients with NHL?

Prime determinant of survival in these patients is histopathological subtype.

Intermediate and high grade lymphomas have better survival than low grade tumours.

Other prognostic factors include:
- Response to therapy (stages I/II have better response)
- FLIPI scale (follicular lymphoma int. prognostic index)
- NOLASH for low grade lymphomas
- >4 nodal areas of involvement
- Abnormal LDH
- Age >60 yrs
- Stage III/IV
- Hb <12 g%
- IPI (international prognostication index) for intermediate/high grade lymphomas
- *APLES*
  - Age >60
  - Performance ECOG >1
  - LDH abnormal
  - Extranodal sites >1
  - Stage III/IV

Table 6.3: Salient features of various subtypes of non-Hodgkin's lymphoma

B cell lymphoma: Low grade	
Small lymphocytic lymphoma	Nodal counterpart of CLL CD5+, CD20+, CD23+
Lymphoplasmacytic lymphoma	Waldenström's macroglobulinemia made up of lymphocytes and plasma cells CD20+ hyperviscosity syndrome
Follicular lymphoma	Grade I: <5 large cells/h.p.f.
	Grade 2: 5–15 large cells/h.p.f.
	Grade 3: >15 large cells/h.p.f
Marginal zone lymphoma	Derived from parafollicular/marginal cells CD20+, CD5–, CD10–MALTomas, splenic lymphomas, monocytoid lymphomas, hairy cell leukaemias
Intermediate and high grade B cell lymphoma	
Mantle cell lymphoma	Mantle zone lymphoma is an indolent variety of MCL
	Adverse prognosis, CD5+, CD20+, CD23–
	Presents in advanced stage with GI tract and BM involvement
Diffuse large B cell lymphoma	Localised presentation
	AIDS related NHL
	Post-transplant lymphoproliferative disorder
	Primary effusion lymphoma (HHV-8/HIV related)
High grade lymphoma	Doubling time may be <24 hours
	Highly aggressive
Burkitt lymphoma	African (endemic)
	Sporadic
	Common in immunosuppressed individuals
B cell lymphoblastic lymphoma	B cell lineage ALL
T cell lymphoblastic leukaemia	Malignancy of immature T cells convoluted nuclei with high mitotic rate Tdt+
	May present as mediastinal mass, effusion or SVC syndrome
Peripheral T cell and NK cell neoplasms	Refers to all T/NK cell neoplasms except TCLL
	Includes mycosis fungoides to aggressive varieties of PTCL
	PTCL affects middle aged to elderly—stage III/IV disease with HSP

- Adult T cell leukaemia/lymphoma
- Aggressive NK cell leukaemia
- T cell pro-lymphocytic leukaemia
- T/NK cell large granular lymphocytic leukaemia
- Anaplastic large cell lymphoma
- Angioimmunoblastic T cell lymphoma
- Nasal type NK cell and T cell lymphoma
- Hepatosplenic T cell lymphoma
- Enteropathy type T cell lymphoma
- Subcutaneous panniculitis-like T cell lymphoma
- Mycosis fungoides and sezary syndrome

Histiocytic and dendritic cell neoplasms	
Malignant histiocytosis hemophagocytic syndrome	Fever, jaundice, HSM, coagulopathy, hemophagocytosis
Langherans cell histiocytosis	Localized—eosinophilic granuloma
	Multifocal unisystem—Hand-Schüller-Christian disease

What is the recommended therapy for aggressive non-Hodgkin's lymphomas?

Non-bulky type IA/IIA with extranodal presentations are managed by 3 cycles of CHOP chemotherapy followed by IFRT 3000 Gy.

Bulky disease is managed using CHOP chemotherapy + rituximab or mBACOD, M-BACOD regime.

Complete restaging is usually done after 3–4 cycles of CHOP f/b 6 more cycles.

CNS prophylaxis using intrathecal chemotherapy +/– cranial irradiation is given in presence of bulky disease. It is also given with: Lymphoblastic lymphoma, primary testicular lymphoma and high grade lymphoma with marrow involvement.

Refractory/relapse lymphomas and high/intermediate grade tumours are given consolidation radiotherapy. If the tumour persists salvage chemotherapy may be followed. Options for salvage chemotherapy include the ICE, MINE, CEPP-B, EVA, EPOCH regimen with or without rituximab. Alternatively high dose chemoradiotherapy with stem cell/BM support may also be given apart from allogenic bone marrow transplant.

What are the recommended treatment options for indolent lymphomas?

The recommended treatment options for patients with indolent lymphomas based on stage are:

True stage I/II

2400–3000 Gy of RT to all known sites of disease

Large fields do not ↑ cure rates, cause chemoresistance

Stage III/IV

Observation with no therapy in advanced tumours

Single agent chemotherapy: Chlorambucil/cyclophosphamide

(2–6 mg/m^2)

Combination chemotherapy: Chlorambucil + steroids.

Fludarabine + Mitoxantrone

(CR/PRs achieved in 60–80% of patients)

Rituximab: Chimeric humanised anti-CD20 monoclonal antibody.

7

Management of Neck Metastasis with Unknown Primary

What is the incidence of unknown primary in metastatic lymph node enlargement?

In about 5–10% of cases which present with metastatic lymph node enlargement the diagnostic work up fails to identify the site of origin. These are also known as carcinoma of unknown primary (CPU).

What are the different histological types in CPU?

The CPU can be
a. Squamous cell carcinoma from head and neck
b. Adenocarcinoma can arise from thyroid, para-thyroid, salivary gland, sinuses, lung or breast.
c. Undifferentiated carcinoma
d. Lymphoma
e. Melanoma

Which groups of lymph nodes are more commonly involved?

The most frequently involved lymph node is level 2 followed by level 3. Levels 1, 4 and 5 are less commonly involved.

How much is the incidence of bilateral lymph node involvement in CPU?

The bilateral lymph nodes are involved in 10% of cases.

Is there any correlation between level of lymph node involved and likely site of primary?

The metastasis in the upper and lower neck is mainly due to head and neck malignancy. Metastasis in the lower neck (supraclavicular lymph nodes) is due to primary malignancies below the clavicle.

What is the mean age at diagnosis and sex preponderance?

The mean age at diagnosis is 55–65 years of age. The majority of patients are males with male: female ratio of 4 : 1.

What are different theories of squamous carcinoma in cervical lymph nodes with unknown primary?

1. The tumour develops in the neck within squamous cells remaining as remnants of branchial cleft cysts. Although this theory is intriguing, a little evidence has been presented to support it, and it has largely fallen out of favour.
2. Others have suggested that these patients have exhibited spontaneous regression of the primary tumour site with persistence of cervical metastases.
3. Current theory is that unknown primary tumours are likely to be primary tumours that exist in the upper aero-digestive tracts or skin but are subclinical at the time of presentation. Thus unknown primary tumours remain undetected but are presumed to be present.
   Anecdotal support of this theory includes the identification of some primary tumours during or after treatment.

What are the most common sites for occult primary cancer?

Common sites are tonsil, base of the tongue, nasopharynx, and pyriform fossa.

The jugulodiagastric lymph node gives suspicion of primary in the oropharynx especially at the base of the tongue or tonsil.

A node in the posterior triangle suggests primary in the nasopharynx.

A node in the supraclavicular region suggests possible infraclavicular primary site, e.g. lung, breast, stomach, or colon.

What are common clinical presentations?

History

a. Complain of lump painless neck mass which may be present for weeks or months.
b. History of previous malignancy both in head and neck or anywhere else in the body should be taken.
c. History of previous radiation.
d. History of any previous cervical or facial skin lesion which has disappeared.
e. History of previous operations like breast, abdomen or chest
f. History of any upper aero-digestive tract symptoms like:
   1. Otalgia or aural fullness for possible site at pharynx, larynx, nasopharynx, or ear.
   2. Dysphagia or odynophagia for esophagus, or oral cavity.
   3. Hoarseness for larynx
   4. Trismus for oral cavity or oropharynx.
   5. Nasal congestion or epistaxis for sinuses and nasal tract.
g. History of tobacco or alcohol consumption.

Physical Examination

a. Inspection and palpation of skin of external ear and scalp in detail with respect to any abnormal skin lesion.
b. Palpate whole of the neck to find out any additional lymphadenopathy.
c. Following points should be noted with respect to swelling:
   1. Size of the neck mass
   2. Consistency
   3. Surface of mass
   4. Exact location of mass in relation to relevant structures, e.g. mandible
   5. Presence or absence of bilateral lymphadeno-pathy.
   6. Complete inspection of oral cavity and nasal vestibule.
   7. Palpation of the oral cavity and oropharynx.
   8. Palpation of the base of the tongue to rule out any sub-mucosal occult primary.
   9. The examination of cranial nerves.

How will you investigate such a patient (Fig. 7.1)?

Fine needle aspiration cytology (FNA) should be performed to confirm the presence of metastatic cancer. If repeated FNA is not conclusive, one should go for core tissue biopsy or excision of lymph node if feasible. Special staining may be employed like PSA, thyroglobulin, or calcitonin.

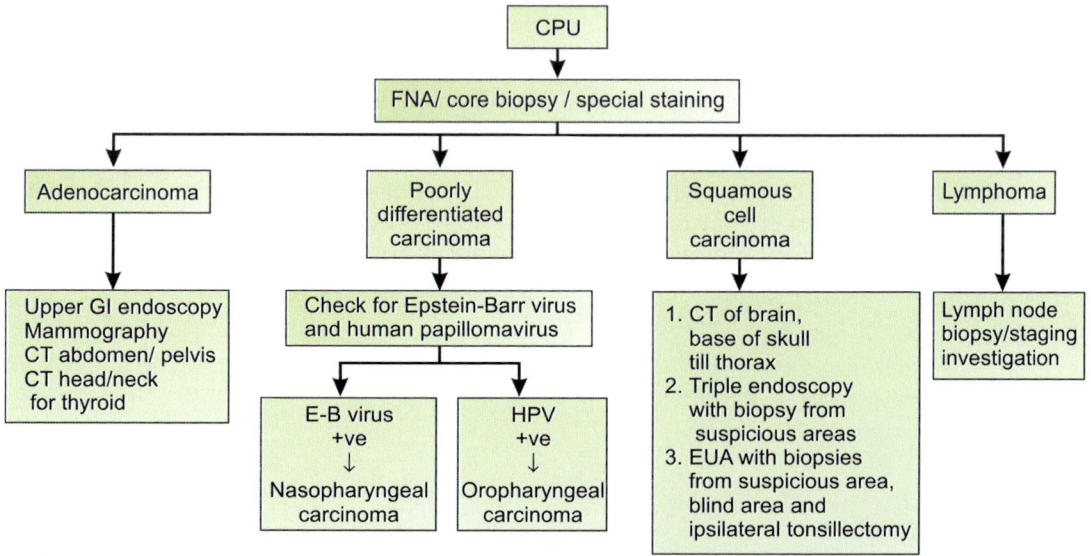

Fig. 7.1: Plan of management with cervical metastasis with primary unknown (CPU)

If FNA demonstrates adenocarcinoma, what is the further work up?

The work up in such patient should include mammography, CT scan of the abdomen and pelvis and GI endoscopies depending on location of node patient age, individual risk factors and result of pelvic/rectal examination.

If FNA demonstrates poorly differentiated carcinoma, what is the further work up?

The detection of Epstein-Barr virus with the use of *in situ* hybridization technique in metastatic lymph node might suggest nasopharyngeal carcinoma. Human papillomavirus (HPV) detected by polymerase chain reaction suggest oropharyngeal cancer.

What is the imaging modalities used if FNA shows squamous cell carcinoma?

Contrast enhanced CT from base of skull till thorax is mandatory. Triple endoscopy which includes bronchoscopy, esophagoscopy and laryngoscopy is carried out in all cases. Biopsies are taken from suspicious areas. PET CT is gaining popularity. It has more sensitivity in histology other than squamous cell carcinoma. It has overall staging accuracy of 69–78%. Tumours of supraglottic region and Waldeyer's tonsillar rings are most difficult to detect by PET scan. PET can detect lesions up to 5 mm.

When to perform examination under anaesthesia (EUA) and describe the technique?

EUA is performed when primary cannot be detected by imaging and triple endoscopy. Biopsies are taken from any suspicious area. Blind biopsies are taken from posterior wall of pharynx near fossa of Rosenmüller. Biopsy is also taken from base of the tongue, post-cricoid region and pyriform sinus. Ipsilateral tonsillectomy is carried out.

How do you manage such cases?

Options available for squamous cilia are:

1. Extensive bilateral neck irradiation (50 to 70 Gy) including head and neck mucosa.
2. If it is N1 disease without extra capsular extension without any history of incisional or excision biopsy neck dissection (Level 1–4) can be carried out. Postoperative radiation is given in cases of extra capsular spread, in cases of previous biopsy or N2–3 disease.
3. Salvage neck dissection is indicated in nodal relapses or after irradiation.
4. Platinum based chemotherapy preceding radiotherapy is recommended for N3 disease.

Poorly Differentiated Carcinoma

The most probable site of origin in these cases is nasopharynx. Treatment consists of radiotherapy to the neck and Waldeyer's ring including nasopharynx. Neck dissection is reserved for residual disease. Concomitant chemotherapy and radiotherapy is reserved for N2 and N3 disease.

Adenocarcinoma

If nodes are located at level 1–3, the possible site of primary is salivary gland. An excision biopsy is carried out in these cases. If clinical and pathological examination cannot identify the source of the primary, there is consensus on neck dissection (level 1–4) including parotidectomy followed by radiotherapy.

If metastatic lymph node is found at level 4 or supraclavicular region, an excision biopsy of the lymph node is carried out and pathologist should make every effort to find out the primary. In case of possible thyroid origin total thyroidectomy and level II–VI dissection should be performed. When the source of primary cannot be detected the tumour is considered as disseminated (M1) and chemotherapy is given.

8

Swelling of Jaw

What are the anatomical characteristics of jaw bones?

a. Jaw bones are mesodermal in origin with membranous ossification.
b. Jaw bones have cartilage at places like pre-maxilla, symphysis mentis and condylar process.
c. Mandible and maxilla contain epithelial elements like embedded tooth germs in their substance not found in any other bone.
d. There are pleuripotent cells in the region of lamina dura.
e. Upper jaw contains maxillary sinus lined by columnar epithelium.
f. Epithelium of the cheek and floor of the mouth are intimately fixed to the mucoperiosteum of the gum.

Describe clinical features of swelling of the jaw.

1. Deformity of face and jaw, including malignment of teeth
2. Recurrent oral or dental sepsis
3. Obstructive features, e.g. epiphora due to nasal obstruction in upper jaw tumour implicating medial wall involvement
4. Past history of trauma, dental extraction, exploitation of teeth or dental sepsis
   Examine upper jaw and lower jaw, teeth, Vth and VIIth nerve, TM joint and lymph nodes.

Enumerate the structures from where jaw tumour can arise from.

a. *Mucoperiosteum*: Swelling arising from alveolar margin of jaw is known as *epulis*.
   The epulis can be:
   1. Fibrous

2. Granulomatous
3. Myeloid
4. Sarcomatous
5. Carcinomatous

b. *From tooth germ*: These swellings are known as odontomes. These can be odontogenic developmental cyst or odontogenic tumours.
   The odontogenic developmental cyst can be:
   1. Dental cyst
   2. Dentigerous cyst
   3. Keratocyst.
   Odontogenic tumours are odontoma or ameloblastoma.

c. *From maxillary antrum*: It can be carcinoma or sarcoma

d. From bone

Classify Jaw Swellings

Epulis

Definition: It is a discrete and localised swelling arising from the alveolar margin of jaw. The term epulis means upon the gum. So epulis is a swelling situated upon the gum. It can originate from:

a. Bone
b. The periosteum
c. Mucous membrane
d. Junction of periodontal membrane with alveolar-mucosa.

What is fibrous epulis?

- Fibrous epulis: It is fibroma and consists of fusiform cells with many new blood vessels and arises as a result of chronic irritation. Initially present as soft, red swelling which later on becomes firm and pink as more collagen is deposited in the central mass. It arises from the periosteum at the neck of incisor or premolar teeth.

Describe clinical features of fibrous epulis.

- More common in females in the age group of thirties.
- Present as slowly growing polypoidal swelling in response to local irritation from sharp margin of teeth or carious cavity. As it grows it separates the teeth and ultimately loosens them.
- It may undergo malignant change, e.g. fibrosarcoma.
- Excision is the treatment of choice. Adjacent tooth or teeth and resection of wedge of bone with its root must be performed to avoid recurrence.

What is granulomatous epulis?

It is also known as false epulis or pregnancy epulis or pyogenic granuloma. It is a mass of granulation tissue around a carious tooth. Similar condition found in pregnancy is known as gingivitis gravidarum which is a temporary condition occurs due to hormonal changes and regresses after child birth. It presents as bright red or pink coloured swelling which is soft, vascular and bleeds easily on touch. It is often associated with a carious tooth, poor oral hygiene and offensive smell of mouth due to infection of the epulis. Draining lymph nodes may be enlarged or tender.

What is the treatment of granulomatous epulis?

The treatment is extraction of a carious tooth and replacement of ill-fitting denture if any. Good oral hygiene should be maintained. The granulation tissue is scraped and sent for histopathology. The mass of granulation tissue is excised by electrocautery.

What is myeloid epulis?

It is a purple pedunculated mass arises from underlying bone. Pathologically it is osteoclatoma. It arises from irritation due to an adjacent infected socket. Microscopically it consists of multinucleated giant cells with fibrocelluar tissue in stroma.

It presents as firm mass arising due to expansion of the marginal bone under cover of the muco-periosteum but the mucosa over the gum is hyperaemic oedematous, soft to touch. Swelling is usually plum coloured due to high vascularity. It is more rapidly growing tumour in comparison to other types of epulis. The adjoining teeth are loosened or separated.

X-ray shows a typical soap bubble appearance.

What is carcinomatous epulis?

It is an epithelioma of the gum arising from the mucous membrane of the alveolar margin. It is an infiltrating tumour which at later stage can fungate to give rise to an ulcerated form. It may present as a lump or an ulcer which can be painful. Soon it may invade the bone and regional lymph nodes are always involved. Biopsy is performed to confirm the diagnosis.

Treatment is adequate excision of growth along with adequate margin of healthy tissue which means excision of maxilla in upper jaw and excision of mandible in lower jaw. Radiotherapy can be tried in selected cases.

What are the tumours arising from tooth germs?

Tumours arising from tooth germs are known as odontomes.

Describe pathology of odontomes.

a. Odontomes are developmental aberrations from tooth germinal layers.
b. They comprise mixture of hard dental tissue, enamely dentine and cementum as burried mass in alveolus.
c. They develop from downward extension of epithelium from enamel organ of tooth, which persist as epithelial rests and give rise to epithelial odontomes.
d. There are projections of dental lamina into ectoderm and mesenchyme.
e. Dental lamina is a layered cap which consists of inner/outer enamel epithelium, stratum inter-medium and stellate reticulum (IEE).
f. The odontoblasts secrete dentin and ameloblasts (from IEE) which leads to formation of enamel.
g. The cementoblasts secrete cementum.
h. Fibroblasts form periodontal membrane.

Diagnosis

Complete history: Pain, loosing of teeth, dental malocclusion, localised jaw swellings and delayed tooth eruption.

Thorough physical examination
Plain radiographs: Panorex, dental radiographs.
  CT for larger, aggressive lesions.
Histopathology: FNA—To rule out vascular lesions, inflammatory.
  Excisional biopsy—smaller cysts, unilocular tumours.
  Incisional biopsy—larger lesions prior to definitive therapy.

What are odontogenic cysts?

- *Inflammatory*
  - Radicular
  - Para-dental
- *Developmental*
  - Dentigerous

Describe dental or radicular cyst?

- Most common (65%)
- Arises from epithelial cell rests of Malassez
- It is the response to inflammation to chronically infected tooth necrotic pulp. The continued irritation stimulates the nests of cells to proliferate. The centre of the mass gets necrosed, liquefied and gets converted into cyst. This type of cyst is usually lined by stratified squamous epithelium. The contents may be fluid or semisolid and usually contains cellular debris, cholesterol crystals and foreign body giant cells.
- The cyst usually appears at the root of normally erupted teeth which is chronically infected or carious.
- Commonly seen in middle age persons.
- More commonly occurs in upper jaw and may attain large size to encroach upon maxillary antrum. It evently open into it.
- With enlargement of cyst there is resorption of adjacent bone thus leading to expansion of jaw. It may fill the maxillary antrum and then it should be differentiated from carcinoma of the antrum.
- When the bone is thinned there will be eggshell crackling and fluctuation will be present if bone is completely destroyed.
- Radiographic findings:
  1. Unilocular oval or circular radiolucent area in relation to the root of a tooth (more often in upper jaw than in lower jaw).
  2. Translucent area may have a thin rim of sclerosed bone.

- *Treatment*—extraction of causative carious teeth and root canal treatment. The cyst is approached intra-orally. The cyst wall is curetted and whole epithelial lining is removed. The soft tissue is pushed into obliterate the residual cavity and wound is sutured.

What is dentigerous (follicular) cyst?

- Most common developmental cyst (24%)
- This is a swelling arising in connection with and containing non-erupted permanent teeth.
- Lesion arises from the follicle of the developing teeth. Follicle contains inner epithelial lining and outer connective tissue covering.
- The cyst is solitary and multilocular.
- Lining of the cyst is usually fibrous but may be stratified squamous or columnar.
- Contents of cyst is thick and viscid containing cholesterol crystals and unerupted teeth.
- The cyst displaces teeth deeper into the jaw and prevents it from erupting. The tooth may lie obliquely free in the cyst cavity or may be embedded in the cyst wall.
- Cyst enlarges with expansion of bone and displacement of teeth to which cyst is attached.
- Fluid between reduced enamel epithelium and tooth crown.
- Radiographic findings:
  - Unilocular radiolucency with well-defined sclerotic margins.
- Histology is non-keratinizing squamous epithelium
  Clinical features: Commonly seen in young adult and children. It may involve the lower or upper jaw. Commonly occur in association with lower third molar or premolar teeth.
  Present with painlessly growing swelling with missing teeth at the site of cyst.
  Treatment: Total excision of cyst via intraoral approach. Other options are enucleation of cyst or decompression if total excision is not possible.

What is odontogenic keratocyst?

- 11% of jaw cysts are odontogenic keratocysts
- May mimic any of the other cysts
- Most often in mandibular ramus and angle
- Radiographically they appear as:
  - Well-marginated, radiolucency
  - Pericoronal, inter-radicular, or pericoronal
  - Multilocular

- *Histology*
  - Thin epithelial lining with underlying connective tissue (collagen and epithelial nests)
  - Secondary inflammation may mask features
- High frequency of recurrence (up to 62%)
- Complete removal difficult and satellite cysts can be left behind
- *Treatment*
  - Depends on extent of lesion
  - Small—simple enucleation, complete removal of cyst wall
  - Larger—enucleation with/without peripheral ostectomy
  - Bataineh *et al.* promoted complete resection with 1 cm bony margins (if extension through cortex, overlying soft tissues excised)
- Long-term follow-up required (5–10 years)

What are odontogenic tumours?

- Ameloblastoma
- Calcifying epithelial odontogenic tumour
- Adenomatoid odontogenic tumour
- Squamous odontogenic tumour
- Calcifying odontogenic cyst.

Describe pathology of ameloblastomas.

- Most common odontogenic tumour which is benign, but locally invasive low grade malignant epithelial tumour with a high rate of recurrences if not removed adequately but do not have any tendency to metastasize.
- Most commonly arise from embryonic enamel organ of tooth. It can also arise from displaced dental epithelial remnants.
- It is clinically and histologically similar to basal cell carcinoma.
- Most commonly occurs in the 4th and 5th decades.
- The tumour enlarges slowly and produces destruction and enlargement of mandible. Once the outer cortex is thinned out tumour ulcerates.
- Spread is mainly local without any lymphatic or blood borne spread. However, endobronchial spread is rarely seen. This apparently arises from ulceration of over lying intraoral mucous membrane over the enlarging either with inhalation of fragmented or detached tumour into the bronchial tree.

- Subtypes of ameloblastoma
  - Multi-cystic (86%),
  - Uni-cystic (13%),
  - Peripheral (extra-osseous—1%)
- Classical radiographic findings are:
- Classically seen as multilocular radiolucency of posterior mandible which is well-circumscribed and known as soap-bubble appearance:
  - Unilocular—often confused with odontogenic cysts
  - Root resorption—associated with malignancy
- *Histology*
  - Two patterns—plexiform and follicular (no bearing on prognosis)
  - Classic—sheets and islands of tumour cells, outer rim of ameloblasts is polarised away from basement membrane
  - Centre looks like stellate reticulum
  - Squamous differentiation (1%)—diagnosed as ameloblastic carcinoma.

What are clinical features of ameloblastoma?

- Commonly seen in females in any age group above 11 years of age but common in 4th and 5th decades.
- Painless progressive swelling in the lower jaw at or near its angle or in the molar region.
- Irregular lobulated surface of the swelling leads to distortion of face and ugly deformity. Swelling grows more towards the cheek with normal medial or lingual side.
- On palpation there is eggshell crackling.
- There is marked protrusion of mandible or malalignment of teeth or malocclusion of teeth. There are no missing teeth.
- No regional lymph nodes palpable.

Describe treatment of ameloblastoma.

According to growth characteristics and type:
- Unicystic
  - Complete removal
  - Peripheral ostectomies if extension through cyst wall
- Classic infiltrative (aggressive)
  - Mandibular—adequate normal bone around margins of resection
  - Maxillary—more aggressive surgery, 1.5 cm margins

- Ameloblastic carcinoma
  - Radical surgical resection (like squamous cell carcinoma)
  - Neck dissection for LAN

What is calcifying epithelial pdontogenic tumour?

- Also known as "Pindborg tumour"
- Aggressive tumour of epithelial derivation
- Impacted tooth, mandible body/ramus
- Chief sign—cortical expansion
- Pain not normally a complaint
- Radiographic findings:
  - Expanded cortices in all dimensions
  - Radiolucent; poorly defined, non-corticated borders
  - Unilocular, multilocular, or "moth-eaten"
  - "Driven-snow" appearance from multiple radiopaque foci
  - Root divergence/resorption; impacted tooth

Histology
- Islands of eosinophilic epithelial cells
- Cells infiltrate bony trabeculae
- Nuclear hyperchromatism and pleomorphism
- Psammoma-like calcifications (Liesegang rings)

Treatment
- Behaves like ameloblastoma
- Smaller recurrence rates
- En bloc resection, hemimandibulectomy partial maxillectomy suggested.

What is adenomatoid odontogenic tumour?

- Associated with the crown of an impacted anterior tooth
- Painless expansion
- Radiographic findings
- Well-defined expansile radiolucency
- Root divergence, calcified flecks ("target")
  Histology
  Thick fibrous capsule, clusters of spindle cells, columnar cells (rosettes, ductal) throughout.
  Treatment: Enucleation, recurrence is rare.

What are other related jaw lesions?

- Giant cell lesions
  - Central giant cell granuloma
  - Brown tumour
  - Aneurysmal bone cyst
- Fibro-osseous lesions
  - Fibrous dysplasia
  - Ossifying fibroma
- Condensing osteitis
- Plastic-like reactive proliferation.

Thorax

Section 2

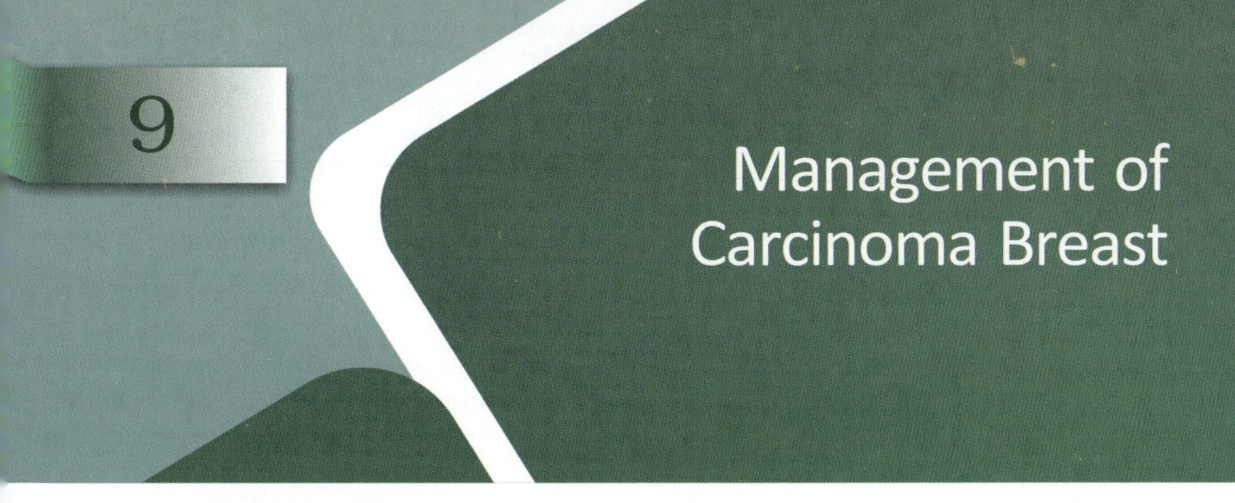

Management of Carcinoma Breast

9

STAGEWISE CA BREAST MANAGEMENT: INVESTIGATIONS AND TREATMENT

What important history should be taken in a lady presenting with breast lump?

Relevant history in women with breast lump comprises the following points:

Breast Lump History

1. Duration of lump
2. Progress of lump or change in size with time
3. Change in lump in relation to menstrual cycle
4. Associated pain with lump
5. Any history of nipple discharge
6. History of hormonal therapy
7. Family history of breast cancer (first or second degree relatives) with age of onset
8. Any past history of breast cancer
9. Any past history of breast lump and biopsies
10. Any recent history of breast trauma or surgery
11. Any recent radiation or chemotherapy
12. Smoking history
13. Age at first childbearing, age at menopause
14. Current lactation status
15. History of breastfeeding

What are the common presenting features of breast cancer?

1. Palpable mass
2. Thickening
3. Pain
4. Nipple discharge
5. Nipple retraction
6. Discolouration of areola
7. Mass or pain in the axillary region
8. Oedema, erythematous changes or ulceration of skin

What is the differential diagnosis of benign breast lumps?

Benign breast masses can be
1. Normal "lumpy" breast tissue
2. Simple (gross) cysts
3. Fibro-adenomas
4. Pseudoangiomatous stromal hyperplasia (PASH)
5. Lipomas (palpable subcutaneous fat lumps)
6. Tubular and lactating adenomas
7. Granular cell tumours, benign vascular lesions
8. Leiomyomas, neurofibromas (all rare)

What is the best time to perform clinical breast examination?

If the breast examination is being performed in premenstrual patients, it should be carried out a week after menses, as during this period breast tissue is least engorged. In postmenopausal patients or in patients presenting with breast lump it can be done at any time.

What are the clinical features of benign breast lump?

Benign breast masses are generally smooth surfaced, have well defined margins, soft to firm in consistency and mobile within the breast tissue. Benign breast lump can be moved in any quadrant of breast and has been often described as breast mouse. They can also present as diffuse symmetric thickening.

What are the clinical features of malignant breast lump?

Malignant breast lumps are:
a. Hard
b. Immobile
c. Fixed to surrounding skin
d. Poorly defined or irregular margins

Why and when should a breast examination be performed?

In the asymptomatic patient: The asymptomatic breast examination is generally performed by the clinician on an annual basis, beginning at the age of 40, which coincides with time of increased risk for development of breast cancer or in younger patients with increased risk of breast cancer. Increased risk of breast cancer is seen in the following conditions:
a. Prior history of breast carcinoma
b. Family history in 1st degree relative (particularly if at a young age)
c. Increasing patient age, and
d. Features that result in prolonged/uninterrupted exposure to oestrogen
   1. Nulliparity
   2. Older age (after 20 years) at first pregnancy
   3. History of benign breast disease especially cystic disease, proliferative type of hyperplasia or atypical hyperplasia.
   4. History of breast cancer
   5. Exposure to ionising radiation
   6. History of breast cancer in first degree relatives
   7. History of hormonal therapy
   8. Obesity (BMI > 30)
      SBE is often recommended on a monthly-to-every-few-months basis.

In the symptomatic patient: The goal of the examination in the setting of symptoms is:
a. To characterize the abnormality,
b. To identify the underlying aetiology, and
c. For additional evaluation and treatment.

What are the common breast related symptoms for which patient presents?

- *Discrete masses* detected by the patient, often concerning for malignancy.
- *Pain*, which can be associated with a number of processes including cyclical in a menstruating woman (reflecting transient hormone induced changes in the breast tissue), occasionally malignancies.

- *Unusual nipple discharge*, which may include:
  - Blood, concerning for malignancy
  - Milk when not pregnant. Suggestive of inappropriate prolactin secretion from the pituitary—(may also be induced by certain medications)
  - Fibro adenoma
  - Hypothyroidism
- *Discolouration or change in the quality of the skin*:
  - Redness suggests infection or inflammation in the post-partum patient; this is often due to mastitis
  - "Peau d'orange" quality—an "Orange Peel" like texture, i.e. caused by a malignancy which causes obstruction of sub-dermal lymphatics leading to oedema of dermis but the fixed points in the dermis where sweat glands are attached cannot swell thus giving an orange peel appearance. This orange appearance can also be seen in chronic breast abscess where lymphatics gets blocked by fibrosis (Fig. 9.1).

If a mass or other abnormality is identified, its location can be described as being in 1 of 4 quadrants (left upper, left lower, right upper, right lower) of the breast. Alternatively, it can be described relative to its position, imagining a clock face was superimposed on the breast (Fig. 9.2).

Detailed Technique of Examination

Getting Started

1. Introduce yourself to the patient (male physician should always have female chaperone during examination.)
2. Carefully explain the procedure of examination and reassure the patient.
3. The examination should be performed at a comfortable room temperature.

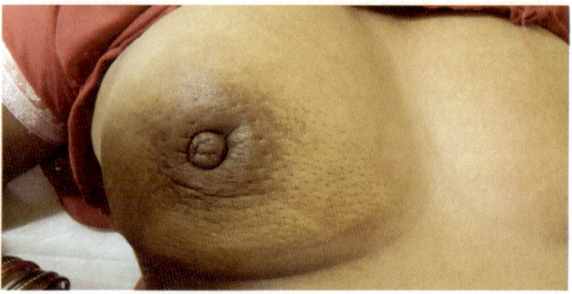

Fig. 9.1: Clinical picture of carcinoma right breast showing peau d'orange appearance

9. Inspection of both the breasts simultaneously while the patient sits up may detect asymmetry or other surface abnormalities, particularly if the person has large breasts (Fig. 9.4).

Inspection to be done in sitting position with arms on the side, with arms raised above head and with the patient leaning forward. During inspection the note is made of asymmetry, nipple discharge, obvious visible lump, skin changes such as dimpling, unilateral nipple retraction or inversion.

Palpation of the breast and axilla: The goal of this examination is to examine the breast in a systematic fashion, such that all of the tissue is palpated.

Palpation Technique in Detail

a. Use the pads of the middle 3 fingers of one hand (Fig. 9.5).
b. Press downward using an circular motion.

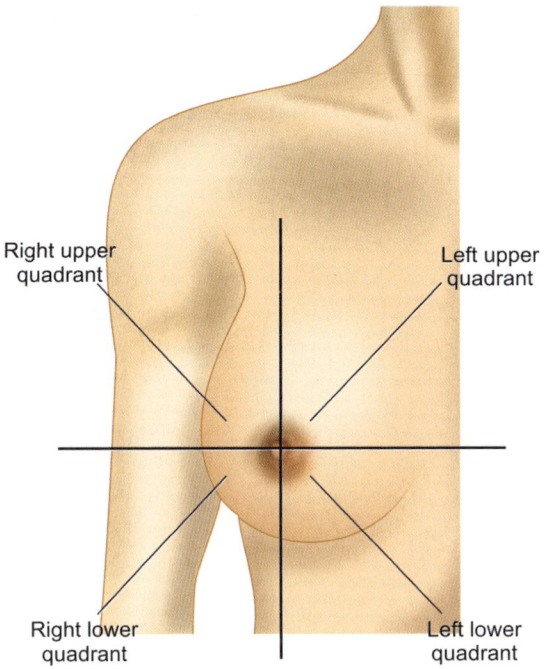

Right upper quadrant

Left upper quadrant

Right lower quadrant

Left lower quadrant

Fig. 9.2: Division of breast into four quadrants

4. Patient should be in a gown with all under-garments (bras, shirts, etc.) removed.
5. The patient should wear the gown in such a manner so that it opens in the front, which makes exposure of one breast at a time a bit easier.
6. Patient should be lying supine on the table.
7. Uncover only the breast to be examined.
8. Inspect the breast, looking for evidence of skin or nipple dimpling/retraction, discolouration, obvious masses or asymmetry (Fig. 9.3).

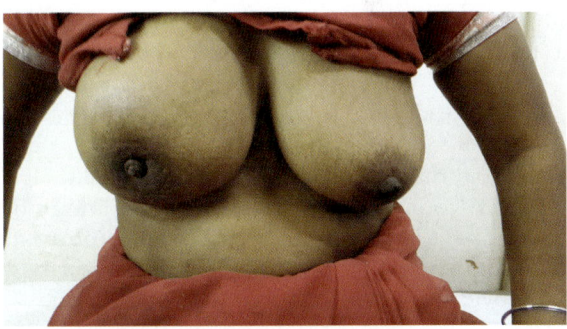

Fig. 9.4: Clinical picture showing a enlarged right breast which is at a higher level in comparison to left

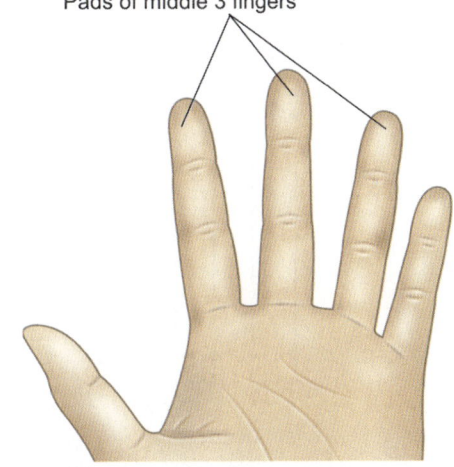

Pads of middle 3 fingers

Fig. 9.5: Technique to palpate the breast with pulps of middle three fingers

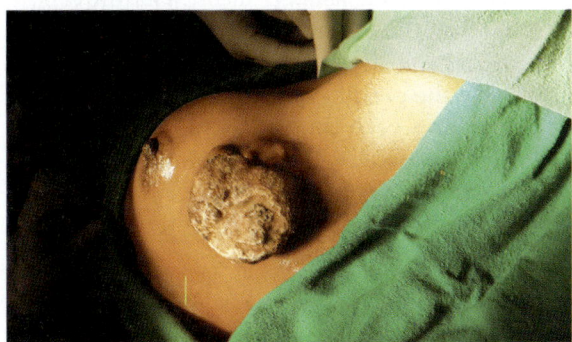

Fig. 9.3: Carcinoma breast with ulcero-proliferative mass involving the upper outer quadrant of the right breast

c. Apply steady pressure, pushing down to the level of the chest wall. Apply enough pressure to palpate to 3 levels of depth: First superficial, then medium, and then deep/to the level of the chest wall.

d. Make sure to palpate the nipple and areolar regions.

What precisely are you trying to identify?

Normal breasts have a lumpy consistency, created by the mix of lobular, ductal and supporting tissue. The CBE (as mentioned above) is largely performed to identify masses consistent with malignancy as described above. It is easier to identify masses in older patients as breast density decreases with age (lobular tissue replaced by fat).

Three Methods for Systematic Examination of the Breast

Method 1—Vertical Stripes (Fig. 9.6)

a. In this technique, the breast is divided into a series of vertical stripes, each of which is evaluated sequentially, moving lateral to medial.

b. Start at the clavicle, adjacent to the axilla

c. Move your hand down in a vertical line until you have reached the area below the breast. Actual palpation technique is as described above.

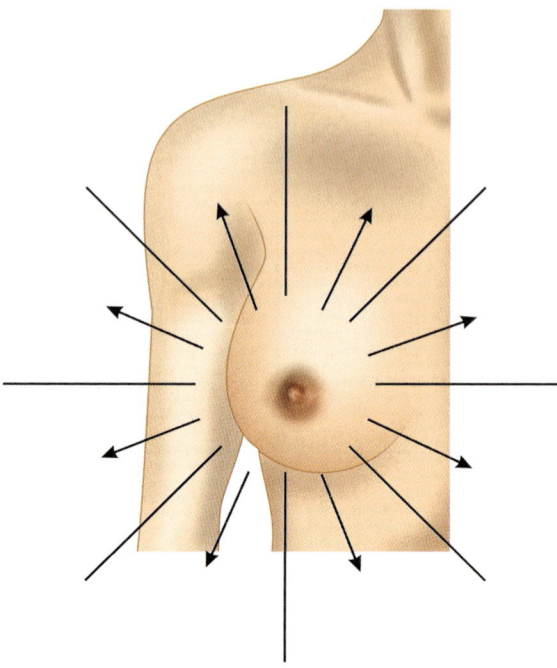

Fig. 9.7: Radial spoke pattern to palpate the breast

d. Then move a bit more medially, and examine while travelling up towards the top of the breast.

e. When you reach the clavicle, move medially and repeat until you have evaluated the entire breast.

f. There is a "tail" of breast tissue that extends from the lateral aspect of the structure towards the axilla. Make sure that you palpate this region as well.

Method 2—Pie or Radial Spoke Pattern (Fig. 9.7)

a. Imagine that the breast is divided into a series of pie-type cone shaped slices, with the nipple at the centre.

b. Start at the nipple, and palpate outwards toward the periphery. Move your hands a few centimetres each time.

c. When you are clearly no longer over the breast, move to the next slice.

d. The "tail" of the breast should be palpated as described above.

Method 3—Circular Pattern (Fig. 9.8)

a. Start at the nipple.

b. Work along in a circular fashion, moving in a spiral towards the periphery.

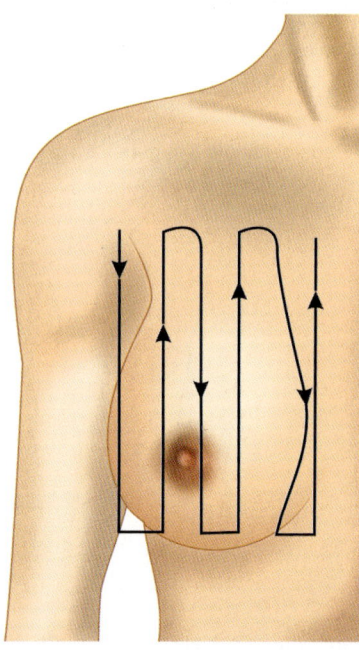

Fig. 9.6: Vertical stripes technique to palpate the breast

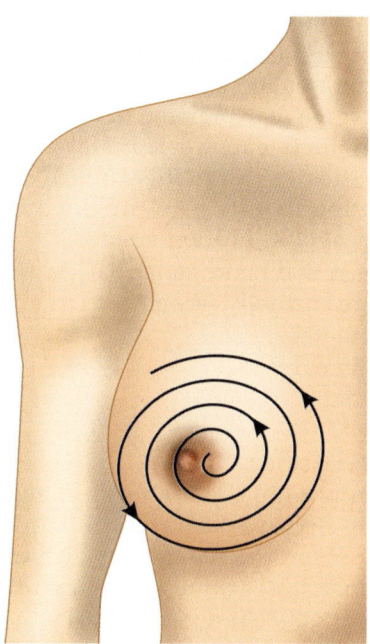

Fig. 9.8: Circular pattern of breast examination

c. Make sure that you palpate the "tail" of the breast as described in above.

After palpation of the breast, the axillary region should be palpated as the axillary lymph nodes are usually the first site of spread in malignancy. To examine axilla the following steps should be followed:

1. Patient sits on a stool or on the edge of examination table
2. Gently raise the arm 20–30 cm away from the patient's body, so that one can gain access to the axillary region.
3. Direct the finger tips of the examining hand (use your left hand when examining the right axilla, and vice versa) toward the top of the axilla.
4. Then direct the palmar aspect of the hand towards the chest wall. Roll the hand downwards on chest wall. You may be able to trap the nodes between your hand and the chest wall, which can then be better characterised.
5. If one feels discrete masses, make note of: Firmness, quantity and degree of mobility. In general, malignancy is associated with: firmness, increased quantity, adherence to each other and/or the chest wall.
6. Similarly attempt is made to palpate nodes behind anterior axillary fold, posterior axillary

fold and the lateral group of nodes. Posterior group of lymph nodes can be palpated from behind of patient.
7. Recognise that adenopathy may not be due to breast disease. For example, infections of the hand can cause acute, painful axillary adenopathy. Similarly, systemic diseases (e.g. lymphoma, sarcoidosis) may also cause lymph node enlargement. Thus, as with all other aspects of the examination, history and findings in other regions are of great importance.

The other breast is then examined

Additional aspects of the exam that can be performed:

1. *Assessment of nipple discharge:* If the patient reports unusual discharge from the nipple, gently palpate the breast near the nipple, with a goal of trying to express and examine any abnormal fluid. Bloody discharge is particularly of concern for cancer. Most discharge, however, will be secondary to benign conditions.
2. *Puckering/dimpling:* This can suggest an underlying mass which is distorting the skin above it. In this setting, careful palpation around the dimpling is often revealing. In addition, if it is unclear whether there is dimpling or asymmetry, observe the breasts while the patient sits up (with hands placed on hips). This may help clarify differences between the 2 sides and accentuate asymmetry.
3. *Nipple retraction:* This is concerning for a mass growing underneath the nipple. In this case, carefully palpate the tissue around and underneath the nipple.
4. *Redness/pain:* Suggestive of inflammation and/or infection. Carefully note the extent of redness as well as temperature differences. Assess for any focal swelling or fluctuance that might suggest underlying abscess.

What follows is directed to the more novice examiner?

- If a clear or a discrete mass is identified, it is considered to be malignant until proven otherwise. In general, determination of final diagnosis requires a tissue diagnosis.
- A dominant breast mass that does not have a corresponding abnormality on mammogram should still be considered malignant until

proven otherwise. This is because not all malignancies generate mammographic findings.

- While uncommon, breast cancer can occur in men. Thus, discrete masses in males should be appropriately evaluated.
- Breast cancer can occur in young women (20s and 30s). Thus, clinically palpable masses in this age group should be appropriately evaluated.
- If one has any doubt or uncertainty, re-examine the finding and seek input from seniors.

How effective is clinical breast examination (CBE)?

Clinical breast examination

a. CBE detects about 60% of mammography detected cancers.
b. CBE finds some cancers not seen on mammography.
c. No randomized trials compare mortality between women offered vs. not offered CBE.

Bimanual palpation should be done to adequately examine all areas in patients with large breasts as these often have an infra-mammary ridge.

What causes skin retraction in breast pathology?

a. In superficial tumours it can be caused by direct extension of tumour into skin or fibrosis.
b. In tumours within the substance of breast tissue, it is caused by involvement of Cooper's ligament.
c. In benign breast disease it is caused by
   1. Granular cell tumour
   2. Traumatic fat necrosis
   3. After surgical biopsy
   4. In thrombophlebitis of the thoraco-epigastric vein (Mondor's disease)

What are the common histopathological types of breast cancer?

1. *In situ* cancer can be of ductal or lobular variety
2. Paget disease of the nipple which can have associated component of invasive ductal carcinoma
3. Invasive carcinoma—80%
4. Invasive lobular carcinoma—10%
5. Uncommon histopathological types—10%
   (a) Medullary, (b) Tubular, (c) Mucinous, (d) Papillary, (e) Squamous
6. Invasive ductal carcinoma (NOS)—80%

What is molecular classification of breast cancer?

Gene expression analysis has demonstrated distinct molecular classes of breast cancers based on the degree of expression of a select number of genes, which can be translated into more prognostically and therapeutically useful information than can be provided by existing histological classification systems.

At least five main molecular classes of breast cancer are currently recognized:
1. Luminal A
2. Luminal B
3. HER2
4. Basal
5. Unclassified

Recently published studies have used five surrogate IHC markers (ER, PR, HER2, CK5/6, and EGFR) for molecular class distinction.

Luminal classes express hormone receptors and have a pattern that agrees with the luminal epithelial component of the mammary gland. They express luminal CK8/18, ER and genes associated with its activation, such as LIV1 and CCND1.

Luminal Type (A)

Luminal A tumours are:
a. ER positive
b. PR positive or negative
c. HER2 negative
d. CK5/6 and EGFR negative
e. Express cytokeratin 8 and 18
f. Luminal A is the most frequent subtype
g. It shows a good prognosis and responds well to hormone therapy. Various studies have reported that ER positive tumours have comparatively poor response to conventional chemotherapy.

Luminal Type (B)

These tumours are similar to luminal type A but they have Ki67 proliferation index of more than 13.25%. Ki67 is a nuclear marker of cell proliferation, and its expression correlates proportionally to poorer clinical outcomes. They tend to have poor prognosis in comparison to luminal type A.

HER2 Positive Tumour

HER2 positive tumours are HER2 positive, ER and PR negative, and CK5/6 and EGFR negative.

Overexpression of HER2 in tumour cells implies a poor prognosis. It also demonstrates the highest sensitivity to neoadjuvant chemotherapy based on anthracyclines and taxanes.

The poor prognosis of HER2 is in the form of high risk of early relapse.

Basal-like Tumours

Basal-like tumours are CK5/6 and/or EGFR positive, ER and PR negative, and HER2 negative. The basal class is named because of its pattern of expression which is similar to basal epithelial cells and normal myoepithelial cells of mammary tissue. This similarity is a product of the lack of ER expression and related genes, low expression of HER2, intense expression of CKs 5, 6, and 17, and the gene expression related with cellular proliferation.

This class has also been called "triple negative" for not expressing ER, PR, or HER2. It has been associated with the BRCA1 mutation. They have characteristic histological features such as solid-pushing borders, geographic areas of necrosis, and dense lymphocytic infiltrates.

Unclassified

Unclassified tumours are ER and PR negative, HER2 negative, and CK5/6 and EGFR negative. They correspond to those triple-negative tumours not exhibiting basal markers. Unclassified cases were initially considered to be synonymous with "normal-like" breast cancers. These tumours cluster with non-tumoural breast cells and exhibit overexpression of PIK3R1 and AKR1C1, in addition to other genomic alterations. The current concept states that the "normal-like" subtype is absolutely different from the unclassified (penta +ve) "ER, PR, HER2, and CK5/6 and EGFR" group, as absent or decreased expression of basal markers is not a feature compatible with the "normal-like" molecular class.

They are very good prognostically and are grouped with the luminals, both of which exhibit low pathologic complete remission rates of 6%.

How will you confirm the diagnosis of breast cancer?

The diagnosis can be confirmed by core tissue biopsy using tru-cut needle or by fine needle aspiration cytology (FNAC).

Advantages of FNAC	Advantages of core needle box over FNAC
Less invasive/traumatic	Can differentiate *in situ* from invasive carcinoma
No local anaesthesia required	Differentiate subtypes of carcinoma
Economical	Differentiate lobular from ductal carcinoma
No cut required	Differentiate giant fibro adenoma from sarcoma
	Application of hormone receptor assay

How do you classify findings on FNAC?

FNAC findings are classified as below:

C1   Insufficient cells for diagnosis. This indicates that FNAC has failed. It requires either repeat FNAC or core biopsy requires.

C2   Benign cells seen

C3   Atypical cells probably benign. In all these cases tissue diagnosis must be obtained.

C4   Atypical cells probably malignant. In this case also tissue diagnosis is required.

C5   Malignant cells seen. It does not necessarily indicate invasive carcinoma as malignant cells can be obtained from DCIS

What metastatic work up you will carry out?

i. Complete blood count (CBC): An abnormal CBC should prompt evaluation of bone marrow for metastatic disease.

ii. Chest X-ray (PA view) for all patients.

iii. CT chest/abdomen reserved for localising symptoms or abnormal lab values suggesting liver involvement or abnormal X-ray chest.

iv. Liver function test including alkaline phosphatase (ALP). Elevated levels of liver enzymes or ALP along with GGT suggest liver secondary. Elevated ALP alone with or without calcium suggests bone secondaries.

v. Bone scan in stage 3 and stage 4, localising symptoms or isolated abnormal ALP.

vi. FDG-PET scan role is still evolving but may be useful to detect occult metastasis but it is not a standard of care.

vii. Evaluation of cardiac systolic function by echocardiography or MUGA scan before and during treatment with anthracyclines-based chemotherapy or during herceptin therapy as both are potentially cardiotoxic drugs.

viii. Mammography for the opposite breast and for the same breast if BCS is being planned.

What is the role of screening by MR mammography instead of digital mammography?

a. A BRCA1 or BRCA2 mutation
b. A first degree relative with BRCA1 or BRCA2 mutation (parent, sibling or child)
c. If the calculated lifetime risk of developing breast cancer is more than 20–25%
d. History of radiation to chest wall between 10 and 30 years of age
e. Germ line p-53 mutation or PTEN mutation as seen in Li-Fraumeni syndrome or in Cowden syndrome
f. If breast biopsy reveals atypical ductal hyperplasia or atypical lobular hyperplasia
g. Very dense breast or unevenly distributed dense breast as determined on mammogram
h. Patient already having breast cancer in one breast.

What is BIRADS system?

The BIRADS acronym stands for Breast Imaging-Reporting and Data System which is a widely accepted risk assessment and quality assurance tool in mammography, ultrasound or MRI. Part of the initial implementation was to make the reporting of mammograms more standardised and comprehensible to the non-radiologist reading the report.

The latest version classifies lesions into 6 categories:

BIRADS 0: The incomplete study—further imaging or information is required, e.g. compression, magnification, special mammographic views, ultrasound. This is also used when previous images not available at the time of reading.

BIRADS I: Negative-symmetrical and no masses, architectural disturbances or suspicious calcifications present.

BIRADS II: Benign findings—interpreter may wish to describe a benign-appearing finding, e.g.
1. Calcified fibroadenomas
2. Multiple secretory calcifications
3. Fat containing lesions such as
   - *Oil cysts*
   - *Breast lipomas*
   - *Galactoceles*
   - *Mixed density hamartomas*
   - *Simple breast cysts*

These all should have characteristic appearances, and may be labelled with confidence; the interpreter might wish to describe intra-mammary lymph nodes, implants, etc. while still concluding that there is no mammographic evidence suggesting malignancy.

BIRADS III: Probably benign—short interval follow-up suggested. The accent is on the word benign.

BIRADS IV: Suspicious abnormality—there is a mammographic appearance which is suspicious for malignancy. Biopsy should be considered for such a lesion.

These can be further divided as

BIRADS IVa: Low level of suspicion for malignancy

BIRADS IVb: Intermediate suspicion for malignancy

BIRADS IVc: Moderate suspicion for malignancy

BIRADS V: There is a mammographic appearance which is highly suggestive of malignancy—action should be taken.

BIRADS VI: Known biopsy proven malignancy. The vast majority of screening mammograms fall into BIRADS I or II

Risk of Cancer

- BIRADS III: ~ 2%
- BIRADS IV: ~ 30%
- BIRADS V: 95%

What is the role of MRI in breast cancer?

1. It can be used as problem solving tool in the setting of equivocal imaging (mammogram or USG) findings or equivocal physical examination findings, when breast cancer is suspected but cannot be established by conventional methods.
2. In the evaluation of patients who have previously undergone excision biopsy for breast cancer.
3. Evaluation of axillary node metastasis and unknown primary: MRI can detect ipsilateral breast cancer in 75 to 86 percent of cases when clinical examination and mammographic examination is normal.
4. In monitoring response to neo-adjuvant chemotherapy in locally advanced breast cancer. Earliest response to chemotherapy is decrease in the contrast enhancement of tumour even before decrease in size.
5. Evaluate breast cancer in a patient with breast implant.

Role in Preoperative Assessment of the Breast

Offer magnetic resonance imaging (MRI) of the breast to patients with invasive breast cancer:

- If there is discrepancy regarding the extent of disease from clinical examination, mammography and ultrasound assessment for planning breast conservation treatment.
- If breast density precludes accurate mammographic assessment
- To assess the tumour size if breast conserving surgery is being considered for invasive lobular cancer.

How to perform staging of the axilla?

Pre-treatment ultrasound evaluation of the axilla should be performed for all patients being investigated for early invasive breast cancer, if morphologically abnormal lymph nodes are identified, ultrasound-guided needle sampling should be offered.

Surgery to the Axilla

Minimal surgery, rather than lymph node clearance, should be performed to stage the axilla for patients with early invasive breast cancer and no evidence of lymph node involvement on ultrasound or a negative ultrasound-guided needle biopsy. Sentinel lymph node biopsy (SLNB) is the preferred technique. In patient with clinically palpable nodes, axillary dissection should be performed.

In which group of patients assessment of bone density is required?

- Patients with early invasive breast cancer should have a baseline dual energy X-ray absorptiometry (DEXA) scan to assess bone mineral density if they:
  - are starting adjuvant aromatase inhibitor treatment
  - have treatment-induced menopause
  - are starting ovarian ablation/suppression therapy

What subgroup of patients will be benefited with chemoprevention by Tamoxifen to reduce breast cancer risk?

1. History of lobular carcinoma *in situ*
2. History of atypical ductal or lobular hyperplasia
3. Premenopausal women with mutation in either BRCA1 or BRCA2 gene
4. Premenopausal women >35 with 5 yr risk of developing breast cancer >1.66% (on Gail model).

How do you stage breast cancer?

TNM staging

- Tx: Primary tumour cannot be assessed (tumour cannot be assessed because either it has been excised previously or disappeared completely due to neo-adjuvant chemotherapy or radiotherapy)
- T0: No evidence of primary tumour (T0 includes tumour which are not clinically palpable but detected on screening mammography)
- Tis: Intraductal carcinoma, lobular carcinoma *in situ*, or Paget disease of the nipple with no associated invasion of normal breast tissue
- Tis (DCIS): Ductal carcinoma *in situ*
- Tis (LCIS): Lobular carcinoma *in situ*
- Tis (Paget): Paget's disease of the nipple with no tumour. [Note: Paget's disease associated with a tumour is classified according to the size of the tumour.]
- T1: 2 cm or less in greatest dimension
- T2: Tumour larger than 2.0 cm but not larger than 5.0 cm in greatest dimension
- T3: Tumour larger than 5.0 cm in greatest dimension
- T4: Tumour of any size with direct extension to (a) chest wall, or (b) skin, only as described below
- T4a: Extension to chest wall, not including pectoralis muscle (chest wall includes ribs intercostal muscles or serratus anterior muscle)
- T4b: Oedema including peau d'orange or ulceration of the skin (Fig. 9.9) of the breast, or satellite skin nodules confined to the same breast

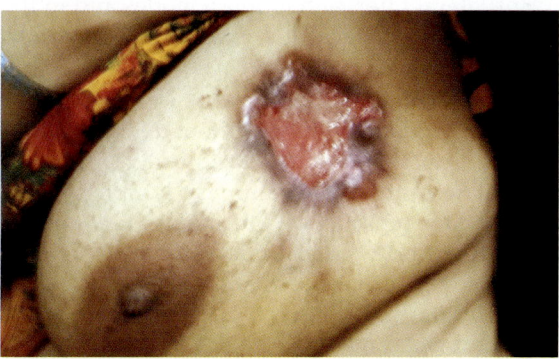

Fig. 9.9: Clinical picture of carcinoma left breast involving the skin

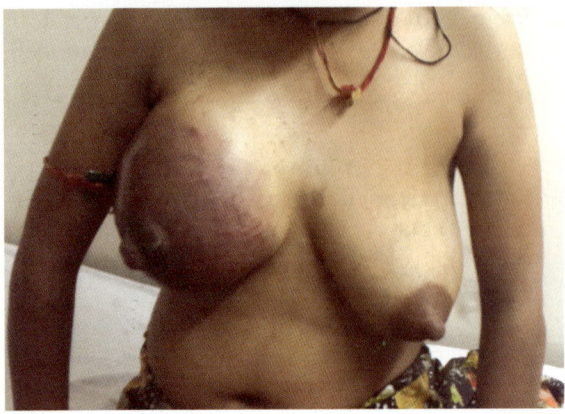

Fig. 9.10: Inflammatory breast cancer fixed to chest wall

- T4c: Both T4a and T4b
- T4d: Inflammatory carcinoma (Fig. 9.10)
- Regional lymph nodes (N)
- Nx: Regional lymph nodes cannot be assessed (e.g. previously removed)
- N0: No regional lymph node metastasis
- N1: Metastasis to movable ipsilateral axillary lymph node(s)
- N2: Metastasis to ipsilateral axillary lymph node(s) fixed or matted, or in clinically apparent* ipsilateral internal mammary nodes in the absence of clinically evident lymph node metastasis

  Clinically apparent internal mammary lymph node means lymph nodes presenting as parasternal mass, or detected on X-ray chest or on CT chest but not on lymphoscintigraphy.
- N2a: Metastasis in ipsilateral axillary lymph nodes fixed to one another (matted) or to other structures
- N2b: Metastasis only in clinically apparent* ipsilateral internal mammary nodes and in the absence of clinically evident axillary lymph node metastasis
- N3: Metastasis in ipsilateral infraclavicular lymph node(s) with or without axillary lymph node involvement, or in clinically apparent* ipsilateral internal mammary lymph node(s) and in the presence of clinically evident axillary lymph node metastasis; or metastasis in ipsilateral supraclavicular lymph node(s) with or without axillary or internal mammary lymph node involvement
- N3a: Metastasis in ipsilateral infraclavicular lymph node(s)
- N3b: Metastasis in ipsilateral internal mammary lymph node(s) and axillary lymph node(s)
- N3c: Metastasis in ipsilateral supraclavicular lymph node

What are AJCC Stage Groupings?

Stage 0
- Tis, N0, M0

Stage I
- T1*, N0, M0

Stage IIA
- T0, N1, M0
- T1*, N1, M0
- T2, N0, M0

Stage IIB
- T2, N1, M0
- T3, N0, M0

Stage IIIA
- T0, N2, M0
- T1*, N2, M0
- T2, N2, M0
- T3, N1, M0
- T3, N2, M0

Stage IIIB
- T4, N0, M0
- T4, N1, M0
- T4, N2, M0

*Stage IIIC***
- Any T, N3, M0

Stage IV
- Any T, Any N, M1

  *T1 includes T1mic.

Discuss treatment of breast cancer: Early/locally advanced/ metastatic breast cancer.

Early breast cancer: Early breast cancer includes stage 1 and stage 2.

Treatment of early breast cancer is appropriate surgery followed by adjuvant chemotherapy or hormonal therapy followed by radiotherapy to chest wall if indicated*

---

*Clinically apparent is defined as detected by imaging studies (excluding lymphoscintigraphy) or by clinical examination or grossly visible pathologically.

What is the aim of adjuvant of chemotherapy

To take care of occult micro-metastasis which over time grow into overt metastasis. Adjuvant chemotherapy is given after the primary surgery. Aim is to increase survival.

Indications of Adjuvant Chemotherapy

a. All node positive patients irrespective of menopausal status or ER status.

CAF × 6 cycles if patient is ER and PR +ve but HER2 negative

Taxane plus anthracycline based regimen (AC × 4 followed by paclitaxel x4), if patient is HER2 positive.

b. Node negative and ER positive, if they fall into high risk category:
   - High grade
   - HER2 gene amplification
   - Size more than 2 cm
   - Young age <45 years

c. Node negative and ER –ve patients if more than 1 cm or less than 1 cm, if HER2 +ve, high grade, or lymph vascular invasion

Adjuvant chemotherapy for node –ve patients can be

- AC × 4 cycles
- CAF × 6 cycles
- Oral or IV CMF (Bonadonna regimen) 6–8 cycles
- Role of Taxane in node negative cancer is not clear.

What is the role of adjuvant trastuzumab therapy?

In patients whose tumour overexpress HER2 as assessed by FISH or are designated 3+ by IHC.

Suggested regimen (ACx4 followed by weekly paclitaxel x12 cycles and trastuzumab for 1 year)

What are surgical options in early breast carcinoma?

- Modified radical mastectomy
- Breast conservation surgery (BCS)
  (Excision of lump along with 1 cm of tumour-free margin all around + axillary lymph node staging)

What are contraindications of BCS?

1. Two or more primary tumour in different quadrants (multi-centric or multi-focal disease)
2. Extensive malignant appearing micro-calcification on mammography
3. Persistent positive margins in spite of repeat re-excision surgery after BCS
4. Previous breast or mantle irradiation
5. Pregnancy
6. History of collagen vascular disease
7. Patients who are positive for BRCA1 or BRCA2 mutation
8. Tumour more than 5 cm
9. Central quadrant tumour

What are indications for radiotherapy (RT) to chest wall in early breast cancer?

i. After BCS, give radiotherapy to the **remaining breast tissue in all cases**

ii. Radiotherapy to **the chest wall to avoid local recurrence after MRM if**:

a. Positive or close (<1 mm) tumour margins in resected specimen

b. Lymph vascular invasion present

c. Tumour: >5 cm in size

d. Lymph nodes: If 4 or more positive LN are present. In these cases radiation field should also include supraclavicular nodes and upper internal mammary nodes

e. In young premenopausal patients with ER –ve tumour

f. RT should be considered in cases even with 1–3 lymph nodes positive in following conditions:

   1. Patient age is less than 35 years
   2. If there is gross extra capsular extension or less than 10 lymph nodes removed
   3. If the tumour is grade 3.

      Aim of RT is to decrease loco-regional recurrence. There is no increase in survival by RT.

      RT should be given after completing adjuvant chemotherapy as concurrent chemotherapy increases the side effects of RT.

What is the management of local advanced breast cancer?

Neo-adjuvant chemotherapy (6 cycles, assess response at 3 cycles): CAF (2nd line is paclitaxel based).

Followed by surgery: MRM (no role of BCS in locally advanced disease).

Followed by radiotherapy to the chest wall in all cases.

What is oncotype DX assay?

This oncotype DX assay quantifies the likelihood of breast cancer recurrence in women with newly diagnosed early stage, lymph node negative ER positive breast cancer. This assay is performed using formalin-fixed paraffin embedded tumour tissue. This assay utilises PCR technique and measures m(SMAU) RNA transcripts of a panel of 16 breast cancer associated genes that correlates with distant metastasis and 5 control genes. Recurrence scores is calculated on a scale of 0–100. Score of more than 31 is taken as high risk, score between 18 and 31 is intermediate and less than 18 is low risk. Patients with high score get statistically significant benefit from adjuvant chemotherapy in comparison to intermediate or low risk.

What is MammaPrint assay?

This test analyses DNA microarray consisting of 70 genes which regulates cell cycle invasion metastasis and angiogenesis. This assay requires the use of fresh tumour tissue preserved in a special buffer designed to preserve RNA integrity. It can be used in ER –ve or ER +ve early stage breast cancers which are lymph node negative.

What is Nottingham prognostic index?

Nottingham Prognostic Index (NPI) is calculated as:

(Tumour size in cm × 0.2) + lymph node stage (1 = no nodes, 2 = 1 to 3 nodes, 3 = 4 or more nodes) + grade (1, 2 or 3)

- Excellent if NPI <2.4
- Good if NPI <3.4
- Moderate 1 if NPI < 4.4
- Moderate 2 if NPI <5.4
- Poor if NPI >5.4

What are the various commonly performed MRM?

Three modifications of MRM are commonly practised:

1. *Patey's type*: Pectoralis minor is removed
2. *Scanlon's type*: Pectoralis minor is detached from coracoid process
3. *Auchincloss type*: Pectoralis minor muscle is retracted. Level III nodes cannot be removed in this modification.

What is thoracic outlet syndrome (TOS)?

Thoracic outlet syndrome is a disease of extrinsic compression of the neurovascular structures within the thoracic outlet. Thoracic outlet obstruction occurs as a result of compression of subclavian vessels and nerves of the brachial plexus in the region of the thoracic inlet. It is more common in middle aged females. It is also known as scalenus anticus syndrome, costoclavicular syndrome or hyperabduction syndrome.

What are different sites of obstruction at various locations (Fig. 10.1)?

a. Inter-scalene triangle which is bounded by scalene anticus anteriorly, scalenus medius muscle posteriorly and first rib inferiorly. Subclavian artery and brachial plexus pass through this space. The area is small at rest and becomes even smaller with certain movements like hyperabduction.

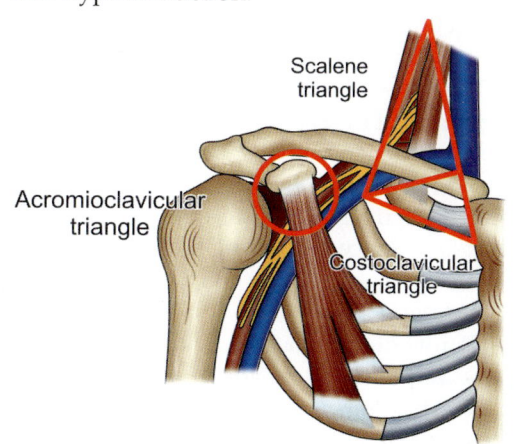

Fig. 10.1: Sites of obstruction in thoracic outlet syndrome

b. *Inter-costoclavicular space*: It is a narrow space between clavicle and first rib and vein can get compressed in this space.

c. *Sub-coracoid space*: It is a space between coracoid process and pectoralis minor tendon. Artery, nerve and vein can get compressed in this space. During hyperabduction axillary vessels and brachial plexus can bend at 90 degree in this area.

What are various causes of TOS?

- *Cervical rib* occurs in 1% of population and produces symptoms in 10% of the population having cervical rib. Symptoms are most commonly seen in thin women with narrow neck in the 3rd or 4th decade. Gradual descent of shoulder girdle due to atrophy of regional muscular is responsible for late onset of symptoms.
- Long transverse process of C7 vertebrae may act as cervical rib.
- Abnormally high placed first rib.
- Scalene anticus muscle hypertrophy may narrow the space in the inter-scalene triangle and cause symptoms.
- Neck hematoma.
- Fibrous bands.
- Bony tumours.

What are boundaries of triangle through which sub-clavian artery and brachial plexus passes?

Subclavian artery and brachial plexus pass through a narrow triangle bounded by:

- Scalenus actinus anteriorly
- Scalenus medius posteriorly
- Base is formed by the first rib.

Enumerate various presentations of TOS.

Neurogenic (95%)

- Pain in the upper limb on the medial aspect
- Radiation of pain to upper back or neck
- Pain becomes worse by the end of the day due to loss of muscle tone
- Tingling, numbness or paraesthesia
- Wasting of small muscles of the hand.

Arterial (4%)

- Compression of the subclavian artery is followed by post-stenotic dilatation or true arterial occlusion can also occur.
- Thrombus may form in the dilated artery due to turbulent blood flow
- Distal embolization can cause distal gangrene of upper limb.
- *Symptoms*
  - Pain is usually diffuse and associated with coldness, weakness, easy fatigability of hand and arm
  - Non-healing ulcers (Fig. 10.2)
- Unilateral Raynaud's phenomenon
  - In 7.5% patients, it is precipitated by hyperabduction or carrying heavy weight.

Venous (1%)

- Subclavian vein thrombosis may cause limb oedema. (Paget-Schroetter syndrome or effort thrombosis)

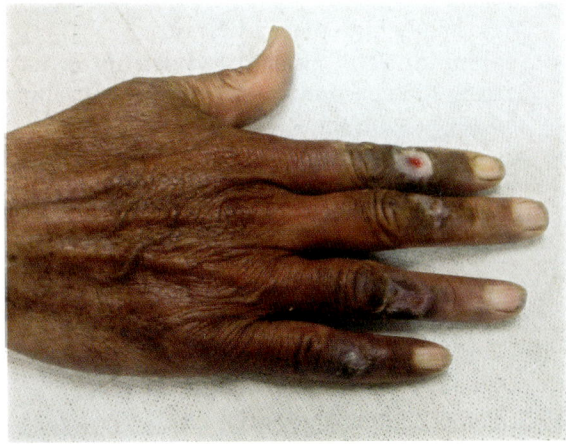

Fig. 10.2: Non-healing digital ulcers in case of thoracic outlet syndrome

How will you examine a suspected case of TOS?

- Look for tenderness in the supra-clavicular fossa and over the scalene actinus
- Look for any bony prominence in the supra-clavicular fossa
- Compression of supra-clavicular fossa to look for pain and paraesthesiae
- Subclavian bruit on auscultation
- *Adson's test*: Patient sits on a stool. Radial pulse is felt in normal sitting posture. Patient is asked to take deep inspiration, extend neck backwards and turn chin towards affected side. The test is positive if deep inspiration, extension of neck and turning the head diminishes the radial pulse because this manoeuvre makes the scalene anterior muscle taut and compresses the subclavian artery.
- *Halsted test (exaggerated military position)*: This test is done to elicit costoclavicular compression. After feeling patients radial pulse in normal posture, patient is asked to throw shoulders backwards and downwards as in exaggerated military posture. This will cause reduction or disappearance of radial as in this posture space between first rib and clavicle is reduced.
- *Wright test (hyperabduction test)*: Patients affected arm is passively hyperabducted to monitor disappearance or diminution of radial pulse. This occurs due to compression of subclavian artery by tendon of pectoralis minor tendon.
- *Roos test*: Patient abducts the arm to 90 degrees and externally rotates the shoulder. This position is maintained and patient opens and closes the hand rapidly for 3 minutes. Positive test will mean reproduction of symptoms.

How will you investigate a case of TOS?

- Skiagram of the cervical spine to detect cervical ribs and degenerative changes.
- CT/MRI to exclude cervical disc lesions specially if osteophytic changes and intervertebral space narrowing are present on plain skiagram.
- Ulnar nerve conduction studies
  - Points of stimulation include:
    - Supraclavicular fossa
    - Middle upper arm
    - Below elbow
    - Wrist

– Normal value across thoracic outlet: 72 m/sec
– Any value <70 m/sec indicates compression
- Doppler study/angiogram is indicated for:
  – Pulsating para-clavicular mass
  – Absent radial pulse
  – Para-clavicular bruit.

Outline the management of TOS.

- *Conservative*:
  – Rest
  – The correction of faulty posture. Simple changes in posture may result in opening the thoracic outlet
  – Muscle stretching/strengthening exercises
  – Short course of analgesics
- *Surgery*:
  – When conservative management fails
  – Rapidly progressing sensory or motor symptoms
  – Presence of abnormal nerve conduction velocity
  – Subclavian vein thrombosis
  – Narrowing of subclavian artery.

Describe various surgical approaches.

- *Trans-axillary approach*: Through trans-axillary approach, first rib is removed and sympathectomy can also be performed. Division of pectoralis minor tendon, if it is causing obstruction can also be carried out through this approach.

- *Supra-clavicular approach*: This approach is employed for removal of first rib or to carry out scalenotomy. Scalenotomy means division of scalenus anticus muscle close to the insertion.

- *Infra-clavicular approach*: This approach is employed for division of pectoralis minor tendon.

- *Posterior approach*: The incision is identical to that of upper thoracoplasty. The subclavian vessels and brachial plexus are easily exposed and displaced anteriorly. This approach provides ample exposure for reconstruction of vessels if it is indicated, e.g. post-stenotic dilatation of subclavian artery. The cervical rib can also be excised through this approach.

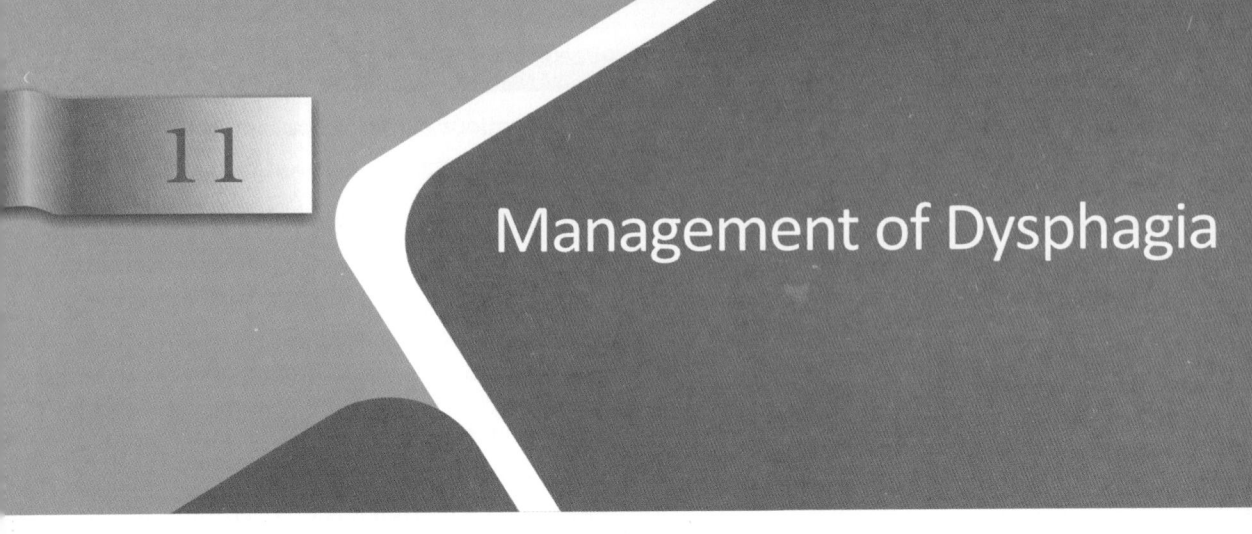

Management of Dysphagia

11

How you define dysphagia?

Dysphagia can be defined as difficulty in initiating the act of swallowing or the sensation of food or liquids getting stuck in the passage from oral cavity to stomach. Basically dysphagia is a feeling of impediment to the normal passage of swallowed food.

What are the types of dysphagia?

Dysphagia can be oro-pharyngeal or esophageal. Oro-pharyngeal dysphagia means difficulty in initiating the act of swallowing. Esophageal dysphagia means feeling of food stuck in the passage from oral cavity to stomach.

Discuss the physiology of swallowing.

Swallowing is controlled by the swallowing center in the medulla and by autonomous peristalsis in the mid-esophagus and distal esophagus

The physiological mechanisms involved in various phases of swallowing are:

a. Oral phase: In this phase food enters the oral cavity and bolus is formed by mastication.
b. Oro-pharyngeal phase: Following sequence of events occurs during this phase:
   1. Tongue is elevated to propel the food bolus into pharynx.
   2. The naso-pharynx is sealed off by elevation of soft palate.
   3. The larynx and hyoid bone moves upwards and anteriorly.
   4. The epiglottis moves in posterior and downward direction to get closed.
   5. The respiration stops for a moment and there is pharyngeal shortening.

c. Esophageal phase:
   1. There is relaxation of upper esophageal sphincter.
   2. The bolus enters the esophagus.
   3. There is segmental contraction of esophagus.
   4. Lower esophageal sphincter relaxes
   5. Food bolus reaches the stomach.

Describe the clinical manifestations of oro-pharyngeal dysphagia.

Oro-pharyngeal dysphagia also known as "high" dysphagia, the pathology most often lies in oral or pharyngeal location. Patients often complain of difficulty in initiating a swallow, and they usually point the cervical area as the trouble area.

Frequent symptoms are
- Difficulty in initiating the act of swallow
- Nasal regurgitation of food
- Coughing during swallowing
- Nasal tone of speech
- Decreased cough reflex
- The sense of choking
- Neurological symptoms like diplopia or slurring of speech may be present in neurologic conditions that cause oro-pharyngeal dysphagia.
- Halitosis may be present in patients with a large residual food collection in food pipe as in Zenker's diverticulum.

Name a few neurological conditions which can cause oro-pharyngeal dysphagia?

Following neurological conditions may be associated with oro-pharyngeal dysphagia:
- Hemiparesis after cardiovascular accident

- In myasthenia gravis
- Parkinson's disease
- Other neurological diseases, e.g. Arnold-Chiari deformity (hindbrain herniation)
- Specific involvement of the cranial nerves involved in swallowing can also lead to the diagnosis of the oro-pharyngeal dysphagia.

What are chief clinical manifestations of eso-phageal dysphagia?

Esophageal dysphagia (also known as "low" dysphagia) with likely pathology in the body or distal esophagus.

Dysphagia, which occurs equally with solids and liquids from the initial stages suggests an eso-phageal motility problem and may be associated with chest pain at intermittent intervals whenever gastro-esophageal reflux occurs.

Dysphagia that begins with solids initially but later progresses to liquids also suggests the possibility of mechanical obstruction with luminal stenosis to diameter <15 mm.

If the dysphagia is progressive, it may be due to peptic stricture or carcinoma. However, patients with peptic strictures usually have a long history of heartburn and regurgitation, but no weight loss. On the contrary patients with esophageal cancer tend to be older men with marked weight loss.

The physical examination of patients with esophageal dysphagia usually does not yield much information although palpable cervical/supra-clavicular lymphadenopathy may suggest eso-phageal cancer. In patients with scleroderma and associated secondary peptic stricture the synd-rome of calcinosis, Raynaud phenomenon, esophageal involvement, sclerodactyly, and telangiectasia (CREST) may be present.

Halitosis may suggest advanced achalasia or long-term obstruction, with accumulation of slowly decomposing residue in the esophageal lumen.

What are the causes of dysphagia?

In order to establish the aetiology of dysphagia, one should make a distinction between causes that mostly affect the pharynx and proximal esophagus (oro-pharyngeal or "high" dysphagia) and causes that mostly affect the esophageal body and esophago-gastric junction (esophageal or "low" dysphagia). However, in many disorders there can be both oro-pharyngeal and esophageal dysphagia. A detailed history-taking including medication use is very important, since drugs may be involved in the pathogenesis of dysphagia.

Oro-pharyngeal Dysphagia

In young patients, the significant causes of oro-pharyngeal dysphagia are:
- Inflammatory, e.g. acute pharyngitis
- Muscle diseases
- Webs and rings in the pharynx

  In older people, it is usually caused by:
  - Central nervous system disorders, including stroke.
  - Parkinson's disease.
  - Dementia.

The clinician should try to make a distinction between mechanical problems and neuromuscular motility or neurological disturbances.

Mechanical and obstructive causes of oro-pharyngeal dysphagia are:
- Cervical lymphadenopathy causing com-pression
- Zenker's diverticulum (with small diverti-cula, the cause may be upper esophageal sphincter dysfunction)
- Reduced muscle compliance (myositis, fibrosis)
- Head and neck malignancies
- Cervical osteophytes impugning upon lumen (rare)
- Oro-pharyngeal malignancy and laryngeal neoplasm are common aetiology for oro-pharyngeal dysphagia.

Neuromuscular Disturbances

- Central nervous system diseases such as stroke, Parkinson's disease, cranial nerve, or bulbar palsy (e.g. multiple sclerosis, motor neuron disease), amyotrophic lateral sclerosis.
- Contractile disturbances such as cricopharyn-geal spasm (upper esophageal sphincter dysfunction) or myasthenia gravis, oculo-pharyngeal muscular dystrophy.
  - Post-stroke dysphagia has been identified in around 50% of cases. The severity of dys-phagia tends to be associated to the severity of stroke.

   – Up to 50% of Parkinson patients manifest some symptoms consistent with oro-pharyngeal dysphagia. Clinically significant dysphagia occurs late in Parkinson's disease. Other unrelated causes can be
  - Poor dentition
  - Oral ulcers
  - Xerostomia
  - Long-term penicillamine use.

What are the causes of esophageal dysphagia?

Three broad groups of conditions can cause esophageal dysphagia

1. Intrinsic diseases involving the esophageal wall which narrow the lumen.
2. Extrinsic diseases outside obstruct the eso-phagus by direct invasion or through lymph node enlargement.
3. Neuromuscular diseases affecting the motility of esophageal smooth muscle by involvement of innervations, causing disruption of peristalsis or lower esophageal sphincter relaxation or both.

   Acute onset dysphagia is usually caused by ingestion of foreign bodies like fish bone, or coins.

Mucosal diseases
- Acid peptic stricture due to gastro-esophageal reflux disease
- Esophageal rings and webs (Plummer-Vinson syndrome)
- Esophageal tumours
- Chemical injury most commonly due to caustic ingestion
- Post-radiation injury
- Infectious esophagitis like Candida infection
- Eosinophilic granulomatous oesophagitis

Diseases causing extrinsic compression
- Tumours (e.g. bronchogenic carcinoma, lymphoma)
- Chronic infections (e.g. tuberculosis, histo-plasmosis)
- Cardiovascular conditions (dilated atrium, thoracic aortic aneurysm causing vascular compression)

Diseases affecting smooth muscle and its innervations
- Achalasia
- Scleroderma

- Post-surgical and iatrogenic (i.e. after fundopli-cation, anti-reflux surgery)

How you will arrive at clinical diagnosis?

A detailed clinical history incorporating all the diagnostic elements can often establish a diagnosis with certainty. It is important to know the location of the site of perceived swallow problem (oro-pharyngeal vs. esophageal dysphagia).

   The timed water-swallow test is an old bedside potentially useful basic screening test to support the evidence obtained by clinical history and physical examination. This test is useful for oro-pharyngeal dysphagia.

   The test comprises the patient drinking 30 ml water from a glass as quickly as possible, with the examiner recording time taken and number of swallows. From these data, the speed of swallowing and the average volume per swallow can be calculated.

   Water swallow test (original version) proposed by Kubota *et al*:

- The patient is asked to sit in a chair, and is handed a cup containing 30 ml of water at normal temperature.
- The patient is then asked to "Please drink this water as you usually do." Time to empty a cup is measured, and the drinking prole and episodes are monitored and assessed.

Drinking prole
1. The patient can drink all the water in 1 gulp without choking.
2. The patient can drink all the water in 2 or more gulps without choking.
3. The patient can drink all the water in 1 gulp, but with some choking.
4. The patient can drink all the water in 2 or more gulps, but with some choking.
5. The patient often chokes and has difficulty drinking all the water.

Drinking episodes
Sipping, holding water in the mouth while drink-ing, water coming out of the mouth, a tendency to try to force himself/herself to continue drinking despite choking, drinking water in a cautious manner, etc.

Diagnosis

Normal: Completed Prole #1 within 5 sec

Suspected: Completed Prole #1 in more than 5 sec, or Prole #2

Abnormal: Any cases of Proles #3 through 5

Modified water swallow test proposed by Saito.

Procedure

The patient is given 3 ml of cold water in the oral vestibule, and then instructed to swallow the water.

If possible, give more water and ask to swallow 2 more times, and the worst swallowing activity is to be assessed. If the patient meets criteria #1 through 4, a maximum of 2 additional attempts (a total of 3 attempts) should be made, and the worst assessment will be recorded as the final result.

Assessment criteria

1. Failed to swallow with choking and/or changes in breathing
2. Swallowed successfully without choking, but with changes in breathing or wet hoarseness
3. Swallowed successfully, but with choking and/ or wet hoarseness
4. Swallowed successfully with no choking or wet hoarseness
5. Criteria #4, plus 2 successful swallowing within 30 sec.

This test is reported to have a predictive sensitivity of >95% for identifying the presence of dysphagia. This test may be complemented by a "food test" using a small amount of pudding placed on the dorsum of the tongue. A water-swallow test can establish dysphagia, however, it fails to identify aspiration in 20–40% of cases when followed up by video fluoroscopy, because of the absent cough reflex.

The video-fluoroscopic swallowing study (also known as the "modified barium swallow") is the gold standard for diagnosing oro-pharyngeal dys-phagia and nasoendoscopy is the gold standard for the evaluation of structural causes of dysphagia. Video-fluoroscopic evaluation may also help to predict the risk of aspiration pneumonia.

Diagnosis and management of esophageal dysphagia

Clinical History

The clinical history should be considered first. The main concern with esophageal dysphagia is to exclude malignancy.

The patient's history can provide many clues; a malignancy is more likely if there is:

- Short duration (<4 months)
- Rapid disease progression
- Dysphagia more for solids than for liquids
- Weight loss

Achalasia is more likely if

- There is dysphagia for both solids and liquids.
- The problem has existed for several months or years.
- There is no weight loss.

Either upper GI endoscopy or barium swallow can be employed as initial to evaluate esophageal dysphagia.

Barium-contrast esophagogram (barium swallow)

The barium esophagogram is carried out with the patient supine and upright. It can outline the irregularities in the esophageal lumen and detect most cases of obstruction, webs, and rings. The barium examination of the oro-pharynx and esophagus during swallowing is the most useful initial test; it can also be helpful in the detection of achalasia and diffuse esophageal spasm, although these conditions are more definitively diagnosed by manometry.

Endoscopy

Endoscopy uses a fiberoptic endoscope passed through the mouth into the stomach, with detailed visualization of the upper gastrointestinal tract. The introduction of the scope into the gastric cavity is very important to exclude pseudoachalasia due to a tumour of the esophagogastric junction.

Other diagnostic tests

- *Esophageal manometry:* This diagnostic method is less commonly used than barium swallow and endoscopy, but has definite place in diagnosing motility disorders. It records the esophageal lumen pressure using either solid-state or perfusion techniques. Manometry is usually performed when an esophageal cause of dysphagia is suspected following an inconclu-sive barium swallow and endoscopy and following adequate anti-reflux therapy (with healing of esophagitis shown endoscopically).

The following conditions can be definitely diagnosed using esophageal manometry are:

a. Achalasia,

b. Scleroderma (ineffective esophageal peristalsis), and

c. Diffuse esophageal spasm.

Radionuclide Esophageal Transit Scintigraphy

The patient ingests a radiolabelled liquid diet (for example, water mixed with ^{99m}technetium sulfur colloid), and the radioactivity within the esophagus is measured. Patients with esophageal motility disorders typically have a delayed disappearance of the radiolabel from the esophagus. The technique is primarily used for research purposes.

Treatment Options

Oro-pharyngeal Dysphagia

The treatment options for oro-pharyngeal dysphagia are not many, as neurological and neuro-muscular disturbances causing dysphagia are not usually amenable to pharmacological or surgical therapy. However, the drug treatment of Parkinson's disease and myasthenia can relieve dysphagia. The management of complications is important and identification of risk factors for aspiration is essential when considering treatment options.

Alternative nutritional support should be considered if there is a high risk of aspiration, or when oral intake does not provide adequate nutritional status.

Alternative nutrition support can be given by following methods:

a. A fine-bore soft enteral feeding tube can be passed down under radiological guidance.

b. Gastrostomy feeding in post-stroke reduces the mortality and improves nutritional status in comparison with nasogastric feeding. Percutaneous endoscopic gastrostomy involves passing a gastrostomy tube into the stomach via a percutaneous abdominal route under guidance from an endoscopist, is usually preferable to surgical gastrostomy. The probability that feeding tubes may be eventually removed is lower in patients who are elderly, suffer a bilateral stroke, or aspirate during the initial video-fluoroscopic study.

Surgical treatments are aimed at relieving the spastic causes of dysphagia.

The cricopharyngeal myotomy, have been successful in up to 60% of cases, but its use still remains unclear. The removal of mechanical impediment to swallowing such as a large, compressing Zenker's diverticulum gives encouraging results.

Swallowing re-education: The following swallowing therapy techniques can be used to facilitate impaired swallowing. These include:

a. Strengthening exercises

b. Biofeedback

c. Thermal and gustatory stimulation.

Management options for esophageal dysphagia are:

Diffuse esophageal spasm and achalasia

- Nitrate, calcium-channel blockers
- Soft food, anti-cholinergics
- Serial dilations or longitudinal myotomy

Scleroderma

Anti-reflux drugs, systemic medical management of scleroderma

Peptic stricture

Anti-reflux drugs (H_2 blockers, proton-pump inhibitors)

Dilation; fundoplication

Infectious esophagitis

Antibiotics (nystatin, acyclovir)

Peptic esophageal strictures

Peptic strictures are usually the result of gastro-esophageal reflux disease (GERD).

The differential diagnosis include

- Caustic strictures after ingestion of corrosive chemicals
- Drug-induced strictures
- Postoperative strictures
- Fungal strictures

The diagnosis is confirmed by endoscopy, the serial dilation is the treatment of choice.

Esophageal strictures should be dilated progressively with bougies or balloons. The choice among dilator types should be based on the experience of physician and the local availability of the dilators in a given hospital.

If dilation is performed with bougies, the first bougie should have a diameter approximately equal to that estimated for the stricture. Bougies of progressively increasing diameter are introduced until first resistance is encountered, after which no more than two additional bougies are passed during any one session. If balloon dilators are used, the initial dilation usually should be limited to a diameter of no more than 45 Fr. The extent of dilation in an individual patient should be based on the symptomatic response to therapy and on the difficulties encountered during the dilation procedure. Most patients experience good relief of dysphagia with dilation to a diameter between 40 Fr and 54 Fr. Strictures generally should not be dilated to a diameter beyond 60 Fr.

Aggressive anti-reflux therapy with proton-pump inhibitors or fundoplication improves dysphagia and decreases the need for subsequent esophageal dilations in patients with peptic esophageal strictures. For patients whose dysphagia persists or returns after an initial trial of dilation and antireflux therapy, healing of reflux esophagitis should be confirmed endoscopically before dilation is repeated. For refractory strictures a trial of steroid injection of the stricture can be considered. Rarely, truly refractory strictures require esophageal resection and reconstruction. Exceptionally endoluminal prosthesis may be indicated in benign strictures. The risk of rupture is about 0.5%. Surgery is generally indicated if frank perforation occurs.

Achalasia

The management of achalasia is largely determined by the surgical risk of the patient. A endoscopic procedure such as botulinum toxin injection, often effective but effect is only short lasting (usually 6 months or less). So this is reserved for patients who are totally excluded from surgery. For those in whom surgery is an option, most physicians advice pneumatic dilation by endoscopy (about 6% risk of perforation) and opt for laparoscopic Heller type myotomy on those in whom two forced dilations fail. Some gastroenterologists prefer to opt directly for surgery without a prior trial of forced dilation (Flowchart 11.1).

Flowchart 11.1: Management of achalasia cardia

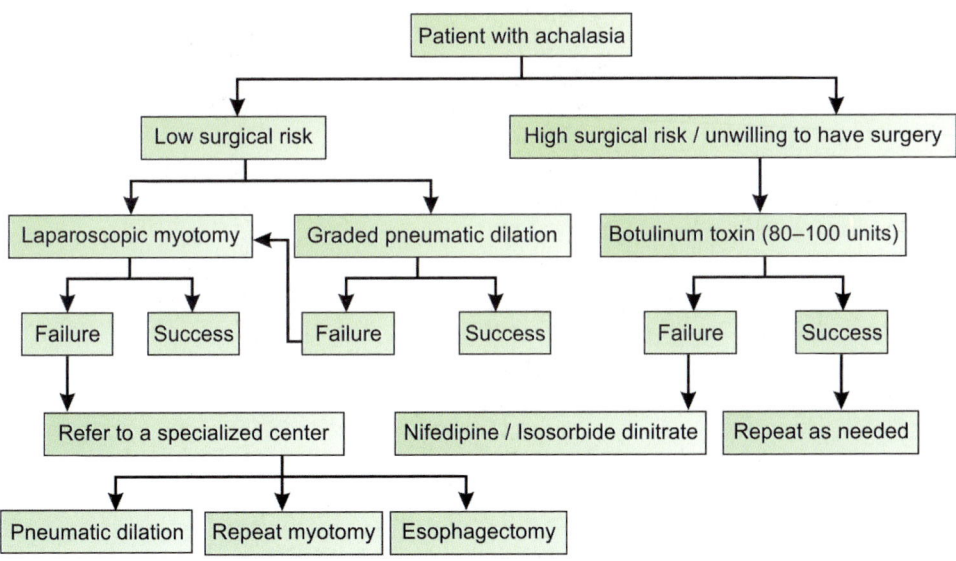

Gastrointestinal

Section 3

12

Gastric Outlet Obstruction

How will you define gastric outlet obstruction?

Gastric outlet obstruction (pyloric obstruction) is not a single entity. It results from clinical and pathophysiological consequences of any disease process that produces a mechanical impediment to gastric emptying. It is usually due to obstruction to gastric emptying due to any cause situated above the ampulla of Vater. Gastric outlet obstruction (GOO) includes obstruction in the antropyloric area or in the bulbar or post-bulbar duodenal segments.

What is the aetiology of GOO?

- Peptic ulcer disease scarring (Fig. 12.1)
- Acid or caustic ingestion
- Carcinoma stomach (Fig. 12.2)
- Extrinsic compression resulting from carcinoma head of pancreas, carcinoma gall bladder

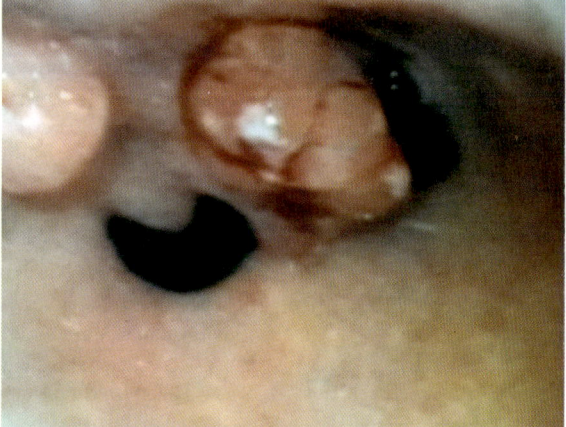

Fig. 12.2: Endoscopic view showing antral growth

- Benign tumours of stomach, i.e. adenoma, GIST, carcinoid
- Inflammatory causes, e.g. chronic pancreatitis like Crohn's disease, eosinophilic gastroenteritis, inflammatory polyp
- NSAID induced strictures/rings
- Post-surgical scarring or anastomotic stricture of gastrojejunostomy
- Postvagotomy due to gastric stasis
- Following endoscopic mucosal resection

Other rare causes

- Tuberculosis, CMV, cryptosporidium
- Annular pancreas causing obstruction above ampulla of vater
- Adult hypertrophic pyloric stenosis
- Duplication cyst of stomach
- Amyloidosis
- Bouveret's syndrome
- Bezoar

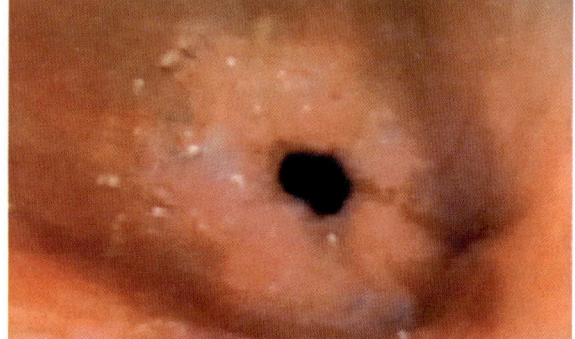

Fig. 12.1: Endoscopic view showing narrowing of pylorus due to healed antral ulcer

What factors lead to GOO in peptic ulcer disease?

In acute peptic ulcer, GOO results from inflammation induced oedema, spasm, tissue deformation and pyloric dysmotility. In chronic disease GOO results from scarring and tissue remodelling. In later stages gastric atony contributes to gastric retention.

What is saline load test?

After gastric decompression, the saline load test is helpful to evaluate mechanical outlet obstruction. The initial role of this test was to evaluate the need for surgery in patients with GOO. A 16 Fr nasogastric tube is placed in the stomach and the stomach contents are emptied with the patient in the right lateral position. 750 mL of 0.9% NaCl is infused through the tube over 3–5 min and is aspirated after 30 minutes to measure the gastric residual volume. Presence of >400 mL is suggestive of definite gastric outlet obstruction, 300–400 mL is probable gastric outlet obstruction, 200–300 mL is indeterminate and less than 200 mL is taken as normal.

Which part of stomach is affected in acid ingestion injuries?

The maximum damage after acid ingestion occurs along the lesser curvature and the pre-pyloric area. Presence of food in the stomach determines the nature of injury. In fasting state most of the damage occurs to the pylorus and antrum while in the fed state the body gets commonly involved causing hour glass deformity.

What are the clinical features of GOO due to peptic ulcer disease?

Vomiting is the principal symptom and is always present. Usually it is preceded by a long history of recurrent dyspepsia. The episodic events coincide with active phases of the ulcer. In half the patients the vomit is copious projectile and effort less. It is free from bile and may contain undigested food taken many hours before.

    Usually the vomiting occurs in the late hours of the evening or in the early hours of the morning. Anorexia and weight loss are the rule. Diarrhea occurs in 20% of cases. Offensive eructation is a diagnostically helpful symptom when it occurs.

Physical Signs

1. A gastric succession splash is a classical finding but it is only significant if at least three hours have passed after meal.
2. Visible gastric peristalsis coursing after intake of food across the abdomen from left to right are of great diagnostic significance.
3. It is possible to see the outline of a grossly distended stomach in epigastrium.
4. Signs of fluid depletion or latent tetany may be found.
5. The normal stomach is empty three to four hours after a meal, but the repeated presence of a large gastric residue, i.e. more than 250 mL. in patients on a normal hospital diet, four or more hours after the last meal, is an almost certain indication of pyloric stenosis.

What is the electrolytes concentration of gastric acid in GOO?

	Benign ulceration	Carcinoma
Sodium	50	55
Potassium	11	11
Chloride	118	50
Acid	56.5	45

All values in mEq/liter

Metabolic Changes

Many patients with pyloric stenosis suffer from the effects of loss of electrolytes and water presenting in its most severe form as gastric tetany due to acidosis.

    The metabolic disturbance of pyloric stenosis is caused by the loss of large amounts of acid and electrolytes.

    The gastric contents as much as four litres per day are lost in severe cases.

The net effects of these losses are:

1. The extracellular fluid and circulating blood volumes are reduced.
2. Serum chloride concentration is low with a corresponding increase in the plasma bicarbonate level due to loss of hydrogen ions.
3. There is a state of hypochloraemic alkalosis.
4. There is hyponatremia, hypokalemia, and hypocalcemia.
5. Initially as a renal compensation to metabolic alkalosis body tries to conserve hydrogen ion and sodium ions are excreted in place of hydrogen ions. As a result, are lost sodium ions instead of hydrogen ions in kidney and hyponatermia gets aggravated leading to renin

angiotensin system activation to preserve intravascular volume and sodium ions. So in later stages hydrogen ions are excreted by kidney and urine is paradoxically acidic even in the presence of metabolic alkalosis.

How will you investigate a case of GOO?

Plain Radiographs of Abdomen

a. Will show an enlarged gastric air bubble which never crosses the midline since lesser curvature is a fixed structure.
b. Small bowel may not show up due to paucity of air.

Contrast Studies with Water Soluble Contrast or Barium (Fig. 12.3)

There is failure of any contrast to pass into the small bowel. In view of risk of aspiration adequate decompression should be done before giving water soluble contrast.

CT Scan

CT scan may reveal additional details, specially the pyloric or gastric wall thickness, lymph nodes or pancreatic lesion not visualized on routine imaging.

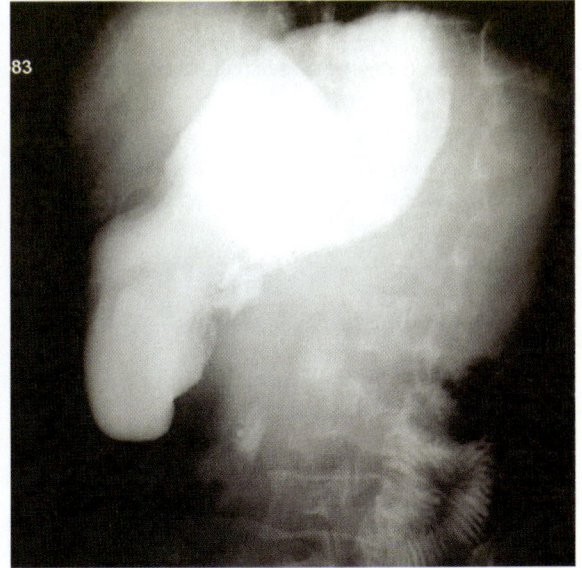

Fig. 12.3: Barium meal upper GI study showing hugely dilated stomach with cut off at the distal half of the first part of the duodenum suggestive of gastric outlet obstruction

Upper GI Endoscopy

Endoscopy is often needed to establish the diagnosis and identify a specific cause along with a therapeutic benefit. Patients should fast for at least four hours before the procedure. Fasting for prolonged periods is not necessary and may increase the amount of retained fluid. Nasogastric tube suction which can minimise the risk of aspiration is recommended before endoscopy. Endoscopic biopsies often allow confirmation or exclusion of a malignant cause of GOO. There is an evolving role for the use of endoscopic ultrasound in the management of these disorders especially in gastric carcinoma.

What are the aims of treatment in GOO?

The aims of treatment are

a. To take care of the pathology causing GOO leading to relief of obstruction. If definitive treatment of aetiology cannot be done then bypass of obstruction should be carried out. Definitive management can be instituted after establishment of diagnosis and correction of underlying metabolic abnormalities.
b. Before carrying out definite treatment, gastric decompression should be carried out using nasogastric tube to take care of gastric atony caused by prolonged obstruction.
c. Metabolic and electrolyte disturbances should be corrected.

What are the advantages of gastric decompression before surgery?

Gastric Decompression

a. Helps in regaining the gastric tone
b. It relieves the discomfort of distension
c. It clears the field for endoscopic procedures
d. It helps in reduction of stomach capacity which is essential for surgery

Aims of Treatment of GOO?

a. To reverse the electrolyte disturbances and metabolic changes to normal. Hypovolemia and hyponatremia is corrected first by normal saline infusion. Once the patient has adequate urine output, then hypokalemia is corrected.
b. To take care of the pathology causing obstruction by definitive surgical procedure is performed.
c. If definitive surgery is not possible, then gastrojejunostomy should be done to bypass the obstruction.

Gastric Cancer

Describe the epidemiology of stomach malignancy.

1. In India, it is the fifth most common cancer in males and seventh most common cancer in females.
2. Highest incidence of gastric cancer in India is seen in Mizoram.
3. It is the most common cancer in Japan.
4. Gastric carcinoma is a disease of elderly with incidence in the seventh decade and carries a very dismal prognosis with an average overall 5-year survival rate of 10%.
5. More than 60% of newly diagnosed cases occur in males.
6. Cancer of stomach is more common in semi-skilled or unskilled people in comparison to professional or executive persons.

What are known risk factors for gastric cancer?

The known risk factors for development of gastric cancer are:

1. *H. pylori gastritis:* The risk of gastric cancer is three times more common in patients with persistent chronic *H. pylori* infection. Gastric cancer develops in 2.9% of patients who are sero-positive for *H. pylori*. *H. pylori* infection leads to atrophic gastritis which in turn progresses to intestinal metaplasia, dysplasia and intestinal type of gastric cancer. Development of gastric cancer in *H. pylori* gastritis is related to virulence of *H.pylori*. Patients infected with positive cytoxan associated gene A (Cag A) are more likely to develop gastric cancer.
2. Consumption of pickled, salted, or smoked food carries high risk of gastric cancer. This type of food contains high level of nitrates. Gastric bacteria which are more commonly seen in conditions of achlorhydria convert nitrates to nitrites. Nitrites are known carcinogen. Preserved food and canned food are rich in nitrates.
3. There is likely a synergistic effect between *H. pylori* infection and dietary factors causing gastric cancer. *H. pylori* increases the growth of bacteria which causes carcinogen production and inhibits its removal. *H. pylori* also decreases the production of ascorbic acid which has scavenging effect on oxygen free radicals.
4. Gastric cancer is more common in following subgroup of patients:

   a. Atrophic gastritis and pernicious anemia
   b. Previous partial gastrectomy after 10 years
   c. *Adenomatous and hyperplastic gastric polyps:* Patients with these types of polyps have 10 times more chance of developing gastric cancer.
   d. Familial polyposis
   e. *Hypogammaglobulinemia:* There is 50 times more chances of developing gastric cancer.
   f. *Blood group A:* Diffuse gastric cancer is more common in patients with blood group A.
   g. Type 3 intestinal metaplasia

5. *Genetic factor:* Most gastric cancers are aneuploid. More than two-thirds of gastric cancers have deletion or suppression of tumour suppressor gene p53 and overexpression of COX-2 gene. Gastric cancers which overexpress COX-2 gene are more aggressive. Germ line mutation in CDH1 gene which encodes E-cadherin is associated with hereditary diffuse gastric cancer and prophylactic total gastrectomy should be considered in these patients as there is 80% lifetime incidence of developing gastric cancer.
6. Smoking has clear association with development of gastric cancer especially of gastric cardia with a hazard ratio (HR) of 4:10.
7. Obesity is clearly associated with development of gastric cancer with 2.3 fold increased chances.

What are the known genetic alterations in gastric cancer?

a. Activation of oncogene; There is overexpression of c-met proto-oncogene which is a receptor for hepatocyte growth factor, k-sam gene and c-erb B2 oncogene.
b. Inactivation of tumour suppressor genes p53 and p16.
c. Reduction of cellular adhesions.
d. Reactivation of telomerase.
e. Presence of microsatellite instability is seen in 20–30% of intestinal type of gastric cancer.

What are different pathological types of gastric cancer?

Various pathological types of gastric malignancy are:

a. Adenocarcinoma (95%)
b. Lymphoma (4%)

c. Malignant GIST (1%)

d. Other rare types include carcinoid, squamous cell carcinoma, blood borne metastasis from other sites, e.g. melanoma or breast or carcino-sarcoma.

What is Borrmann's classification?

This classification divides gastric cancer into five types based on gross appearance. It was described way back in 1926 but still used these days for describing endoscopic findings.

Five types are

a. Protruding type or polypoidal type: The lesion is elevated above the surrounding mucosa (type 1)

b. Ulcerated type with sharply demarcated margins (type 2)

c. Ulcerated without definite limits with infiltration into surrounding walls (type 3)

d. Diffusely infiltrating without significant ulceration (type 4)

e. Non-classifiable (type 5)

What is Lauren classification?

Lauren in 1965 classified gastric cancer into two types, i.e. intestinal and diffuse. These are two distinct entities in terms of pathology, epidemiology and prognosis.

Intestinal Type

a. Majority of cases are associated with intestinal metaplasia.

b. Commonly occurs in the setting of precancerous condition like gastric atrophy.

c. Males are more commonly affected.

d. Involves older age group of patients.

e. Usually they are well differentiated with glandular structure formation.

f. Blood borne metastasis leading to distant spread is more common.

g. Genetic abnormality commonly seen in intestinal type of gastric cancer are microsatellite instability and mutation of genes like APC and inactivation of tumour suppressor gene like p53 or p16.

Diffuse Type

a. Usually not associated with intestinal metaplasia.

b. Most of the time genetic factors play a major role in its causation and are familial in nature.

c. Females are more commonly affected.

d. Occurs in younger age group in comparison to intestinal type.

e. There is no glandular structure formation and is poorly differentiated with a lot of signet ring cells.

f. Metastasis is mainly lymphatic and trans-mural.

g. There is decreased E-cadherin formation.

What are signs and symptoms of gastric carcinoma?

1. Signs and symptoms in initial stages are non-specific and includes recent onset "As", i.e. anemia, anorexia, asthenia in a middle aged person and malignancy itself remain silent.

2. Recent onset of non-specific dyspepsia which is insidious in onset in an elderly person.

3. Patient may present with epigastric lump which is a late feature. This palpable lump is either due to bulky antral tumour or due to omentum involvement with secondary in the lymph nodes. It is known as omentum caking.

4. Patient may present with obstructive symptoms like dysphagia in carcinoma of cardia or gastric outlet obstruction in pyloric tumours.

5. Distant metastasis, e.g. ascites, umbilical nodule (Sister Joseph nodule), left supraclavicular lymph node enlargement (Virchow's lymph node).

6. A bulky antral tumour or lymph node enlargement may lead to jaundice due compression of common bile duct in hepato-duodenal ligament.

How to define early gastric cancer?

Early gastric cancer is defined as cancer confined to mucosa or sub-mucosa irrespective of lymph node involvement. Prognosis is very good in early gastric cancer as the incidence of lymph node involvement is very low in comparison to late carcinoma. Incidence of lymph node involvement is 10–15%. The 5-year survival rate after adequate resection is 80 percent. Early gastric cancer can be classified as protruding, superficial or excavating type on the basis of endoscopy. Superficial type can be of elevated type, flat type or depressed type.

What investigations will you perform for pre-operative staging?

Following investigations are performed for pre-operative staging:

a. *Flexible endoscopy and endoscopic ultrasonography:* It provides complete visualisation of tumour and tissue diagnosis. It can be used therapeutically in treatment of early gastric cancer confined to mucosa by performing endoscopic mucosal resection known as EMR. If patient presents late with gastric outlet obstruction and not fit for surgery endoscopic dilatation and stent insertion can be done to relieve obstruction. Endoscopic ultrasound is the investigation of choice for accurate T staging and for assessment of peri-gastric lymph nodes. On endoscopy ultrasound is performed with 7.5 to 12 MHz ultrasonic transducer with stomach distended with water. The stomach appears as five alternating hypo-echoic and hyper-echoic layers.

b. *Computed tomography:* It is mainstay for evaluation of intra-abdominal metastatic disease. It can also be used for locoregional staging; however, its accuracy is less than endoscopic ultrasonography.

c. *Positron emission tomography (PET):* PET has no role in the primary staging work up as only 50% of gastric cancers are PET avid. However, in patients with advanced disease who are given neoadjuvant chemotherapy PET can be used to monitor the response of neoadjuvant chemotherapy if they were positive for PET initially. PET response can be seen within 14 days.

d. *Laparoscopy:* Staging laparoscopy is a part of standard protocol for the preoperative work up of carcinoma stomach. It can detect peritoneal deposits and secondary liver not picked up on CT.

Describe the treatment of gastric carcinoma.

Curative surgical resection remains the mainstay for treatment. Recently addition of adjuvant or neoadjuvant chemotherapy or combination with radiotherapy has been shown to increase the cure rate and disease free survival in appropriately selected cases.

NCCN guidelines recommend neoadjuvant chemotherapy for any patient without metastatic disease if node positive or staged T2 or more on preoperative staging. Chemotherapy which has been used is epirubicin, cisplatin, and 5-fluorouracil. This preoperative chemotherapy leads to significant increase in survival and reduced disease progression as shown in MAGIC (Medical Research Council Adjuvant Gastric Infusional Chemotherapy) trial.

Adjuvant chemotherapy: There is clear advantage of 5 FU based adjuvant chemotherapy in R1 resction or R0 resection with T2 or greater disease or node positive disease.

The principal of surgical resection is removal of tumour with 5 cm of normal stomach beyond the palpable margins with R0 resection which means resected margins are free on microscopic examination. R1 resection means whole of the disease has been removed macroscopically but resected margin are not tumour free microscopically.

For nodal dissection all peri-gastric lymph nodes should be removed and resected specimen should contain at least 15 lymph nodes.

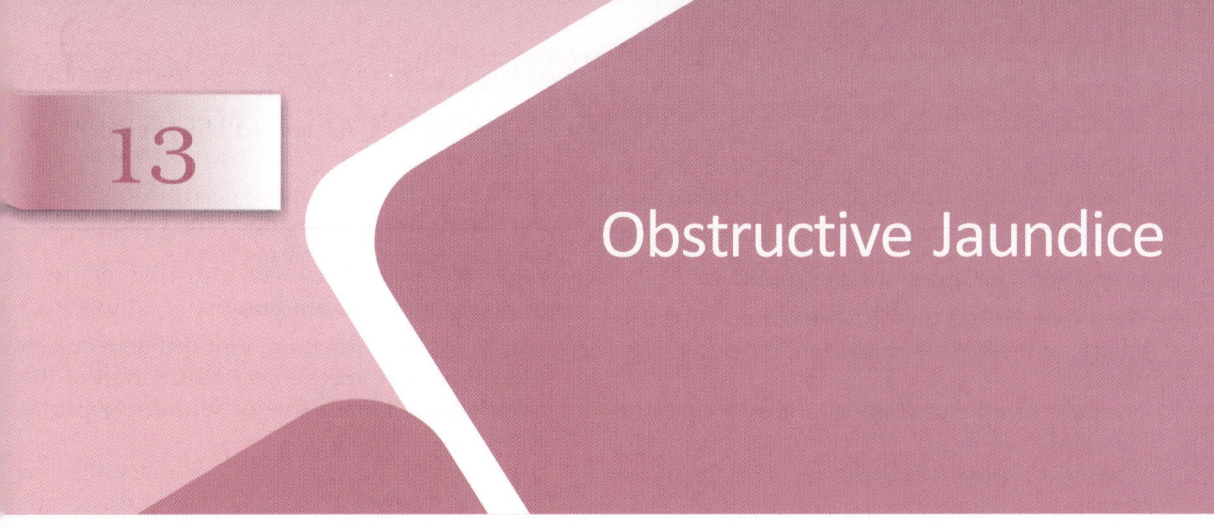

13

Obstructive Jaundice

What is the definition of Jaundice?

The term Jaundice is derived from French word 'jaune' meaning yellow. Another word for jaundice is icterus (Latin word for jaundice) means yellowish staining of the skin, sclera and mucous membranes by deposition of bilirubin (a yellow orange bile pigment) in these tissues. Jaundice indicates excessive levels of conjugated or un-conjugated bilirubin in the blood and is clinically apparent when the bilirubin level exceeds 2 mg/dl (34.2 mmol per L).

Historical Aspect

Jaundice was also known as the "morbus regius" (the regal disease) because it was thought only the touch of a king could cure it.

Where to look for Icterus?

It is most apparent in natural sunlight. In fact, it may be falsely absent in artificial or poor light. If natural light is not available, one should look for it in the white light.

In fair-skinned patients, jaundice is most noticeable on the face, trunk, and sclera; in dark-skinned patients, it is noticeable on the hard palate, sclera, and under surface of tongue, skin creases and in nails.

Icterus first appears in sclera due to high content of elastic tissue in it which has a high affinity for bilirubin.

Pseudo-jaundice may be found
1. In black patients with pigmented sclera,
2. In beta hypercarotenemia

3. In uremia (a sallow yellowish pallor),
4. In patients on quinacrine therapy (a yellow-green colour).
5. Malingering with Picric acid. Picric acid gives yellow discoloration when applied to skin.

Icterus first appears in sclera, followed by hard palate, under surface of tongue then on skin creases, nail bed and rest of the skin.

Causes of jaundice can be classified into pre-hepatic, hepatic or post-hepatic.

In this chapter, our focus is on post-hepatic causes of jaundice (obstructive or surgical cholestasis) as this is more relevant to surgeons.

Describe the development and surgical anatomy of the hepatobiliary system?

Embryology

The liver, gallbladder, and biliary tree develop as a ventral bud (hepatic diverticulum) from the most caudal part of the foregut early in the fourth week. This ventral bud divides into two parts while growing between the layers of the ventral mesentery. From the larger cranial part (pars hepatica), the primordium of the liver develops and from the smaller caudal part (pars cystica), the gallbladder and the cystic duct develops. The initial connection between the hepatic diverticulum and the foregut narrows, thus forming the bile duct. As a result of the positional changes of the duodenum, the entrance of the bile duct is carried around the dorsal aspect of the duodenum.

Gross Anatomy

The biliary system can be broadly divided into two components, the intra-hepatic and the extra-hepatic tracts.

Intra-hepatic Component Comprises

1. The secretory units of the liver, i.e. hepatocytes, biliary epithelial cells, including the peribiliary glands
2. The bile canaliculi, bile ductules (canals of Herring)
3. The intra-hepatic bile ducts make up the intra-hepatic tract.

   The extra-hepatic system comprises:
   1. The hepatic ducts (right and left)
   2. The common hepatic duct
   3. The cystic duct
   4. The gallbladder
   5. The common bile duct biliary tree.

   The cystic and common hepatic ducts join to form the common bile duct (CBD) which is approximately 8 to 10 cm in length and 0.4 to 0.8 cm in diameter.

   The CBD can be divided into three anatomic segments:
   a. Supra-duodenal portion
   b. Retro-duodenal portion
   c. Intra-pancreatic portion

   The common bile duct then enters the medial wall of the duodenum, courses tangentially through the submucosal layer for 1 to 2 cm, and terminates in the major papilla in the second portion of the duodenum. The distal portion of the duct is encircled by smooth muscle that forms the sphincter of Oddi. The common bile duct may enter the duodenum directly (25%) or join the pancreatic duct (75%) to form a common channel, termed the ampulla of Vater.

   The biliary tract is supplied by a complex peri-biliary vascular plexus. Afferent vessels of this plexus derive from hepatic arterial branches, and this plexus drains into the portal venous system or directly into hepatic sinusoids.

Define Cholestasis

Cholestasis is reduction or stoppage of bile flow. It can be intra-hepatic or extra-hepatic
- Intrahepatic:
  - Nonobstructive (disorders that impair the body's ability to eliminate bile)
  - Obstructive (widespread blockage of small ducts)
- Extra-hepatic (obstructive jaundice): Obstruction to the flow of bile in the extra-hepatic biliary tree or at the porta-hepatis.

What is Obstructive Jaundice?

- Failure of the normal amount of bile to reach intestine due to mechanical obstruction of the extra-hepatic biliary tree or within the porta-hepatis.

Physiological Facts

- Total bile flow: 600 ml/day (500–1000 ml/day)
- Hepatocyte component—450 ml/day. Which can be bile salt dependent or bile salt independent due to biliary glutathione and ductular bicarbonate secretion
- Cholangiocyte component—150 ml/day. It depends upon secretin stimulation
- Total serum bilirubin 0.3 to 1.2 mg per dl
- The normal conjugated bilirubin level is less than <15 percent of total.
- 1 mg/dl of bilirubin =17 mmol /L

Types of Biliary Tract Obstruction

- Complete obstruction
- Intermittent obstruction
- Chronic incomplete obstruction
- Segmental obstruction

Complete Obstruction

- Always presents as jaundice

Common Causes

- Head of pancreas tumour
- Common bile duct ligation
- Cholangiocarcinoma
- Parenchymal liver tumours causing complete obstruction

Intermittent Obstruction

- Clinical symptoms and typical biochemical changes. The symptoms can be itching, pain, bouts of high grade fever with chills and rigors suggestive of cholangitis
- Clinically jaundice may or may not be present.

Causes

- CBD stones

- Peri-ampullary tumours
- Duodenal diverticulum
- Choledochal cyst
- Biliary parasites
- Hemobilia

Chronic Incomplete Obstruction

- With or without classical symptoms or bio-chemical changes
- Pathological changes in bile ducts or liver

Causes

- Strictures of common bile duct
- Stenosis of biliary—enteric anastomosis
- Chronic pancreatitis
- Cystic fibrosis
- Sphincter of Oddi stenosis

Segmental Obstruction

One or more segment of intra-hepatic biliary tract obstructed.

Causes

- Traumatic
- Intra-hepatic stones
- Sclerosing cholangitis
- Cholangiocarcinoma in a segment of intra-hepatic biliary tract

Physiological Effects of Bile Duct Obstruction

- Normal secretory pressure of bile is 15–25 cm of water
- At 35 cm of water there is suppression of bile flow
- High pressure leads to cholangio-venous and cholangio-lymphatic reflux of bacteria
- Dilatation of bile duct and intra-hepatic biliary radicals (IHBR)
- IHBR dilatation is absent if there is secondary hepatic fibrosis or cirrhosis.

Functions of Bile

Bile has multipurpose spectrum of functions:
1. Intestinal digestion
2. Absorption of lipids
3. Elimination of environmental toxins, carcinogens, drugs, and their metabolites (xenobiotics)
4. Serves as the primary route of excretion for a variety of endogenous compounds and metabolic products, such as cholesterol, bilirubin, and many hormones.

Effects of Bile Duct Obstruction

a. The absence of bile constituents (most importantly, bilirubin, bile salts, and lipids) in the intestines, and their backup, which causes spillage into the systemic circulation.
b. Stools are often pale because less bilirubin reaches the intestine.
c. Absence of bile salts can produce malabsorption, leading to steatorrhea and deficiencies of fat-soluble vitamins (particularly A, K, and D); vitamin K deficiency can reduce prothrombin levels.
d. In long-standing cholestasis, concomitant vitamin D and Ca malabsorption can cause osteoporosis or osteomalacia.
e. Bilirubin retention produces mixed hyperbilirubinemia. Some conjugated bilirubin reaches and darkens the urine.
f. High levels of circulating bile salts are associated with, but may not cause pruritus.
g. Cholesterol and phospholipid retention produces hyperlipidemia despite fat malabsorption (although increased liver synthesis and decreased plasma esterification of cholesterol also contribute); triglyceride levels are largely unaffected.
h. The lipids circulate as a unique, abnormal, low-density lipoprotein called lipoprotein X.
i. Cholestatic liver diseases are characterized by accumulation of hepatotoxic substances, mitochondrial dysfunction and impairment of liver antioxidant defense.
j. The storage of hydrophobic bile acids has been indicated as the main cause of hepatotoxicity with alteration of some important cell functions, such as the mitochondrial energy production. Both mitochondrial metabolism impairment and hydrophobic bile acids accumulation are associated with increased production of oxygen free radical species and development of oxidative damage.

Other Pathological Changes

- Increase in biliary pressure leads to
  - Disruption of tight junctions between hepatocytes and bile duct cells with increased permeability leads to reflux of bile contents in liver sinusoids.
  - Neutrophil infiltration, increased fibrinogenesis and deposition of reticulin fibers in the portal triad

- Reticulin fibres gets converted into type 1 collagen
- Laying down of collagen fibres leads to hepatic fibrosis, obstruction of sinusoids, secondary biliary cirrhosis and portal hypertension
- Fibrosis can also lead to atrophy of obstructed liver.

Changes in Liver Blood Flow

- Acute obstruction: Increase in hepatic arterial blood flow.
- No change in portal venous blood flow.
- Chronic bile duct obstruction leads to decrease in total liver blood flow, dilation of sinusoids and elevation of portal pressure.

Wound Healing

- Delayed wound healing
- High incidence of wound dehiscence
- Decreased activity of enzyme propyl hydroxylase in the skin
- This enzyme helps in incorporation of proline in collagen leading to defective synthesis of collagen in jaundice

Cardiovascular Effects

- Decreased cardiac contractility
- Reduced left ventricular pressure
- Impaired response to beta agonist drugs
- Decreased peripheral vascular resistance
- Net result
  - Hypotensive patient
  - Exaggerated hypotensive response to bleeding
  - More prone to postoperative shock

Renal Failure

- 10% incidence with 70% mortality
- Factors responsible
  - Depressed cardiac function
  - Increased levels of ANP resulting in hypovolemia
  - Direct effect of bile salts on kidney mediated by increased prostaglandin E2
- Endotoxemia (50%)
  - Renal vasoconstriction
  - Shunting of blood from cortex
  - Activation of complement system—peritubular and glomerular fibrin deposition
- Leading to tubular and cortical necrosis

Immune System

- Defects in cellular immunity
  - Impaired T cell proliferation
  - Decreased neutrophil chemotaxis
  - Defective bacterial phagocytosis
  - Depressed function of RE system i.e. Kupffer cells

Coagulation Factor Defects

- Prolongation of prothrombin time
- Loss of calcium
- Endotoxin induced damage to factor XI and XII, platelets
- Low grade DIC with increased fibrin degradation products
- Thrombocytopenia from hypersplenism

Biochemical Effects

- Bilirubin rise by 25–43 micromol/litre/day
- Mechanism of hyperbilirubinemia due to biliary venous and biliary lymphatic regurgitation due to disruption of tight intracellular junction.
- Transhepatocytic regurgitation due to reversal of the secretory polarity of hepatocytes
- Rupture of dilated canaliculi into sinusoids due to necrosis of hepatocytes.

Alkaline Phosphatase

- Most sensitive indicator
- Factors responsible are:
  - Biliary compartment regurgitation
  - Increase in hepatic synthesis

Clinical Features

History

- Previous dyspepsia, fat intolerance
- Jaundice: Onset, course, itching
- Pain
- Pyrexia
- Weight loss
- Dark urine and clay colored stools
- Travel to endemic area
- Contact with jaundice patient
- History of upper abdominal operation
- History of plasma or blood transfusion
- Drug intake, i.e. anti-tubercular drugs
- History of injection in preceding six months.

Jaundice

- Yellowing of sclera at 3 mg%
- Yellowing of skin and mucous membrane at 6 mg%.
- Bilirubin level rise up to three weeks to stabilize
- **Why bilirubin levels plateau**
  - Increased excretion of bile pigments by-products other than bilirubin not giving diazo reaction.
  - With increasing levels of conjugated bilirubin, a portion gets covalently bonded to serum albumin. This protein bound bilirubin (Delta bilirubin) is not measurable by routine technique.

Itching

- Retained bile salts.
- Levels does not correlate well with level of bile salts.
- Itching disappears in terminal liver failure but bile salt level still increased.
- Other theory of itching
  - Due to endogenous opiate peptides inducing opioid receptor mediated scratching activity of central origin.

Clinical Examination

- *Age:* Middle or old age goes in favour of malignancy
- *Anemia:* It can be present in haemolytic anaemia, malignancy or cirrhosis
- *Gross weight loss:* Malignancy
- *Hunched up position:* Chronic pancreatitis or cancer head of pancreas
- *Fetor, flapping tremors, personality changes:* Impending hepatic coma
- *Skin changes:* Bruising, purpuric spots, vascular spiders, palmar erythema, white nails, and loss of secondary sexual characters. These are all stigmata of chronic liver disease.
- Scratch marks, melanin pigmentation, finger clubbing, xanthoma on eyelids, extensor surface, palmar creases
- Malignant skin nodules, e.g. umbilical nodule also known as Sister Joseph nodule
- *Multiple venous thrombosis:* Pancreatic body carcinoma
- *Ankle oedema:* Indicates cirrhosis or IVC obstruction due to hepatic or pancreatic malignancy.

Abdominal Examination

- *Dilated peri-umbilical veins:* Cirrhosis and portal collateral circulation. Normal flow of blood in peri-umbilical region is away from umbilicus. Reversal of flow indicates IVC obstruction.
- *Ascites:* Cirrhosis or malignant disease
- *Nodular liver:* Secondaries in the liver.
- Smooth surfaced liver enlargement can be due to back pressure changes leading to hydro-hepatosis.
- *Courvoisier's law:* Palpable non-tender distended gallbladder in jaundice patient indicates— malignant biliary obstruction, e.g. carcinoma head of pancreas, peri-ampullary carcinoma, cholangio-carcinoma or carcinoma gallbladder. In case of obstructive jaundice, etiology of CBD obstruction because of stone in the CBD is highly unlikely as gall bladder becomes fibrotic without any ability to distend due to past attacks of cholecystitis. Additionally obstruction due to stone in CBD is not complete so enough pressure will not be generated to distend the gall bladder even if the gall bladder is capable of distension.
- Exceptions to Courvoisier's law are:
  - *Double impaction of stones:* Impaction at neck of gall bladder causes mucocele of gall bladder and impaction of stone in CBD causes jaundice.
  - Impaction of pancreatic calculus at ampulla of Vater
  - Mirizzi's syndrome, i.e. big impacted stone at neck of gall bladder causing extrinsic compression.

Investigations

a. Biochemistry and Haematology

Liver function tests are carried out to confirm that it is obstructive jaundice on biochemical basis.

Elevated serum bilirubin level with a preponderance of the conjugated fraction is the rule.

The serum gamma glutamyl transpeptidase (GGT) level is also raised in obstructive jaundice.

The alkaline phosphatase is markedly elevated (more than one and half times of upper limit of normal). The transaminases (SGOT and SGP) may be normal or mildly raised (less than 10 times of upper limit) in obstructive jaundice.

Elevated WBC may be present in cholangitis. Tumour markers like CA 19-9, CEA and CA-125 are usually elevated in pancreatic cancers, cholangiocarcinoma and peri-ampullary cancers, but they are non-specific and may be elevated in other benign diseases of the hepatobiliary tree.

b. Imaging

The goals of imaging are:

1. To confirm the presence of an extra-hepatic obstruction
2. To determine the level of the obstruction
3. To identify the specific cause of the obstruction
4. To provide complementary information relating to the underlying diagnosis (e.g. staging information in cases of malignancy).

Ultrasonography can Reveal

1. The dilated CBD and size of the bile ducts,
2. It may identify the level of the obstruction,
3. It may discover the cause and other information related to the disease (e.g. hepatic metastases, gallstones, hepatic parenchymal change).

It identifies bile duct obstruction with 95% accuracy though results are largely operator dependent. It will also show stones in the gall bladder and dilated bile duct, but it is unreliable for small stones or strictures in the bile ducts. It may also demonstrate various other pathologies like tumours and cysts, in the pancreas, liver, and surrounding structures.

- **Computed tomography (CT)** of the abdomen provides excellent visualization of the liver, gall bladder, pancreas, and retroperitoneum. It can differentiate between intra- and extra-hepatic obstruction with 95% accuracy. However, CT may not define incomplete obstruction caused by small gallstones, tumours, or strictures. Contrast-enhanced multi-slice CT is very useful for assessment staging of biliary malignancies and carcinoma head of pancreas. Contrast agents given orally or intravenously are used and imaging is done in unenhanced, arterial and venous phases.
- **Magnetic resonance cholangiopancreatography (MRCP)** is a non-invasive technique for visualization of the biliary and pancreatic ductal system. Excellent visualization of biliary (Fig. 13.1) anatomy is possible without the invasiveness of ERCP (endoscopic retrograde

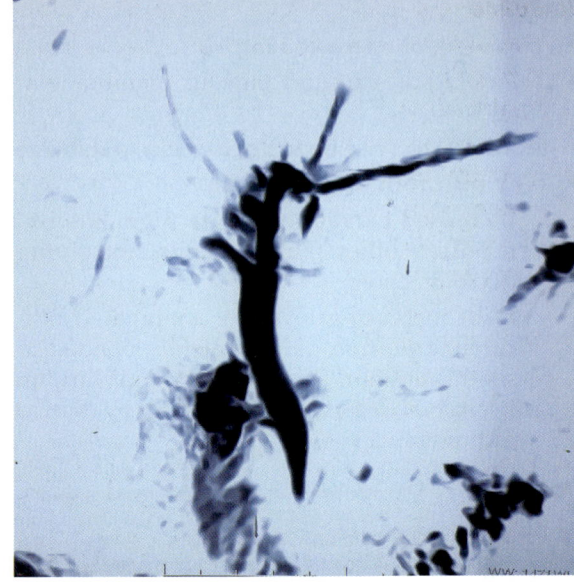

Fig. 13.1: Magnetic resonance cholangiopancreatogram showing normal common bile duct without any filling defect

cholangio pancreatography). Unlike ERCP, it is purely diagnostic. Its sensitivity and specificity in detecting CBD is as good as ERCP. MRCP has almost replaced ERCP for diagnosis of CBD stones (Fig. 13.2).

- **ERCP and PTC (Percutaneous transhepatic cholangiography)** provide direct visualization of the level of obstruction. However, they are invasive and associated with complications like cholangitis, biliary leakage, pancreatitis and bleeding. These are not used diagnostic modalities but are great therapeutic tools in management of CBD stones and in relieving bild duct obstruction.

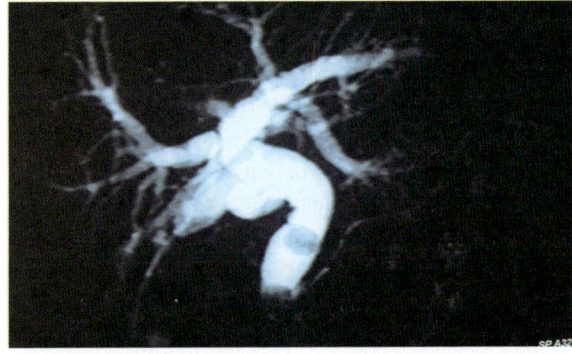

Fig. 13.2: Magnetic resonance cholangiopancreatogram showing dilated common bile duct with filling defect

- **Endoscopic ultrasound:** Endoscopic ultrasonography though not widely available has various applications, such as staging of gastrointestinal malignancy, evaluation of submucosal tumours, and has grown to be an important modality in evaluating the pancreaticobiliary system. With regard to the biliary system, EUS is useful for the detection and staging of ampullary tumours, detection of microlithiasis, choledocholithiasis and evaluation of benign and malignant bile duct strictures. It can further evaluate relationships to vascular structures. It may help define benign lesions mimicking cancer (e.g. sclerosing pancreatitis) if there is diagnostic doubt. Endoscopic ultrasound enables the aspiration of cysts and biopsy of solid lesions, but is operator-dependent. This facility is not readily available in most centres in developing countries. Role of endoscopic ultrasound is highly specific and is not required in routine management of obstructive jaundice.

Approach to the Jaundiced Patient

Is it direct or indirect hyperbilirubinemia on the basis of history and clinical examination?

Dark urine, pale stools and other features such as pruritus or cholangitis, are suggestive of direct hyperbilirubinemia, while normal colour urine and stool reflect unconjugated hyperbilirubinemia. In majority of cases, clinical findings alone will be sufficient to differentiate conjugated from unconjugated hyperbilirubinemia.

Is it hepatic or post-hepatic jaundice?

Clinical features of hepatic jaundice include history of alcohol abuse, acute hepatitis, and stigmata of chronic liver disease like palmar erythema, caput medusae, ascites and Dupuytren's contracture.

Post-hepatic jaundice usually present with abdominal pain, itching and palpable liver more than 2 cm below the costal margin.

Using clinical approach and simple biochemical tests (total serum bilirubin, alkaline phosphatase and gamma glutamyl transferase levels) clinician can have a good judgement on whether the jaundice is hepatic or post-hepatic.

What is the level of the obstruction?

Imaging is the main method to determine the level of obstruction. Ultrasonography can identify the level of obstruction in about 90% of cases. Other imaging facilities like MRCP, CT scan are used where ultrasonography cannot determine the level of the obstruction.

What is the cause of the obstruction?

The commonest causes of obstruction in India are:

1. CBD stones
2. Bile duct stricture which may be due to varied etiology, e.g. postoperative, inflammatory
3. Carcinoma head of pancreas
4. Periampulary carcinoma
5. Cholangiocarcinoma
6. Carcinoma gall bladder
7. Ascaris or round worm in the CBD

How to evaluate the extent of the disease (staging) clinically?

While obvious metastases may be present by a palpation of a nodular enlarged liver or other evidence of widespread disease like ascites, nodule at the umbilicus, deposit in the pouch of Douglas or palpable left supraclavicular lymph node. Fever and elevated WBC are indicative of cholangitis.

How to decide the resectability of malignancy?

Assessment of the resectability of a tumour usually performed by contrast enhanced multislice triple phase CT. The involvement of the superior mesenteric vein, the portal vein, the superior mesenteric artery, and the porta hepatis indicate non-resectable tumour. The evidence of significant local adenopathy or extra-pancreatic extension of tumour also denotes advanced disease. Optimal evaluation is achieved with a triple-phase (arterial phase, portal and venous phase) CT.

What are different methods of palliation of jaundice in non-resectable tumours?

a. *Upper third obstruction*: Surgical palliation is best achieved with a left (segment 3) hepaticojejunostomy (the long extrahepatic course of the left hepatic duct makes it more accessible).

b. *Middle third obstruction*: Surgical palliation used is hepaticojejunostomy.

c. *Lower third obstruction*: Surgical palliation performed is Roux-en-Y choledochojejunostomy. Cholecystojejunostomy carries a high risk of complications and subsequent jaundice.

Discuss treatment of obstructive jaundice.

Extra-hepatic biliary obstruction always requires mechanical decompression. Decompression of extra-hepatic biliary obstruction can be achieved by any of these three methods:

1. Surgical bypass
2. Resection of obstructing lesions
3. The percutaneous insertion of stents
4. The endoscopic insertion of stents.

General Considerations

Pruritus usually subsides when biliary obstruction is relieved. 2 to 8 gm of oral cholestyramine twice daily can be tried which binds bile salts in the intestine. However, this does not work in complete biliary obstruction. The hypoprothrombinemia usually subsides after use of (vitamin K_1) 5 to 10 mg sc once/day for 5 days. Ca and vitamin D supplements, with or without a bisphosphonate, slow the progression of osteoporosis in long-standing irreversible cholestasis. Vitamin-A supplements prevent deficiency and severe steatorrhea can be minimized by replacing some dietary fat with medium-chain triglycerides.

Jaundiced patients undergoing surgery are prone for following complications in the post-operative period.

These include
- Infections (cholangitis, septicaemia, wound infections)
- Bleeding (due to non-coagulant carboxyl derivatives of vitamin K dependent factors)
- Renal failure
- Fluid and electrolyte abnormalities

Preparation for surgery is important because of the associated perioperative morbidity. The specific measures required in all patients are:
- Parenteral administration of vitamin K analogues—to normalise prothrombin time.
- Intravenous fluid to correct electrolyte abnormalities and catheterization of the urinary bladder.
- Forced diuresis by mannitol with induction of anaesthesia to avoid renal failure.

- Antibiotic prophylaxis against gram-negative aerobes—using a three-dose regimen.

Specific Treatment based on causes

CBD stones

There are various options available. The options should be determined on the following factors:
- Physical condition of the patient including co-morbidity, performance status and medical history
- Previous history of cholecystectomy
- Availability of equipment/theatre/anaesthetist/expertise of interventionist
- Patient preference.

Open Exploration of the Common Bile Duct: Involves

- Cholecystectomy, if gall bladder *in situ* present.
- The supraduodenal longitudinal opening in CBD
- Extraction of calculi by Fogarthy balloon, Desjardins forceps or Dormia basket and irrigation with saline.
- Confirmation of duct clearance superiorly and inferiorly by choledochoscopy and/or intra-operative cholangiography.

Where facilities for choledochoscopy and intraoperative cholangiogram are not available, to avoid the risk of leaving retained duct stones, a T-tube is usually inserted to confirm clearance of the duct by a postoperative cholangiogram after seven to ten days. The T-tube is removed after two weeks, when an epithelialzed tract has formed to avoid bile leak into the peritoneal cavity.

In developing countries where there may be no facilities for intraoperative cholangiogram or intraoperative choledochoscopy, T-tube placement should be a standard approach.

Other Procedures in Difficult Cases

Removal of common bile duct calculi may be difficult in the following situations:
- Impacted stone when all efforts to remove it have failed
- Multiple large stones

In these cases choledochoduodenostomy may be done by anastomosis of a dilated common bile duct to the duodenum.

In a non-dilated duct, a transduodenal sphincteroplasty can be performed by first carrying out an open sphincterotomy and stone extraction, then suturing the mucosa of the duct and duodenum together to keep the lower end patent. Percutaneous stenting or nasobiliary drainage may be done in an unfit patient with common bile duct stones that cannot be removed by ERCP.

ERCP and sphincterotomy: A cholangiogram is performed after the cannulation of ampulla of Vater to confirm the anatomy and presence of stones. An adequate sphincterotomy is undertaken and the duct cleared using a balloon catheter or Dormia basket. Confirmation of duct clearance should be established with a radiograph. If the stones are very big, they can be crushed *in situ* using a mechanical lithotripter. Other techniques include extracorporeal shockwave lithotripsy, contact lithotripsy, laser under direct vision. These are, however, time consuming, resource intensive and are limited to a few specialized centres.

Endoscopic placement of a stent, or temporary naso-biliary drainage should be used if the stones are multiple or too large for extraction. This relieves obstruction and prevents impaction of stones at the ampulla of Vater.

Success rate after ERCP±sphincterotomy is about 90% with low complications in experienced hands. Complications include perforation, acute pancreatitis, and bleeding from damage to a branch of the superior pancreatico-duodenal artery.

ERCP may be considered the definitive treatment for some unfit patients, but most will require cholecystectomy to remove remaining gallstones and prevent further complications.

Endoscopic balloon dilation is used for elderly and frail patients as an alternative to sphincterotomy, because of the advantages of preserving the sphincter of Oddi.

Laparoscopic exploration of the common bile duct can be done through the cystic duct (if the gall bladder has not been previously removed) or common bile duct via a choledochotomy. Stones are extracted under fluoroscopic guidance using balloon catheters or Dormia basket.

Medical dissolution of common bile duct stones: Flushing with normal saline; infusion of bile salts, monooctanoin, methyl tert-butyl ether (MTBE), or other solvents into the CBD through a T tube are medical remedies for choledocholithiasis that have been reported. However, the low efficacy of these therapies have made them unattractive and are rarely used. The principal drawback of bile acid infusion are the prolonged period of hospitalization, the unsatisfactory handling of distal occluding stones and those on the hepatic side of the T-tube, the high incidence of side effects, and the rather unpredictable outcome.

Cholangiocarcinoma

Cholangiocarcinomas are malignancies of the cholangiocytes and they can occur at any site of the biliary tree. They are broadly classified into intra-hepatic tumours (extra-hepatic), hilar tumours and (extra-hepatic) distal bile duct tumours.

Hilar cholangiocarcinoma accounts for two-thirds of all cases of extra-hepatic cholangiocarcinoma.

Intra-hepatic and distal extra-hepatic cholangiocarcinomas are less common, but surgical resection remains the only chance of cure consisting of liver resection and pancreaticoduodenectomy, respectively. The majority of these tumours are unresectable, surgery is the only curative option for cholangiocarcinoma. The recent trends of treatment in these patients are accurate pre-operative staging with an aggressive onco-surgical approach involving en-bloc hilar or hepatic resections.

Currently, cholecystectomy, lobar or extended lobar hepatic and bile duct resection, regional lymphadenectomy, and Roux-en-Y hepatico-jejunostomy are the treatments of choice for hilar cholangiocarcinoma.

Systemic therapy/palliative therapy: The majority of patients with cholangiocarcinoma present at an advanced stage or have associated co-morbidity that make them unfit for surgery. The goal of treatment for these patients is to obtain adequate palliation. Biliary endoprosthesis (stent) placement is a useful option for palliation of jaundice. The approach can be either by ERCP or the trans-hepatic route may be used.

Photodynamic therapy, radiation and chemotherapy are all available as palliative options. Several chemotherapeutic agents have been evaluated with limited results. Gemcitabine or 5-fluorouracil are the two common agents used as a single agent or in combination with other drugs.

Ampullary Tumours

Peri-ampullary cancers can be defined as tumours arising within 1 cm of the ampulla of Vater and include ampullary, distal bile duct, pancreatic, and duodenal cancers.

Surgical excision is the mainstay of treatment for peri-ampullary cancers. Proper preoperative staging and assessment of respectability is crucial. If the tumour is resectable, the procedure of choice is a pancreaticoduodenectomy.

The classical approach is Whipple's procedure described by Kausch and Whipple. The more conservative approach (pylorus preserving Whipple resection described by Watson in 1943 and later popularized by Traverso and Longmire is another technique that is gradually gaining more poularity. Pylorus-preserving pancreatico-duodenectomy is easier and less time-consuming operation with less blood loss and a shorter-hospital stay. However, no differences in the recurrence rate and patient survival exist between two procedures.

For unresectable tumours, palliative treatment is carried out depending on availability of resources and expertise for endoscopic treatment.

Biliary bypass procedures can be done operatively, laparoscopically, endoscopic stenting or by percutaneous transhepatic approaches.

Gastric bypass procedures may also be indicated in patients with gastric outlet obstruction. The role of prophylactic gastric bypass procedures is controversial.

Pancreatic Cancer

Pancreatic carcinoma is one the most lethal GI malignancy with an overall 5-year survival rate of less than 4%. Factors responsible for this poor prognosis are:

1. Clinical symptoms in the early stage are usually absent or nonspecific resulting in late diagnosis, with only 15–20% of tumours being resectable at presentation.
2. Clinically, aggressive growth with retro-peritoneal and perineural infiltration, angio-invasion, high rates of local relapse, formation of metastases.

3. Resistance to most of the available treatment regimens.

The only cure for this malignancy is surgery, but only less than 20% are resectable. The acceptable operative mortality rate for resection is less than or equal to 5% when performed at experienced or high volume centers with high volume centres.

The role of adjuvant therapy in advanced pancreatic cancer is controversial as most of the trials show limited benefits. Gemcitabine, 5FU are agents that has shown some promise.

Pain palliation: Patients who present with severe pain must receive NSAID and opioids. Oral Morphine is generally the drug of choice. Parenteral routes of administration should be considered for patients who have impaired swallowing or gastrointestinal obstruction. Percutaneous celiac plexus blockade can be considered, especially for patients who experience poor tolerance of opiate analgesics.

Biliary Strictures

Biliary strictures can be benign or malignant. The majority of benign strictures are iatrogenic—as a result of operations on the gall bladder and the biliary tree. Noniatrogenic causes of benign strictures include inflammatory conditions and subsequent fibrosis related to chronic pancreatitis, cholelithiasis, choledocholithiasis, sclerosing cholangitis, stenosis of the sphincter of Oddi, or infections of the biliary tract.

The options for the management of benign biliary strictures include:

a. Percutaneous dilation and stenting
b. Endoscopic dilation and stenting
c. Surgical biliary drainage, most commonly by a Roux-en-Y hepaticojejunostomy.

The choice of treatment modality is based on the following considerations:

1. Location and severity of the stricture
2. Presence of biliary-enteric continuity
3. Degree of infection
4. Overall health of the individual patient.

14

Right Hypochondrial Lump

From which structures lump in the right hypochondrium can develop?

It can arise from:
a. Right lobe of liver
b. Gall bladder
c. Right kidney
d. Right adrenal gland
e. From hepatic flexure of colon.

Name the different lumps of hepatic origin which can arise from liver and are of surgical importance.

It can be **congenital, infective, or neoplastic origin.**

Congenital origin includes polycystic disease or solitary cyst of liver. Common infective pathology includes amoebic liver abscess, pyogenic liver abscess, and hydatid cyst of liver. Hepatic masses of neoplastic origin comprises focal nodular hyperplasia, adenoma, hemangioma, hepatoma, and secondary to liver. Metastatic lesions can arise from colon, stomach, ovaries, neuroendocrine tumour, breast and lungs. 50% of the patients with a primary malignancy will eventually develop metastases in the liver; primary tumours that drain into portal circulation are more likely to develop hepatic metastasis.

What are the benign tumours of liver?

Epithelial

Hepatocellular
a. Focal nodular hyperplasia
b. Hepatocellular adenoma
c. Regenerative nodule

Cholangiocellular
a. Biliary adenoma
b. Biliary cystadenoma
c. Simple cyst

Other Epithelioid Leiomyoma

Mesenchymal

- *Endothelial*
  a. Haemangioma
  b. Haemangioendothelioma (adult, infantile)
- *Mesothelial*
  Solitary fibrous tumour (benign mesothelioma, or fibroma)
- *Adipocyte*
  a. Lipoma
  b. Myelolipoma
  c. Angiomyolipoma

Other Tumour

Biliary hamartoma

Pseudotumour

a. Focal fatty infiltration
b. Adrenal neoplasm
c. Inflammatory pseudotumour

What are the features of liver enlargement?

The mass is in continuity with liver dullness.
- The mass moves well with respiration.
- One cannot insinuate finger between costal margin and lump.
- The renal angle is free.

- The lump is not ballotable or bimanually palpable.
- It may have well defined lower margin (rounded or sharp.)

What are the causes of gall bladder enlargement?

Gall bladder enlargement can be due to:

a. Distended gall bladder due to malignant obstruction at the lower end of CBD, e.g. carcinoma head of pancreas, periampullary carcinoma, cholangiocarcinoma at the lower end of CBD or due to pancreatic duct calculus impacted at lower most end of CBD.

b. Mucocoele of gall bladder due to stone impacted at the neck of gall bladder or due to malignancy at the neck of gall bladder causing obstruction to the flow of bile at the neck. If there is obstruction at the neck, bile in the gall bladder gets absorbed and secreted bile by gall bladder mucosa gets accumulated. Normally gall bladder secretes 20 ml of bile per day. So mucocoele of gall bladder can be defined as aseptic dilatation of gall bladder due to accumulation of mucus resulting from obstruction at the neck of gall bladder.

c. Empyema of gall bladder results if mucocoele gets infected.

d. *Gall bladder mass resulting from acute cholecystitis*: This gall bladder mass results when the surrounding structures like omentum, colon, duodenum try to wall off infection in acute cholecystitis. The gall bladder mass is inflammatory comprising gall bladder and surrounding structures like omentum, small gut or duodenum.

e. Gall bladder malignancy gives rise to a hard nodular fixed mass with irregular surface.

What are the characteristics of gall bladder lump?

Gall bladder lump is:

a. Globular or pear shaped.

b. It is in continuity with liver dullness.

c. It moves with respiration.

d. It has well defined lower margin and side margins but upper margin is not palpable as it merges with liver.

e. It is mobile side-to-side.

f. It is not ballottable or bimanually palpable.

What is Courvoisier's law regarding palpable gall bladder in obstructive jaundice?

If in a case of obstructive jaundice gall bladder is palpable, the cause of jaundice is unlikely because of obstruction due to CBD stone because the previous attacks of chronic cholecystitis would have rendered the gall bladder fibrotic and not capable of distension. Another reason that gall bladder is not palpable in a case of CBD stone obstruction is that CBD stone does not produce complete obstruction and there is not enough pressure for the gall bladder to distend.

In other words, palpable gall bladder in a case of obstructive jaundice usually means that the cause is malignant, e.g. carcinoma head of pancreas, periampulary carcinoma, or cholangiocarcinoma.

What are the exceptions of Courvoisier law?

The exceptions to Courvoisier's law are:

a. *Double impaction of stone*: One stone in the CBD causing jaundice and another stone impacted at neck of gall bladder causing distended gall bladder or mucocoele (Mirizzi syndrome).

b. Pancreatic duct stone impacted at ampulla of Vater.

c. Big stone impacted at neck of gall bladder causing mucocoele and extrinsic compression on CBD leading to jaundice.

What are the different presentations of carcinoma gall bladder?

- Patient may be asymptomatic.
- The patient can present due to signs and symptoms of gall stones as 80% of carcinoma gall bladder have associated stones. Malignancy can be detected as incidental finding on histopathology of gall bladder specimen removed for gall stones.
- Patient may present with obstructive jaundice.
- Patient may present with hard mass in right hypochondria.
- Advanced cases may present with signs of metastatic disease.

What is the mechanism of obstructive jaundice in patients of carcinoma gall bladder?

30–50% percent of patients with carcinoma gall bladder present with obstructive jaundice. The cause may be:

1. If the growth is in the neck of gall bladder there can be sub-mucosal extension of tumour via cystic duct in CBD lumen and patient can present with jaundice.
2. There can be extrinsic compression of CBD by malignant gall bladder mass.
3. Extrinsic compression by pericholedochal lymph nodes.

Enumerate different organisms which can cause hydatid disease of liver?

There are four forms of hydatid disease:
a. *Echinococcus granulosis (EG)* is the most common and gives rise to cystic hydatid disease (CHD).
b. *Echinococcus multilocularis* is uncommon and causes alveolar hydatid disease (AHD), which is far more aggressive and frequently mimics malignancy.
c. The rarest clinical form is *Echinococcus vogeli* or polycystic hydatid disease (PHD).
d. *Echinococcus oligarthus* causes primarily muscular type of disease.

What is the classification of hydatid cyst?

Gharbi classification of hydatid cysts

Type description
  I. Pure fluid collection.
 II. Fluid collection with a detached membrane.
III. Fluid collection with multiple septa and/or daughter cysts.
IV. Hyper-echoic with high internal echoes.
 V. Cyst with reflecting calcified thick wall.

What are different layers in hydatid cyst of liver?

The different layers of hydatid cyst are

a. *Endocyst*: The endocyst comprises the germinal layer inside and laminated membrane outside. The germinal layer is the living component of parasite and has undifferentiated cells. The germinal layer produces invaginations inside the cyst cavity and these are known as brood capsules. These brood capsules get detached from germinal layer and produce daughter cysts. The germinal layer has absorptive function for nutrition of cyst and secretes hydatid fluid. The laminated membrane is totally acellular and protects the cyst from host enzyme, bacteria and bile.

b. *Ectocyst*: It is also known as pericyst and is the reaction of host **tissue surrounding endocyst. This pericyst is present only in liver and spleen hydatid cyst but absent in lung and brain.**
   The fluid in the hydatid cyst has same level of sodium, chloride and bicarbonate as those of patient plasma but lower levels of potassium and calcium. The fluid is sterile bacteriologically and pressure can reach up to 70 cm of water thus explaining the chances of rupture due to trauma or surgical manipulation. The right lobe of the liver is more commonly involved and in the right lobe segments 7 and 8 are more commonly involved.

Describe clinical features of hydatid cyst of liver.

Many hydatid cysts remain asymptomatic throughout. The size of the cysts and its location determine the degree of symptoms. A history of living in or visiting an endemic area must be established. Many patients give history of exposure to the parasite through the ingestion of foods or water contaminated by the feces of a definitive host.
Symptoms can be produced:
a. By mass effect
b. By complications.
   • Symptoms due to pressure usually take a long time to manifest and usually appear when the cyst is larger than 5 cm.
   • Organs commonly involved by *E. granulosis* are the liver (63%), lungs (25%), muscles (5%), bones (3%), kidneys (2%), brain (1%), and spleen (1%).
Pressure effects include:
a. Non-specific pain, cough,
b. Low-grade fever, and
c. The sensation of abdominal fullness.
d. As the mass grows, the symptoms become more specific because the mass impinges on or obstructs specific organs.
e. Obstructive jaundice can occur due to pressure effect or due to communication of cyst with intrahepatic bile duct leading to passage of daughter cyst in CBD and obstruction. With biliary rupture or communication, the classic triad of biliary colic, jaundice, and rash is observed. Passage of hydatid membranes in the emesis and passage of membranes in the stools may be noted.
   • Involvement of the lungs produces chronic cough, breathlessness, pleural chest pain, and blood in the sputum.

Headache, dizziness, and neurological symptoms may signify cerebral involvement.

Secondary complications may occur as a result of infection of the cyst or leakage of the cyst.

- Major rupture leads to a full-blown anaphylactic reaction.
- A rupture into the biliary tree can lead to obstruction by the daughter cysts, producing cholangitis.
- Rupture into the bronchi can lead to expectoration of daughter cysts and fluid.
- Infection of the cyst can occur either as a primary infection or as a secondary infection. Following an episode of a leak into biliary tree symptoms range from mild fever to full-blown sepsis.
- Extremity pain with or without neurologic deficit is a sign of either bone or muscle involvement.
- *Abdomen*
  - The most common sign is hepatomegaly or a mass.
  - Tenderness is a sign of secondary infection of the cyst or indicates impending rupture if associated with fever and chills.
  - Ascites is rare.
  - Splenomegaly can be the result of either splenic echinococcosis or portal hypertension.

How will you investigate a suspected case of hydatid cyst of liver?

- Eosinophilia is present in 25% of all persons who are infected.
- The indirect hemagglutination test and the enzyme-linked immunosorbent assay (ELISA) have a sensitivity of 80% and are the initial screening tests of choice.
- Immunodiffusion and immunoelectrophoresis can detect antibodies to antigen 5 and provide specific confirmation of reactivity.
- The ELISA test is useful in follow-up to detect recurrence.

  Ultrasound
  - Ultrasonography helps in the diagnosis of hydatid cysts when the daughter cysts and hydatid sand are demonstrated.
  - The accuracy of ultrasound evaluation remains operator-dependent.

  CT scan
  - CT scan has an accuracy of 98% and a high sensitivity to demonstrate the daughter cysts.

- It is the best test for the differentiation of hydatid from amoebic and pyogenic cysts in the liver.

What is the medical management for hydatid cyst and the indications?

- Chemotherapy in hydatid cyst is indicated in patients with primary liver or lung cysts that are inoperable (because of location or medical condition), patients with cysts in 2 or more organs, and peritoneal cysts.
- *Chemotherapeutic agents*: Albendazole and mebendazole. Albendazole is administered in several 1-month oral doses (10–15 mg/kg/d) separated by 14-day intervals.

The optimal period of treatment ranges from 3 to 6 months, with no further increase in the incidence of adverse effects if this period is prolonged. Mebendazole is also administered for 3–6 months orally in dosages of 40–50 mg/kg/d. Limited data are available on the weekly use of praziquantel, an isoquinoline derivative, at a dose of 40 mg/kg/wk, especially in cases in which intraoperative spillage has occurred.

Monitoring: Monitor patients for adverse effects of agents every 2 weeks with a CBC count and liver enzyme evaluation for the first 3 months and then every 4 weeks. Monitoring albendazole and mebendazole serum levels is desirable, but a few laboratories are capable of performing this measurement. Imaging studies are required for follow-up on the morphologic status of the cyst.

What is PAIR treatment for hydatid cyst?

- The Puncture Aspiration Injection Reaspiration (PAIR) technique is performed using either ultrasound or CT guidance involves aspiration of the cyst contents followed by injection of a scolicidal agent for at least 15 minutes, and then reaspiration of the cystic contents. This is repeated until the return is clear. The cyst is then filled with isotonic sodium chloride solution. Perioperative treatment with a benzimidazole is mandatory (4 d prior to the procedure and 1–3 months after).
- The PAIR technique can be performed on liver, bone, and kidney cysts.
- It is contraindicated on lung and brain cysts.

Indications for PAIR
- The cysts should be larger than 5 cm in diameter.

- Type I or II according to the Gharbi ultrasound classification of liver cysts.
- PAIR can be performed on type III cysts as long as it is not a honeycomb cyst.
- Inoperable patients; patients refusing surgery; patients with multiple cysts in segment I, II, and III of the liver; and relapse after surgery.

Contraindications

a. Early pregnancy,
b. Lung cysts,
c. Inaccessible cysts,
d. Superficially located cysts (risk of spillage),
e. Type II honeycomb cysts,
f. Type IV cysts, and
g. Cysts communicating with the biliary tree (risk of sclerosing cholangitis from the scolecoidal agent)
   Outcome: The reduced cost and shorter hospital stay associated with PAIR compared to surgery make it desirable.

The risk of PAIR:

a. Spillage and anaphylaxis especially in superficially located cysts.
b. Sclerosing cholangitis (chemical) and biliary fistulas are other risks.

What are the indications of surgery for hydatid cyst?

Indications

a. Large liver cysts with multiple daughter cysts;
b. Superficially located single liver cysts that may rupture (traumatically or spontaneously);
c. Liver cysts with biliary tree communication or pressure effects on vital organs or structures;
d. Infected cysts; and
e. Cysts in lungs, brain, kidneys, eyes, bones, and all other organs are indications for surgery.

Contraindications

a. General contraindications to surgical procedures (e.g. extremes of age, pregnancy, severe pre-existing medical conditions)
b. Multiple cysts in multiple organs
c. Cysts that are difficult to access
d. Dead cysts
e. Calcified cysts; and very small cysts are contraindications.

Choice of surgical technique

a. Radical surgery (total pericystectomy or partial affected organ resection, if possible),

b. Conservative surgery (open cystectomy), and
c. Simple tube drainage of infected and communicating cysts are choices for surgical technique. The more radical the procedure, the lower the risk of relapses but the higher the risk of complications. Patient care must be individualised accordingly.

The basic steps of the procedure are:

a. Mechanical removal.
b. Sterilisation of the cyst cavity by injection of a scolicidal agent.
c. Protection of the surrounding tissues and cavities.

- Scolicidal agents include:
  a. Formalin,
  b. Hydrogen peroxide,
  c. Hypertonic saline,
  d. Chlorhexidine,
  e. Absolute alcohol, and
  f. Cetrimide.
- 0.5% cetrimide solution provides the best protection with the least complications. Other good scolicidal agents are 70–95% ethanol and 15–20% hypertonic saline solutions.
- At surgery, the cyst is identified and correlated with the radiologic findings. The surrounding tissues are protected by covering them with scolicidal-soaked pads. The cyst is then evacuated using a strong suction device, and scolicidal is injected into the cavity. This procedure is repeated until the return is completely clear. The scolicidal agent is instilled and allowed to remain for 10 minutes, after which it is evacuated, and the cavity is irrigated with isotonic sodium chloride solution. This ensures both mechanical and chemical evacuation and destruction of all cyst contents. During this process, care is taken to ensure no spillage occurs to prevent seeding and secondary infestation.
- The cavity is then filled with isotonic sodium chloride solution and closed. Rarely, omentum is needed to fill the cavity. The cyst fluid is inspected for bile staining at the end of the evacuation and irrigation process. The inside of the cyst is inspected, and any bile duct communication is sutured. In case of infected cysts with biliary communication, closed suction drainage is required.

What are the primary tumours of liver?

Primary tumours of the liver are derived from hepatocytes, biliary epithelium, endothelial cells, and cells of the connective-tissue stroma.

Hepatocellular carcinoma (HCC) is a common malignancy and is responsible for one million deaths per year worldwide.

Describe the epidemiology of HCC.

Hepatocellular carcinoma is most common in Mozambique, Zimbabwe, and Southeast Asia, with the estimated of 30 cases per 100, 000 population per year. High prevalence is also seen in Japan, Greece, and Africa. Intermediate risk areas include Spain, Italy, France, and the Pacific with the incidence rate ranging between 5 and 10 per 100, 000 population per year.

What are the risk factors for development of HCC?

Hepatic cirrhosis: 70% of HCCs develop in cirrhotic livers with the annual incidence of developing HCC in cirrhosis is 3 to 5%. The mechanism for the development of HCC in cirrhosis probably is increased cellular turnover in chronic inflammation which leads to the development of dysplasia and invasive malignancy in a manner similar to that seen in conditions involving other organs.

Hepatitis B viral infection: As high as 25% of patients with HCC are hepatitis B surface antigen positive. Hepatitis B virus causes genetic damage and there is integration of viral DNA with host genome.

Hepatitis C viral infection: HCV infection may promote HCC development through the induction of chronic inflammation and hepatic fibrosis.

Metabolic disorders: The primary and secondary hemochromatosis is associated with increased incidence of HCC. The autosomal recessive metabolic conditions like tyrosinemia, Alpha 1 antitrypsin deficiency, Wilson's disease, hypercitrullinemia, and Porphyria cutanea tarda are also associated with increased incidence of HCC.

Other risk factors for HCC are
a. Chronic venous obstruction
b. Aflatoxins
c. Alcohol
d. Androgens
e. Radiation
f. Other chemical carcinogens.

What are the different pathological types of HCC?

1. *Intrahepatic*
   a. *Expanding type*: In this type of growth there is sharp demarcation between the lesions and the surrounding compressed non-malignant liver tissue.
   b. *Spreading type*: Lack of demarcation between tumour and surrounding liver tissue characterises the spreading type of HCC.
   c. *Multifocal type*: Multifocal tumours occur as multiple small nodules spread throughout the liver either as a result of synchronous multi-centric tumour development or intrahepatic portal venous dissemination. This class accounts for between 5 and 17% of all HCCs.
   d. *Indeterminate*: HCC which cannot be assigned to any of above category.
   e. *Fibro lamellar type*: Fibro lamellar HCC is a distinct variant characterised by well-differentiated large polygonal tumour cells embedded in a fibrous stroma, forming lamellae. Special features of this variety are:
      1. It is common in young males.
      2. It is not commonly associated with raised alpha fetoprotein or background of cirrhosis
      3. Appears to have better prognosis than other subtypes.
      4. Portal lymph node metastasis more common than other subtypes.
      5. Up to 75% of fibro lamellar variants of HCC are resectable in contrast to less than 30% of non-fibrolamellar variety.

2. *Pedunculated type*: The pedunculated lesions are characterised by a predominantly extra-hepatic pattern of growth, with much of the tumour mass visible outside the liver capsule, usually with the formation of a distinct pedicle.

What is TNM classification of HCC?

T (Primary Tumour)

T1   Solitary tumour 2 cm or less in diameter without vascular invasion

T2   Solitary tumour 2 cm or less in diameter with vascular invasion or

Multiple tumours limited to one lobe, none more than 2 cm in diameter without vascular invasion

Solitary tumour greater than 2 cm in diameter without vascular invasion

T3 Solitary tumour greater than 2 cm in diameter with vascular invasion

Multiple tumours limited to one lobe, none more than 2 cm in diameter with vascular invasion

Multiple tumours limited to one lobe, any more than 2 cm in diameter with or without vascular invasion

T4 Multiple tumours in more than one lobe, or tumours involving a major branch of the portal or hepatic veins

N (Regional lymph nodes):

N0 No regional lymph node metastases

N1 Regional lymph node metastases

M (distant metastases):

M0 No distant metastases

M1 Distant metastases

Stage grouping

Stage I: T1 N0 M0

Stage II: T2 N0 M0

Stage III:

T1 N1 M0

T2 N1 M0

T3 N0 M0

T3 N1 M0

IVA T4 N any M0

IVB T4 N any M1

Source: AJCC cancer staging manual. 5th edn.

What are clinical features of HCC?

a. Incidental finding on radiological investigation.

b. Many times raised serum alpha fetoprotein is the only abnormality.

c. Patient can present with unexplained weight loss, upper abdominal distension, pain, jaundice, ascites and fever.

d. Patient may present with signs of chronic liver disease.

e. Spontaneous rupture with haemoperitoneum is seen in 5% of cases.

f. There can be associated paraneoplastic syndromes like increased erythropoietin secretion, hypoglycemia and hypercalcemia.

How will you investigate a case of HCC?

a. Ultrasonography

b. Dual phase CT with separate imaging of hepatic arterial and portal venous phase. As a result most HCC appears as enhancing mass against the background of minimally enhancing liver in arterial phase. However, this is not true in HCC less than 2 cm in diameter as these have predominantly portal venous supply. Lipiodol-enhanced CT scanning has sensitivity of 93 to 96% in the detection of HCC, although this decreases to fewer than 90% in patients with lesions 3 cm or less in diameter. Lipiodol-enhanced CT may be falsely positive in haemangioma, hyperplasic nodules and metastatic lesions.

c. *MRI*: Hyperintense lesion on T2-weighted images is diagnostic of HCC.

What are different modalities of treatment of HCC?

a. Percutaneous transarterial particle embolization using polyvinyl alcohol particles, particles of gelatin, ivalon, gelfoam, or lipiodol either alone or in combination with chemotherapeutic agents (adriamycin, mitomycin-C, or cisplatin). Combining cytotoxic drugs with lipiodol, an iodised oily agent that remains selectively in HCC for long periods, may enhance their antitumour effect. A combination of lipiodol and chemotherapeutic agents (usually Adriamycin) has been used for palliation in patients with unresectable lesions.

b. Percutaneous alcohol injection has a role in HCC of less than 5 cm. This injection is carried out under CT guidance. This can lead to ablation of tumour foci. This procedure can be carried out in several sittings and can be combined with embolisation. The acetic acid may be a more effective agent since it has better diffusion characteristics in the cirrhotic liver as suggested by current studies.

c. *Cryotherapy*: It is safe technique with less mortality and morbidity in comparison to liver resection. Recently cryotherapy has been used through laparoscope.

d. *Radio-frequency ablation*: In this technique an ultrasonic electrode is positioned into centre of

HCC percutaneously and is connected to a radio-frequency generator. The surrounding tissue is ablated through coagulative necrosis by heating the electrode tip. This therapy is useful for small HCCs (<4 cm in diameter) located in the periphery of the liver. The "post-embolisation syndrome" does not occur in this method and the technique can be used percutaneously, resulting in a much shorter hospital stay.

Surgery: Hepatic resection has remained the standard therapy for HCC. Patients with lesions <5 cm in diameter have a better 5-year survival (57%) in comparison to patients with lesions >10 cm in diameter (32% survival). Patients with no cirrhosis have a better prognosis following resection. Adverse prognostic factors following resection are:

1. The presence of a positive surgical margin (relative risk, 2.0),

2. Serum α-fetoprotein >2,000 ng/mL (relative risk, 0.5), and

3. Vascular invasion (relative risk, 1.7).

Resection in patients with HCC and cirrhosis can be facilitated by a segment-orientated approach which optimizes preservation of functional liver tissue and allows the surgeon to plan the extent of resection by selective division of portal and arterial inflow to specific hepatic segments.

This technique is also useful in patients undergoing repeat resections for recurrent disease. It can be combined with cryotherapy to further reduce the incidence of positive margins.

The use of intra-arterial iodine-131 (^{131}I)-labelled lipiodol after resection results in decreased rate of local recurrence and significantly longer disease-free and overall survival.

Currently, the role of transplantation versus resection has yet to be clarified, and transplantation is reserved for a select group of young patients with small HCC associated with cirrhosis.

15

Left Hypochondrium Mass

What is the differential diagnosis of left hypochondrial mass?

Left hypochondrial mass can arise from:
1. Spleen
2. Left kidney
3. Splenic flexure of colors
4. Tail of pancreas colors
5. Left adrenal gland
6. Para-aortic lymph nodes.

What do you understand by the word splenomegaly?

The word splenomegaly means abnormal enlargement of spleen.

Describe basic anatomy of spleen.

- The spleen lies in the left hypochondria
- The dimensions of spleen can be remembered by odd numbers (1, 3, 5, 7, 9–11):
  - It is 1 inch thick
  - Its breath is 3 inches
  - It is 5 inches long
  - It weighs 7 ounces
  - It underlies from 9 to 11 ribs
- *Orientation*: Spleen lies obliquely along long axis of 10th rib; directed downward, forward and laterally
- Arterial supply is by splenic artery from celiac trunk
- Venous drainage is via splenic vein which forms portal vein along with superior mesenteric vein
- *Lymphatic drainage*: It drains into lymph nodes at hilum of spleen which further drains into celiac (para-aortic) nodes

- *Nerve supply*: Sympathetic from celiac plexus

Histological examination: It comprises red pulp and white pulp. The red pulp contains sinuses and white contains lymphoid follicles.
- *Red pulp*: Sinuses lined by endothelial macrophages and cords (spaces).
- *White pulp*: Structure similar to lymphoid follicles.

How do you define splenomegaly?

The normal sized spleen weight can vary from 50 to 250 g, and this decreases with age.

The clinical finding of a palpable spleen can be fallacious. In up to 16% of patients palpable spleens are found to be of normal size on radiological assessment. Patients with emphysema and low diaphragms commonly have palpable but normal-sized spleens. While clinical examination can be convincing in massive spleen enlargement, radiology is often needed to confirm the diagnosis. A single radiological definition of normal spleen size has not been adopted, and the assessment is often partly subjective.

On ultrasound examination various definitions of spleen enlargement are commonly used. Craniocaudal length of spleen measured in right decubitus position. Normal values varies from 11 to 14 cm (normal = a maximum cephalocaudal diameter of 13 cm). This value correlates well with spleen volume.

Spleen normally becomes palpable only when 2–3 times enlarged. Enlargement takes place in a superior and posterior direction before it becomes palpable subcostally.

What are the different mechanisms involved in enlargement of spleen?

The spleen is a lymphoreticular organ which can get enlarged due to the following mechanisms:
Spleen usually enlarges or hypertrophy occurs due to excessive load of its normal function.

a. Immune response due to various foreign antigens as seen in sub-acute bacterial endocarditis or infectious mononucleosis.
b. RBC destruction as seen in various hemolytic anemias such as hereditary spherocytosis or thalassemia major.
c. Congestive spleen enlargement due to portal hypertension or splenic vein thrombosis.
d. Myelo-proliferation as seen in chronic myeloid metaplasia.
e. Infiltration by various substances as seen in sarcoidosis or lipid storage disorders.
f. Neoplastic disorders as seen in lymphoma or chronic lymphocytic leukemias.

What are functions of spleen?

Functions of spleen can be hematological or immune functions:

Hematological functions are:
a. Acts as site of quality control for red blood cells
b. Removes old damaged or fragmented erythrocytes from circulation.
c. Remodels the surface of maturing RBC and maintains normal relationship between membrane surface area and volume. After removal of spleen, target cell with high ratio of membrane to intracellular hemoglobin appear in the circulation.
d. By process known as pitting intra-erythrocyte inclusions are removed from spleen. They form Howell-Jolly bodies.
e. *Hematopoiesis*: From one and half to six and half months of intrauterine life, it is site of production of myelocytes and platelets. From three and half to five months, it also produces red blood cells which can get reactivated in children if the bone marrow compensatory activity is exceeded.

Immune functions are:
a. It is the site for production of IgM, opsonins and tuftsins.
b. Spleen is the site of filtration of encapsulated bacteria and foreign antigen through macrophages and reticuloendothelial system through phagocytosis.

c. It is the storage site for iron.
d. It is the site for sequestration of 30% of circulating platelets.

What are the grades of splenomegaly?

Grading of splenomegaly is done by Hackett's grading. This method was adopted by WHO for usage in malaria surveys and can be used for routine clinical examination also.

Class 0: The spleen not palpable even on deep inspiration.

Class 1: The spleen just palpable below costal margin on deep inspiration.

Class 2: The spleen palpable but not beyond a horizontal line half way between the costal margin and umbilicus.

Class 3: The spleen palpable more than half way to umbilicus, but not below a line running horizontally through umbilicus.

Class 4: Spleen palpable below umbilicus but not below a horizontal line between umbilicus and pubic symphysis.

Class 5: Extending lower than class 4.

Hackett's classes 1 and 2 are considered as mild splenomegaly, class 3 as moderate splenomegaly, and class 4 and 5 are considered as massive splenomegaly.

Grading of splenomegaly based on length of enlargement

- Chronic myeloid leukemia (CML)
- Myelofibrosis
- Chronic malaria, chronic kala-azar
- Gaucher's disease
- Tropical splenomegaly syndrome or hyperactive malarial splenomegaly (HMS)

Moderate (4–8 cm or 2–4 Fingers)

- Hemolytic anemia
- Portal hypertension
- *Lymphoproliferative disorders*: Lymphoma, chronic lymphoid leukemia (CLL)

Mild (<4 cm or <2 Fingers)

- Causes of moderate splenomegaly
- Infectious hepatitis
- Infectious mononucleosis (IM)

- Sub-acute bacterial endocarditis (SBE)
- Idiopathic thrombocytopenic purpura (ITP)
- Amyloidosis
- Sarcoidosis
- Felty's syndrome

What are the important points in the history with spleen enlargement?

1. *History suggestive of splenomegaly*
- Patient complain of pain and a dragging (heaviness) sensation in left upper quadrant of abdomen which can radiate to back.
- This pain and heaviness is not associated with any urinary symptoms and radiating to back.
- Pain can radiate to left shoulder tip in splenic infarction.
- Feeling of early satiety in massive splenomegaly.

2. *History suggestive of associated disease*
- B symptoms, i.e. fever, night sweats, or weight loss (neoplastic, SBE and other infections)
- Bone pain (acute myeloid leukaemia, sickle cell disease, Gaucher's disease)
- Fatigue, dyspnoea, bruising and/or petechiae (hemolytic)
- Joint pains (rheumatoid arthritis, SLE)
- Pruritus (Hodgkin lymphoma, polycythemia)
- Epigastric or generalised abdominal pain (splenic vein thrombosis, e.g. pancreatitis)
- Cough and dyspnoea (sarcoidosis)
- History of alcoholism, liver disease (liver cirrhosis)
- History of pancreatitis (splenic vein thrombosis)
- Personal or family history of haemoglobinopathy, lysosomal storage disorder, rheumatoid arthritis
- History of neonatal umbilical vein sepsis (portal vein thrombosis)
- Recent infections including malaria
- History of recent dental work or blood transfusions (SBE).

What are the causes of asymptomatic spleen enlargement?

Causes of asymptomatic splenomegaly are:
1. Liver disease with portal hypertension
2. Splenic vein thrombosis
3. Agnogenic myeloid metaplasia (myelofibrosis)

4. Gaucher's disease
5. Splenic cysts
6. Sarcoidosis
7. Amyloidosis
8. Mild hereditary spherocytosis
9. Early stages of polycythemia vera.

How to palpate spleen and describe findings?

Palpation of spleen is done by the following methods:

Palpation is done by right hand which is kept still and the patient is asked to take a deep breath through the mouth so that one can feel spleen edge when it is being displaced downwards. Move right hand up diagonally starting from right iliac fossa, towards left upper quadrant on expiration. So palpation is done during deep inspiration and the hand is gradually moved upwards towards left hypochondrium during expiration. The left hand can be placed around patient's lower rib and which are depressed down so that the spleen is pulled forward.

If there is strong suspicion of splenomegaly on the basis of history but spleen is not palpable, then roll the patient on to the right lateral position with flexion of left hip and knee and examine as before. If gross ascites is present, then dipping method is used to palpate the spleen.

Percussion
- Examine the spleen with the patient holding the breath during full inspiration; and percuss from both below and then above the left costal margin from resonant to dull area.

Castell's sign: With the patient supine, the percussion in the lowest inter-costal space in the anterior axillary line (8th or 9th) is done. It produces a resonant note if the spleen is normal in size both during expiration or full inspiration. A dull percussion note on full inspiration suggests spleen enlargement.

The palpable spleen should be described under following headings

- *The grade of enlargement*: Measured below from the left costal margin along the spleen axis in centimeters/inches or number of fingers. Splenic axis is in a line from midpoint of left costal margin to right anterior superior iliac spine.
- The splenic notch is usually felt on its lower medial border.

- *The anterior margin*: Usually have a sharp anterior margin.
- *The consistency*: It can be firm or hard.
- *Tenderness*: Tenderness goes in favour of abscess, infective pathology or recent infarct.
- *Surface*: The surface can be smooth or irregular.
- *Movement with respiration*: The spleen always moves downwards and medially with respiration.
- *Finger insinuation*: One cannot insinuate fingers between spleen and ribs.
- *Palpable spleen rub*: It may be present or absent.

The *palpable spleen is distinguished from palpable left kidney mass by*

- Not bimanually palpable and not ballottable.
- Renal angle free (no obliteration or tenderness) in case of spleen enlargement.
- Upper limit cannot be reached in spleen but in kidney one may be able to reach upper limit if kidney is pushed down.
- Kidney lump grows downwards but spleen enlarges obliquely.
- Notch on lower medial border with sharp anterior margin.
- Fingers cannot get between spleen and ribs (in kidney enlargement one can insinuate finger between costal margin and ribs).
- Dull on percussion in case of spleen but in renal lump there may be band of colonic resonance anteriorly.

Differential diagnosis of spleen enlargement

1. Enlarged left kidney
2. Enlarged left lobe of liver
3. Carcinoma of stomach arising from fundus or from greater curvature
4. Carcinoma of splenic flexure of colon
5. Omental mass (TB or malignancy)
6. Malignancy of tail of pancreas
7. Ovarian tumour in females

Normal sized spleen may be palpable in:
- Chronic emphysema
- Low diaphragm.

What is the other relevant examination you will like to perform in case of splenomegaly?

Auscultation: Venous hum or a friction rub may be heard.
Percussion: Palpation is confirmed by dullness as spleen is dull to percussion.

Other relevant findings in physical examination

a. *Skin*
- *Pallor with spleen enlargement can suggest*: Chronic Malaria, Chronic Kala-azar, leukemia, lymphomas, cirrhosis, hemolytic anemia, hypersplenism.
- *Icterus in a case of splenomegaly can point towards*: Hemolysis (hemolytic anemias, acute malaria, lymphoma), Budd-Chiari syndrome (hepatic vein obstruction), chronic liver disease.
- *Plethora of bacteria with palpable spleen*: Polycythemia vera.
- *Skin infiltration, nodules and masses along with palpable spleen points towards*: AML or ALL.
- *Associated butterfly rash*: SLE.
- *Presence of Janeway's lesion*: SBE.
- *Spider naevi and palmar erythema*: Portal hypertension due to chronic liver disease.
- *Haemorrhagic spots*: Acute leukaemia, SBE, SLE, ITP, Felty's syndrome, blast crisis of CML or CLL.

b. *Generalised lymphadenopathy*
- *Autoimmune disorders*: RA, Felty's syndrome, SLE, sarcoidosis.
- *Infection*: Infectious mononucleosis, AIDS, toxoplasmosis, CMV, disseminated TB.
- *Neoplasm*: Lymphomas and leukaemias.

c. *Fever*
- *Infections*: Malaria, kala-azar, enteric fever, SBE, miliary TB, acute viral hepatitis.
- *Neoplasm*: Acute leukemias, CML, lymphoma.
- Collagen vascular diseases.

d. *Extremities*
- *Digital ischaemia/gangrene or thrombosis*: Essential thrombocytosis.
- *Joint deformities*: RA, Felty's syndrome, SLE.
- *Lower extremity oedema*: Amyloidosis.

e. *Abnormal neurological examination*:
- Essential thrombocytosis
- Non-Hodgkin's lymphoma (NHL).

Diagnostic approach to isolated splenomegaly

1. **Step one is to rule out known illness that causes splenomegaly**
   - Infections, e.g. Malaria, Kala-azar, Infectious and mononucleosis, etc.
   - Hematological, e.g. haemolytic anaemias, haemoglobinopathies, malignancies and myelo-proliferative disorders.
   - Hepatic, e.g. portal hypertension, splenic or portal vein thrombosis

2. Step two is to search for any occult disease
- Infections, e.g. infective endocarditis
- Hematological, e.g. hereditary spherocytosis and polycythemia vera
- Hepatic, e.g. cryptogenic cirrhosis
- Autoimmune, e.g. systemic lupus erythematosus
- Storage disease, e.g. Gaucher's disease
- Miscellaneous, e.g. sarcoidosis, amyloidosis, tropical splenomegaly and splenic cysts
  If found manage appropriately.

3. Diagnostic splenectomy if
- Systemic symptoms are present and suggests malignancy
- Focal replacement of the spleen on imaging studies
- No other sites are available for biopsy.

4. Monitor closely and repeat studies until the splenomegaly resolves or a diagnosis is apparent.

How will you investigate?

1. *Initial investigations*
- White cell count with differential count:
  - *Leucocytosis*: It is seen in bacterial infections, Leukaemia. In leukaemia immature WBC are often seen in peripheral smear.
  - *Leucopenia*: Seen in malaria, kala-azar, enteric fever, Felty's syndrome.
  - *Pancytosis*: Polycythemia
  - *Pancytopenia*: Hypersplenism
- ESR:
  - *Increased*: Chronic infection, SLE, lymphoma, severe anaemia
  - *Decreased*: Polycythemia
- Peripheral blood smear (PBS):
  - Abnormal cell morphology with immature cells: Leukaemia, hereditary spherocytosis, thalassemia
  - Peripheral smear for parasites: Malaria, kala-azar
  - Reticulocyte count is done in anaemic patients
  - *Increased*: Haemolytic anaemias
- Blood cultures is often done in febrile patients.
  - It can diagnose SBE, enteric fever
- Liver function tests:
  - Hyperbilirubinemia: Often seen in haemolytic anaemia, hepatitis, chronic liver disease.

2. *Based on disease suspected by clinical and/or initial laboratory findings following investigations may be carried out:*
- Haemoglobin electrophoresis to detect increased levels of HB F in β-thalssemia
- Coombs' test is used to differentiate between autoimmune haemolysis and hereditary (+ve in autoimmune haemolysis and –ve in hereditary spherocytosis)
- Red cell enzyme testing in suspected cases of G6PD deficiency
- Osmotic fragility testing in hereditary spherocytosis
- Flow cytometry for lymphoproliferative profile (CLL, hairy cell leukaemia, lymphomas)
- Erythropoietin level in polycythemia vera
- Coagulation test (chronic liver disease, DIC in AML, SLE)
- Paul-Bunnell test (infectious mononucleosis)
- Congo red test (amyloidosis)
- Serum ACE (sarcoidosis)
- Napier's aldehyde test (chronic kala-azar)
- Anti-nuclear antibodies (SLE)
- Rheumatoid factor (RA, Felty's syndrome)

3. *Bone marrow aspiration and biopsy*
- Myeloproliferative diseases
- Lymphomas
- Immunological diseases (sarcoidosis, SLE, Felty's syndrome, amyloidosis)
- Gaucher's disease

4. *Lymph node biopsy*
- Tuberculosis
- Sarcoidosis
- Lymphoma

5. *Splenic biopsy*
- Diagnosis of lymphoma
- Niemann-Pick's disease (large foamy cells)
- Amyloidosis (large hyaline masses)

6. *Liver biopsy*
- Alcohol induced liver disease
- Hepatic steatosis
- Hemochromatosis

Imaging
Role of radiology in evaluation of spleen enlargement:

A. Confirmation of splenic size;
B. Evaluation of splenic architecture;

C. Assessment of other organs affecting the differential diagnosis; and

D. In certain patients, radiologically-guided biopsy.

1. *To evaluate splenomegaly*
   - Ultrasonography
   - CT scan
   - Splenoportography
   - Spleen liver colloid scan
   - MRI
   - Angiography

2. *Confirming suspected diagnosis*
   - Chest X-ray:
     - Miliary TB
     - Lymphoma
     - Sarcoidosis
     - Extramedullary hematopoiesis in thalassemia
   - Bone X-ray:
     - Mosaic pattern in small bones of hand: Thalassemia
     - Increased bone density: Myelofibrosis or myelosclerosis
     - Erlenmeyer flask sign in distal femur: Gaucher's disease
   - Skull X-ray:
     - 'Hair on end' appearance in thalassemia

Investigations should be based on disease suspected by clinical and/or initial laboratory findings.

Splenectomy

What are the indications of splenectomy?

- Hodgkin's lymphoma (for staging the extent of disease) not indicated these days
- Massive splenomegaly (for control of symptoms)
- Traumatic or iatrogenic splenic rupture (for disease control)
- Hypersplenism or immune-mediated destruction of one or more blood cell line (for correction of cytopenias)

Causes of splenic rupture:
- Trauma
- Infectious mononucleosis
- Leukaemias
- Myelofibrosis
- Congestive splenomegaly

What are the common problems after splenectomy?

- Immediate: Increased platelet count may lead to thromboembolic phenomenon
- Long-term: Increased risk of infection with capsulated organisms (like *Streptococcus pneumoniae, Neisseria meningitidis, H. influenzae* or *E. coli*), malarial parasites, Babesia.

What are the causes of asplenism or hyposplenism?

- Asplenia: Absence of spleen
- Surgical: Splenectomy
- Diminished function: Sickle cell disease, celiac disease, dermatitis herpetiformis with enteropathy

What is the required prophylaxis for post-splenectomy infection?

- Vaccinate 2–3 weeks before elective splenectomy: Pneumococcal vaccine, *Haemophilus influenzae* type B (Hib) vaccine, meningococcal group C vaccine, influenza vaccine.
- Lifelong antibiotic prophylaxis: Long-term penicillin V 500 mg 12 hourly (erythromycin if allergic to penicillin).
- Revaccination of pneumococcal vaccine: In every 5 years and influenza vaccine anually.
- Antimalarial chemoprophylaxis: If needed (travel to endemic area).

What are the post-splenectomy hematological features?

- *Thrombocytosis*: Persists in 30% cases
- *WBC count*: Usually normal but there may be mild lymphocytosis and monocytosis
- *Red cell morphology*: Howell-Jolly bodies (nuclear remnants), Pappenheimer bodies (contain sideroblastic granules), Heinz bodies (denatured haemoglobin), target cells, nucleated erythrocytes (occasionally).

What is tropical splenomegaly syndrome?

The condition more appropriately known as **hyperreactive malarial syndrome (HMS)**. This is one of the important causes of massive splenomegaly.

Following conditions should be fulfilled before labeling a patient as HMS:

1. The patient should be resident of malaria endemic area.

2. Presence of chronic massive splenomegaly as per WHO criteria.
3. Serum IgM levels at least 2 standard deviations (SD) above local mean.
4. High malarial antibody titer.
5. Presence of hepatic sinusoidal lymphocytosis.
6. Clinical and immunological response to antimalarial drugs prophylaxis.

What is the pathophysiology of HMS?

a. There is an exaggerated stimulation of polyclonal B-lymphocytes, leading to excessive and partially uncontrolled production of immuno-globulin M (IgM) due to exposure to malarial antigen (the initiating event).
b. These IgM antibodies are polyclonal and not specific for any one particular malaria species
c. As there is defective regulatory control of B-lymphocytes by suppressor or T-lymphocytes, there is increase in B-lymphocytes and a decrease in T-lymphocytes in the peripheral blood.
d. There is T-cell infiltration of the hepatic and splenic sinusoids.
e. An increase occurs in serum cryoglobulin levels, autoantibody levels, and high-molecular-weight immune complexes which lead to anemia, deposi-tion of large immune complexes in Kupffer cells in liver and spleen, reticuloendothelial cell hyperplasia, and hepato-splenomegaly.

What are clinical features of HMS?

a. Usually occurs in young or middle persons. It is rare before the age of 8 years.
b. Chronic abdominal dragging pain and swelling are most common features.
c. Intermittent fever is rare and the presence of fever should raise the possibility of alternative diagnosis.
d. Moderate or massive splenomegaly is the hall-mark.
e. Majority have accompanying hepatomegaly.
f. Blood examination reveals anaemia, leucopenia and thrombocytopenia.
g. Peripheral smear does not show presence of malarial parasites.

What is the treatment of HMS?

1. Antimalarial drugs for prolonged period.
2. Treatment has to be continued for one year.
3. The response is monitored by serum IgM levels, spleen size, improvement of anaemia and general improvement.

16

Right Iliac Fossa Mass

What is the etiology of right iliac fossa mass (RIF)?

It can arise from structures normally present in RIF

- Terminal ileum
- Caecum
- Appendix
- Right ovary and fallopian tube (in females)
- Ureter
- Lymph nodes
- Iliac vessels
- Psaos muscle with sheath
- Iliac bone

It can also arise from structures which can be present in RIF

- Undescended testis
- Unascended kidney
- Fundus of gall bladder
- Liver in massive enlargement

Cause of RIF mass can be

1. Infective
2. Neoplastic
3. Inflammatory
4. Vascular
5. Miscellaneous

Infective causes are

- Appendicular lump
- Appendicular abscess
- Ileocaecal tuberculosis (hyperplastic type)
- Amoeboma of caecum
- Actinomycosis
- Pyogenic psoas abscess
- Tubercular psoas abscess (Fig. 16.1)
- Infective iliac lymphadenitis
- Pyosalpinx in females
- Tubo-ovarian mass due to pelvic inflammatory disease in females

Neoplastic causes are

- Carcinoma caecum/ascending colon
- Secondary in iliac lymph nodes
- Lymphoma of iliac lymph node
- Tumors of iliac bone like chondroma
- Tumour arising in an undescended testis, e.g. seminoma
- Ovarian cyst or ovarian tumour
- Fibroid uterus

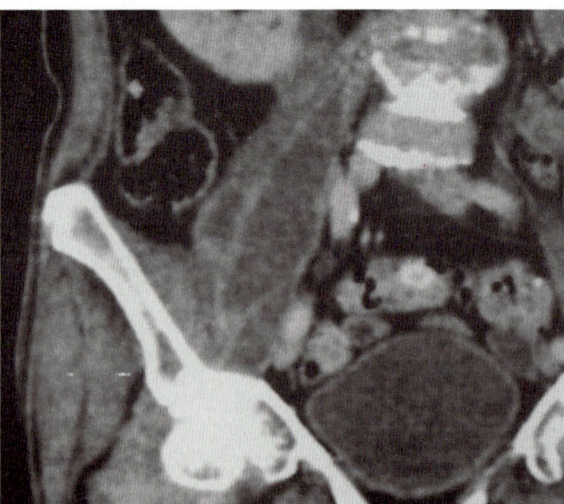

Fig. 16.1: CT scan showing right psoas abscess

Inflammatory causes are

- Crohn's disease
- Sarcoidosis

Vascular aetiology causes

- Iliac artery aneurysm
- Haematoma following ruptured inferior epigastric artery

Miscellaneous causes

- Spigelian hernia
- Kidney transplant
- Pelvic kidney
- Ileo-colic intussusception

What are the relevant points in the history?

- H/o mass without any symptoms
- 3A's: **A**norexia, **a**naemia and **a**sthenia in carcinoma caecum
- Altered bowel habits with alternate diarrhoea with constipation in tuberculosis
- Colicky abdominal pain
- Constitutional symptoms in lymphoma or tuberculosis
- Urinary symptoms in pelvic kidney with some pathology like hydronephrosis
- Restricted mobility of hip joint in psoas abscess
- History of absence of testis since childhood in case of undescended testis
- Lower limb swelling in case of iliac lymphadenitis.

Describe the relevant general physical examination.

- Poor nutritional status
- Pallor
- Lymphadenopathy in case of lymphoma
- Pedal oedema in case of iliac lymphadenitis
- Flexion deformity of hip joint in case of psoas abscess

Describe points in local examination.

Inspection

- Shape and extent of swelling if it is visible
- Visible peristalsis or bowel loops
- Decide if the swelling is parietal or intra-abdominal by Valsalva manoeuvre or forceful coughing or leg raising test (Carnett's test). If swelling becomes less prominent, it is intra-abdominal.

Palpation

- Look for tenderness
- Confirm findings of inspection
- Check for mobility of swelling
- Describe the swelling in detail like size shape, margins, consistency
- Genitalia examination
- *Groove sign:* Look for space between iliac crest and swelling. If it is present, it points towards swelling of ileocecal origin or appendix. If absent, it points towards psoas abscess.
- Per rectal examination
- Per vaginal examination

Percussion

Shifting dullness and fluid thrill for free fluid.

Auscultation

Increased bowel sounds

Describe the plan of investigations.

Aims of investigations are
- To establish anatomical diagnosis
- To establish the pathological diagnosis
- To assess the extent of disease
- To assess fitness for surgery

Ultrasonography

- First investigation to be performed
- It is non-invasive/cost effective
- Indicates organ of origin
- Can decide diagnosis in many conditions like psoas abscess, appendicular abscess.
- It can detect free fluid
- Iliac lymph nodes greater than 1.5 cm in diameter can be detected
- In females pathology of adenexa can be visualised

Colonoscopy is performed in suspected cases

- Carcinoma caecum
- Ileocecal tuberculosis or terminal ileitis

Spiral CT abdomen with or without Virtual colonoscopy.

- 3D reconstruction of whole colon is possible
- Small mucosal lesions can be detected.
- Unnecessary diagnostic colonoscopy can be avoided.

- Staging of ileocecal malignancy can be carried out.
- Kidney pathology can be detected.

Image-guided FNAC of mass is indicated in

- Psoas abscess
- Lymph node enlargement

Discuss the treatment plan.

- Appendicular lump
  - Conservative management followed by interval appendicectomy 6 weeks later.
  - Ochsner-Sherren regimen
- Outcome can be summarised as: 3S as the lump can
  - **S**ubside
  - **S**uppurate means appendicular abscess form. This situation needs surgical intervention.
  - **S**pread means lump increases in size also needs operative intervention.

Appendicular Abscess

Drain abscess

In hyperplastic Ileocecal Koch

If no features of obstruction, then treat patient with

- Liquid or semisolid diet with small meals at a time
- Anti-tubercular therapy (ATT) for 6 months

In case of recurrent or acute intestinal obstruction which does not get relieved on conservative management patient needs surgery (limited resection) with ATT.

Carcinoma Caecum

- Confirm diagnosis and rule out synchronous lesions by colonoscopy and biopsy
- Stage the disease by CT
- Right hemicolectomy is perfomed
- Chemotherapy if indicated

Amoeboma

- Emetine or dihydroemetine
- If it does not regress, then surgery

Psoas Abscess

- **Pyogenic**
  - Drain abscess
  - Antibiotic therapy
- **Tubercular**
  - ATT
  - If large, then drain by catheter
  - Bedrest if spine involved

Unascended Kidney

- If normal no pathology in kidney, then no intervention needed
- If hydronephrotic kidney, then treat the cause.

What are the common differential diagnosis of rectal carcinoma?

Common differential diagnosis of rectal carcinoma is:
a. Lipoma
b. Carcinoid
c. Lymphoma
d. GI stromal tumour
e. Leiomyoma
f. Leiomyosarcoma
g. Metastatic neoplasm
h. Colitis cystic profunda (benign dilated mucus filled sub-mucosal glands)
i. Pneumatosis cystoides intestinalis (air in the bowel)
j. Lymphoid polyp
k. Rectal endometriosis

How does patient with rectal cancer present?

1. Rectal cancer usually present to the surgeon after definitive endoscopic diagnosis. As many of the patients are initially asymptomatic and diagnosed on surveillance colonoscopy.
2. Patient may complain of rectal bleeding, change in bowel habit or constant sense of rectal pressure.
3. The constant sensation to empty the bowel, i.e. Tenesmus is present.
4. Constant anal pain or pain with defecation suggests involvement of anal canal.
5. Digital rectal examination (DRE) is very important part of examination. On DRE fixation of lesion to anal sphincter, rectal wall and pelvic wall should be evaluated. The relation of the tumour with respect to ano-rectal ring should be noted.

6. With the help of DRE and rigid sigmoidoscopy one should decide how much normal rectum lies below the lower margin of tumour. This information is crucial to decide whether sphincter saving surgery is possible or not.

What are the genetic syndromes associated with rectal cancer?

Genetic syndromes associated with colorectal cancer are:
a. Familial adenomatous polyposis (FAP)
b. Attenuated familial adenomatous polyposis (AFAP)
c. Hereditary nonpolyposis colon cancer (HNPCC) or Lynch's syndrome
d. Familial colorectal cancer

FAP is an autosomal dominant condition accounting for less than 1% of all colorectal cancers. The genetic abnormality is mutation in the APC gene located on chromosome 5q. Seventy five percent of patients with FAP give positive family history. Clinically patients develop hundreds to thousands of polyps throughout the colon soon after puberty. All most all patients develop colonic malignancy by the age of 50 years. First degree relatives of FAP should be tested for APC mutation and if positive flexible sigmoido-scopy should be performed every year beginning from 10 years of age. FAP patients are also prone to develop adenoma anywhere in the gastro-intestinal tract particulary in duodenum. These patients are also have high risk of developing peri-ampullary carcinoma.

FAP can also be associated with extraintestinal manifestations like:
a. Congenital hypertrophy of retinal pigmental epithelium (CHRPE)

b. Desmoid tumours and epidermal cysts

c. Mandible osteomas

FAP associated with above extra intestinal manifestations constitute Gardner's syndrome

FAP associated with CNS tumours is known as Turcot's syndrome.

AFAP is a variant of FAP with patients presenting later in life and fewer polyps (10–100) and predominantly located in right colon. Colorectal cancer develops in about 50% of cases around 55 years of age. APC gene mutation is present in only 30% of patients and in remaining of the patients mutation of MYH gene result in AFAP phenotype.

Hereditary nonpolyposis colon cancer (HNPCC) or Lynch's syndrome is more common than FAP but still a rare diseases seen in 1–3% of all cancers. The genetic defect associated with HNPCC is defect in mismatch repair. The colorectal cancer develops at an early age (40–45) and 50% of affected individuals develops colorectal cancer located in the proximal colon. There is very high risk of synchronous or metachronus malignancy as high as in 40% of cases. It may be associated with extra colonic malignancies like endometrial carcinoma, ovarian pancreatic, small bowel, and biliary tree malignancy. The diagnosis is based on family history by the Amsterdam criteria which consist of clinical diagnosis of colonic cancer in three relatives out of which one must be first degree relative. Two successive generations should be involved with one patient diagnosed before the age of 50. The presence of other HNPCC carcinoma raises the suspicion of this syndrome.

HNPCC results from mutation in mismatch repair gene. The mutation in PMS2 or MSH6 results in more attenuated form of HNPCC. The MSH6 inactivation results in higher risk of endometrial carcinoma.

Familial colorectal cancer which is non-syndromic is seen in 10–15% of patients with colorectal cancer. The risk of developing colorectal cancer increases significantly to 12%, if one first degree relative is affected and 35%, if two first degree relatives are affected.

What are the investigations necessary in the workup of a patient with rectal malignancy?

1. Colonoscopy should be done in every case before surgical resection. The colonoscopy helps in establishing the diagnosis by biopsy. Synchronous benign polyps are seen in 13–62% of cases of rectal cancer. Synchronous cancers are seen in 2–8% of cases.

2. Endo-rectal ultrasound (ERUS) is used to determine the T stage and N stage. The accuracy of ERUS is 62–92% in T staging and 64 to 88% for N staging. The drawbacks of EURS are steep learning curve, not accurate in near obstructing lesions and in downstaged tumours after chemo-radiation. Currently it is considered as the most accurate method in local staging of rectal cancer.

3. *CT*: The role of CT in assessment of locoregional disease is limited. CT is done to rule out metastatic disease prior to surgical resection.

4. *MRI*: Endorectal coil MRI and phased array MRI are more accurate in determining the extent of tumour mesorectal involvement and T staging. The traditional body coils MRI are much more inferior to ERUS to determine T staging. The limitations of endorectal coil MRI are relatively small field of view, expensive and uncomfortable to the patient. It has a role in detecting whether the mesorectal fascia has been breached by tumour or not.

5. PET scan has a role in evaluation of post-operative recurrences if the patient has rising CEA levels.

What is CEA and what is its role in patients with carcinoma colon?

Carcinoembryonic antigen (CEA) is a glyco-protein's involved in cell adhesion is found in the embryonal endodermal epithelium. CEA is normally produced in gastrointestinal tissue during fetal development, but the production stops before birth. Therefore, CEA is usually present only at very low levels in the blood of healthy adults. However, its level is raised in primary colon malignancy, pancreatic breast, lung and liver malignancy. It can be elevated in benign conditions like diverticulitis, peptic ulcer, bronchitis, liver abscess and alcoholic cirrhosis.

Use of CEA in clinical practice:

a. In monitoring postoperative recurrences in colorectal cancer.

b. The preoperative elevation is an indicator of poor prognosis.

c. The determination of CEA is the most cost effective approach in detecting metastasis. The postoperative CEA monitoring should be done every 3 months for 3 years in stages 2 and 3 colorectal cancer.

d. May be useful in assessing the effectiveness of chemotherapy or radiation treatment.

e. May be useful in detecting or screening cancer but it is not recommended.

What is Duke's staging?

Cuthbert Duke in 1932 described a classification for staging rectal cancer, which was later adapted to include colon cancer. The initial staging system only included the three stages, but later on stage D was added for advanced disease.

Stage A: Tumour confined to the mucosa. (90%, 5-year survival)

Stage B: Tumour infiltrating through muscle. (70%, 5-year survival)

Stage C: Lymph node metastases present. (30%, 5-year survival)

Stage D: Distant metastases.

Astler and Coller (1954) adapted the original Duke's system as follows:

• *Stage A*—limited to mucosa

• *Stage B1*—extending into muscularis propria but not penetrating through it; nodes not involved

• *Stage B2*—penetrating through muscularis propria; nodes not involved

• *Stage C1*—extending into muscularis propria but not penetrating through it. Nodes involved

• *Stage C2*—penetrating through muscularis propria. Nodes involved

• *Stage D*—distant metastatic spread.

What is the TNM staging for colonic cancer?

TNM classification for colon cancer:

Primary tumour (T)

Tx	Primary tumour cannot be assessed
T0	No evidence of primary tumour
Tis	Carcinoma *in situ*: Intraepithelial or invasion of lamina propria
T1	Tumour invades submucosa
T2	Tumour invades muscularis propria
T3	Tumour invades through the muscularis propria into the pericolorectal tissues
T4a	Tumour penetrates to the surface of the visceral peritoneum
T4b	Tumour directly invades or is adherent to other organs or structures

Regional lymph nodes (N)

Nx	Regional lymph nodes cannot be assessed
N0	No regional lymph node metastasis
N1	Metastasis in 1–3 regional lymph nodes
N1a	Metastasis in 1 regional lymph node
N1b	Metastasis in 2–3 regional lymph nodes
N1c	Tumour deposit(s) in the subserosa, mesentery, or non-peritonealised pericolic or perirectal tissues without regional nodal metastasis
N2	Metastasis in 4 or more lymph nodes
N2a	Metastasis in 4–6 regional lymph nodes
N2b	Metastasis in 7 or more regional lymph nodes

Distant metastasis (M)

M0	No distant metastasis
M1	Distant metastasis
M1a	Metastasis confined to 1 organ or site (e.g. liver, lung, ovary, non-regional node)
M1b	Metastases in more than 1 organ/site or the peritoneum

Stage	T	N	M
0	Tis	N0	M0
I	T1	N0	M0
	T2	N0	M0
IIA	T3	N0	M0
IIB	T4a	N0	M0
IIC	T4b	N0	M0
IIIA	T1–T2	N1/N1c	M0
	T1	N2a	M0
IIIB	T3–T4a	N1/N1c	M0
	T2–T3	N2a	M0
	T1–T2	N2b	M0
IIIC	T4a	N2a	M0
	T3–T4a	N2b	M0
	T4b	N1–N2	M0
IVA	Any T	Any N	M1a
IVB	Any T	Any N	M1b

What is the surgical management of carcinoma rectum?

Surgical management of carcinoma rectum can be local excision or radical excision.

What is the risk of lymph node involvement in rectal cancer?

The risk of lymph node involvement in rectal cancer depends upon T stage. It is 0–12% for T1 cancer. For T2 tumours it is 12–28% and for T3 malignancy, it is 36 to 79%.

What are the indications for local excision in carcinoma rectum?

Local excision is carried out in patients who found to be T1 on EURS without any adverse factors or distant metastasis. The adverse factors are poorly differentiated tumour, vascular invasion or neural invasion.

What is the incidence of recurrence after local excision?

After local excision even in a case without adverse factors chances of recurrence are 20%. The recurrence rate is much higher in patient with adverse pathological factors. T1 tumours with adverse pathological factors are treated by radical resection.

Discuss the treatment of T2, N0, M0 carcinoma rectum.

These patients are treated by radical resection. If pathologically no lymph nodes are found to be involved, these patients are observed. If lymph nodes are found to have metastasis on pathological examination, these patients are given chemo-radiotherapy.

What is the treatment for T3 /T4 or node positive disease?

These patients are treated by preoperative chemo-radiotherapy followed by radical surgery on the principals of Total Mesorectal Excision (TME).

What are the different aims of treatment for carcinoma rectum?

The aims of treatment for carcinoma rectum are:
- Local control
- Long-term survival
- Preservation of anal sphincter, bladder and sexual function.
- Improvement in quality of life

What is total mesorectal excision (TME)?

TME involves sharp dissection and removal of entire rectal mesentery including distal to the tumour as an intact single unit. The rectal mesentery is removed under direct vision by sharp dissection to avoid any injury to autonomic pelvic nerves and without violation of mesorectal envelope. Its rational is based on the assumption that rectal cancer spread is limited to this envelope. TME results in reduction of positive radial margins from 25% in convention surgery to 7%. The patients with positive radial margins are three times more likely to die and 12 times more likely to local recurrence. TME requires precise sharp dissection in areolar plane between the visceral fascia that surrounds the rectum and mesorectal pelvic fascia that overlie the pelvic wall structures. Properly done TME helps in removing the intact mesorectum along with draining lymph nodes and preservation of pelvis autonomic nervous system. There should be negative circumferential resected margin (CRM) and distal margin at the end of properly carried out TME. Negative CRM should be more than one mm. Distal resected negative margin of 2 cm is sufficient as distal spread beyond 1 cm occurs only in 10% of cases that too in node positive or poorly differentiated carcinoma.

What is the importance of negative CRM?

Patient with negative CRM more than 1 mm had 5% recurrence rate at 29 month follow up in comparison to 20% local recurrence with negative CRM less than 1 mm.

What are the indications for performing abdominoperineal resection (APR) and what all structures are removed in this procedure?

Abdominoperineal resection of the rectum commonly known as APR needs creation of a permanent end colostomy, is therefore, not a favourable operation. It may still be required in following situations:

1. Carcinoma of the lower one-third of rectum if tumour free distal margin of 2 cm cannot be obtained or if the carcinoma is involving the anal sphincter.

2. Squamous cell carcinoma of the anal canal when chemoradiotherapy (combined modality) has failed or if there is a recurrence after combined modality treatment.

3. Adenocarcinoma of the anal canal arising *de novo* within the anal canal is treated by APR. Adenocarcinoma in anal canal can arise either from anal glandular epithelium or within a long-standing complex anal fistula.
4. Malignant melanoma of the anal canal is treated primarily by surgery, specially in a young patient irrespective of size.
5. Sarcoma of levator ani muscle involving the anal canal.
6. Chordomas of presacral region.
7. Locally advanced bulky tumours of rectum.
8. Recurrent rectal carcinomas if resectable, should be treated by APR.

APR involves removal of the following structures:
1. Distal 10 cm of sigmoid colon.
2. Whole of rectum and anal canal along with perianal skin.
3. Ischiorectal fat.
4. As much of levator ani muscles as possible.

APR involves en bloc resection of the tumour as well as the surrounding lymph nodes and the anal sphincters resulting in a permanent colostomy. Oncological and functional results are better if principle of total mesorectal excision (TME) and autonomic nerve preservation are followed.

How is a patient planned for colonic surgery prepared?

Clear fluid liquid diet 1–3 days prior to surgery with one of the following modality:
- Laxatives and enemas
- Whole gut irrigation with saline via nasogastric tube
- Mannitol solution
- Polyethylene glycol (PEG) based lavage solutions. PEG solutions are found to be most reliable.

What is the role of antibiotic prophylaxis?

The antibiotic prophylaxis is used to decrease the incidence of postoperative septic complications as mechanical cleansing reduces the stool load from colon but does not reduce the concentration of bacteria per ml of effluent.

What is the traditional antibiotic prophylaxis regimen?

The traditional antibiotic prophylaxis regimen for colon surgery is known as Nichols/Condon preparation. It comprises:

Neomycin and Erythromycin 1 gm each orally at 1.00 PM, 2 PM, and 11 PM on the day before surgery.

Many surgeons have replaced erythromycin with metronidazole 500 mg as it is found to be more bactericidal against greater percentage gut anaerobes.

What is the difference in approach for colonic resection for malignancy vs inflammatory disease?

In colonic resection for malignancy the vascular pedicle is ligated at the origin. The aim is to remove whole of the mesentery and all draining lymph nodes. In resection for inflammatory conditions the vessels are ligated near the gut and it is not mandatory to remove whole of the mesentery. Colonic resection for malignancy aims to achieve 5 cm of negative resected margins on both sides but for inflammatory conditions only involved portion of gut is removed.

What are the indications for adjuvant chemotherapy in carcinoma colon and what are the various regimes available?

For stage 1 colon cancer adjuvant chemotherapy is not indicated.

For stage 2 cancer following patients should be given adjuvant chemotherapy:
1. When the no. of sampled lymph nodes are small (less than 13) and hence considered inadequately staged (as per National Cancer Data Base Guidelines). If more than 13 lymph nodes are analysed, then chances that patient has residual disease are less.
2. T4 lesions
3. Patients with bowel obstruction on presentation or perforation at the tumour site
4. Poorly differentiated tumour
5. Peri tumoural lymphovascular involvement
6. Tumours with low frequency micro-satellite instability (MSI-L)

For stage 3 all patients receive adjuvant chemotherapy.

Adjuvant chemotherapy regimens are

5-FU + LV (Roswell Park Regimen)

5-FU 500 mg/m^2 IV bolus 1 hr after the start of leucovorin

Leucovorin 500 mg/m^2 IV over 2 hrs

Qw × 6 weeks every 8 wks for 3–4 cycles

5-FU + LV (Mayo clinic regimen)

5-FU 370–425 mg/m^2/d IV bolus d1–5
Leucovorin 20–25 mg/m^2/d IV bolus d1–5
Q4w × 6 cycles

Uracil-Tegafur + Leucovorin

Uracil-Tegafur (UFT) 100 mg/m^2 po every 8 hours
× 4 weeks
Leucovorin (LV) 30 mg po every 8 hours × 4 weeks
Avoid food 1 hour before and 1 hour after each
dose
Q5w

Capecitabine

Capecitabine (Xeloda) 1250 mg/m^2 po bid × 14
days
Q3w × 8 cycle × 5 cycles

FOLFOX4

Leucovorin 200 mg/m^2 IV over 2 hrs before 5-FU,
d1 and d2
5-FU 400 mg/m^2 IV bolus and then 600 mg/m^2 IV
over 22 hrs, d1 and d2
Oxaliplatin (Eloxatin) 85 mg/m^2 IV d1
Q2w × 12 cycles

FOLFOX6

Leucovorin 400 mg/m^2 IV over 2 hrs before 5-FU d1
5-FU 400 mg/m^2 IV bolus d1 followed by 2400
mg/m^2 IV over 46 hrs
Oxaliplatin (Eloxatin) 100 mg/m^2 in 500 ml
dextrose 5% IV over 2 hours d1
Q2w × 12 cycles

How are patients with carcinoma colon followed up?

First Year after Treatment

- Physical examination and CEA testing every
  three to six months
- Abdominal and chest CT scan each year (every
  6 to 12 months for patients with a high risk of
  recurrence)
- For patients with rectal cancer, pelvic CT scan
  every 6 to 12 months

- Colonoscopy one year after surgery
- Rectosigmoidoscopy every six months for
  patients with rectal cancer who did not have
  radiation therapy to the pelvis.

Second Year after Treatment

- Physical examination and CEA testing every
  three to six months
- CT scan each year (every 6 to 12 months for
  patients with a high risk of recurrence)
- For patients with rectal cancer, pelvic CT scan
  every 6 to 12 months
- Rectosigmoidoscopy every six months for
  patients with rectal cancer who did not have
  radiation therapy to the pelvis.

Third Year after Treatment

- Physical examination and CEA testing every
  three to six months
- CT scan each year (every 6 to 12 months for
  patients with a high risk of recurrence)
- For patients with rectal cancer, pelvic CT scan
  every 6 to 12 months
- Rectosigmoidoscopy every six months for
  patients with rectal cancer who did not have
  radiation therapy to the pelvis.

Fourth Year after Treatment

- Physical examination and CEA testing every
  three to six months
- For patients with rectal cancer, pelvic CT scan
  each year
- Rectosigmoidoscopy every six months for
  patients with rectal cancer who did not have
  radiation therapy to the pelvis.

Fifth Year after Treatment

- Physical examination and CEA testing every
  three to six months
- For patients with rectal cancer, pelvic CT scan
  each year
- Rectosigmoidoscopy every six months for
  patients with rectal cancer who did not have
  radiation therapy to the pelvis.

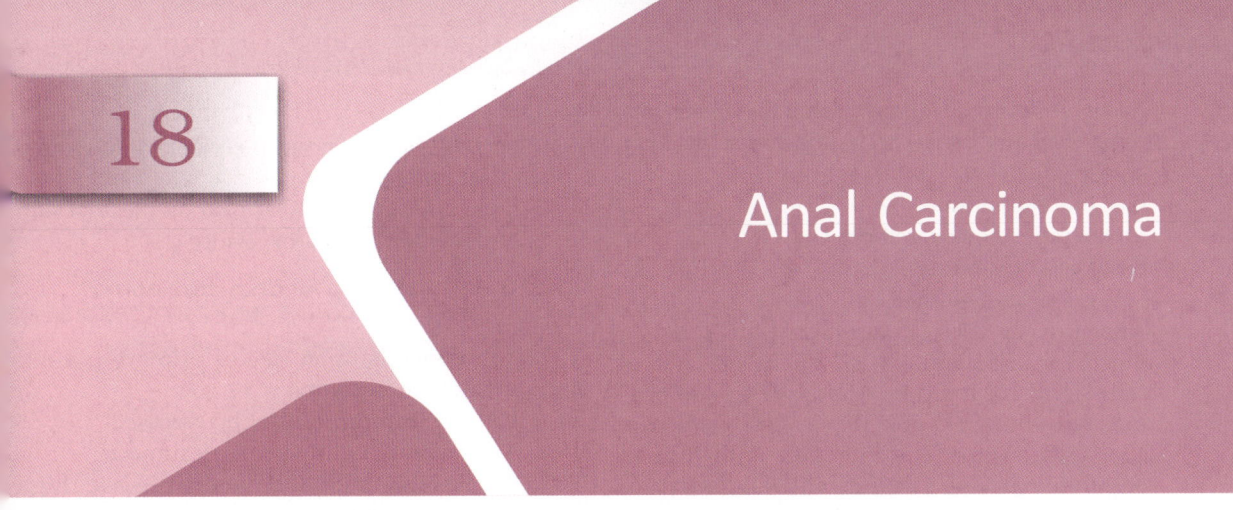

18

Anal Carcinoma

MALIGNANT LESION OF THE ANUS AND ANAL CANAL

What is anatomical anal canal and surgical anal canal?

The anatomical anal canal extends from anal verge to the dentate line. The surgical anal extends from pelvic floor till anal verge. The surgical anal canal corresponds to the length of the internal sphincter. The length of anal canal varies from 3 to 6 cm in males and 2 to 4 cm in females. The anal verge is the junction of specialized anoderm of distal anal canal with the normal squamous epithelium of the anal margin.

What is the lymphatic drainage of anal canal?

Above the dental line the lymphatics follow the superior haemorrhoidal artery and drain in to the pre-aortic and para-aortic nodes. The area around dentate line drains into internal pudendal, hypogastric and obturator nodes. The area below the dentate line drains in to inguinal nodes via inferior haemorrhoidal vessels.

What are the risk factors for development of anal canal cancer?

The risk factors for development of anal carcinoma are:

1. History of immunosuppression
2. Human papillomavirus (HPV) infection. HPV is seen in 70 percent of patients with invasive anal carcinoma. HPV 16 and HPV 18 are most commonly associated with anal canal carcinoma.

3. *Smoking:* There is increased anal carcinoma among smokers.
4. Men who have sex with men (MSM). Homosexual men are 20 times more likely to develop anal cancer in comparison to heterosexual men. Presence of HIV further increases the predisposition to carcinoma anal canal in MSM.

Describe epidemiology of anal carcinoma.

1. The age adjusted incidence rate has been found to be 8.9 per million population in Europe.
2. The incidence of anal cancer is increasing along with the increase in the incidence of HIV.
3. Anal canal cancer is found to be more in geographical areas with high incidence of penile, vulvar and cervical cancer.
4. It is seen three times more commonly in females with peak incidence around 60 years of age.
5. Anal canal carcinoma accounts for 3–5 percent of all large gut malignancies.

What are different histological types?

• Squamous cell carcinoma (Fig. 18.1)

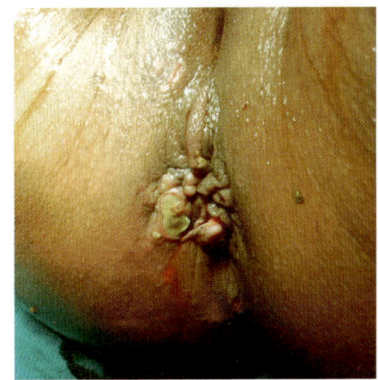

Fig. 18.1: Clinical picture of anal carcinoma

- *Adenocarcinoma:* It accounts for less than 10% cases of all anal canal carcinoma and arises from anal glands
- Basiloid carcinoma
- Mucoepidermoid carcinoma
- Basal cell carcinoma
- Malignant melanoma
- Anal intraepithelial neoplasia (AIN). It is a precursor of squamous cell carcinoma of anal canal and its incidence is high in patients infected with HIV and those with history of anal condyloma. The infection with human papillomavirus is a significant risk factor for development of AIN.

How AIN is graded?

The AIN is graded into three grades.

Grade 1: In grade 1 nuclear changes are seen only in the lower 1/3rd of epithelium

Grade 2: The nuclear changes are seen in the lower 2/3rd of epithelium.

Grade 3: The nuclear changes are seen in the whole of the epithelium.

   The grade 1 is defined as low grade and grade 2–3 are described as high grade.

What is the incidence of anal carcinoma?

- 2% of all colorectal cancer
- Usually in 6th and 7th decade of life
- 70% anal tumours arise from the anal canal (the anal canal is 4 cm in length extending from anal margin till anorectal ring).
- 30% anal tumours arise from anal verge (the anal verge starts from anal margin and includes 4 cm of the peri-anal skin all around)

Describe clinical features.

Symptoms

- Rectal bleeding
- Mucus discharge
- Tenesmus
- Sensation of lump in the anus
- Change in bowel habit
- The incontinence due to involvement of anal sphincter.
- Pelvic pain
- Patient can also present as rectovaginal or rectovesical fistulae.
- Inguinal lymph node enlargement due to metastasis

Signs

- Ulcerating hard, tender, bleeding mass in anal canal or at anal verge
- Lesions can fungate and appear on the anal skin
- Can present as fistula or fissure

What is AJCC staging for anal carcinoma?

T staging

T staging depends upon size of primary tumour in its greatest dimension.

Tx   Primary tumour cannot be assessed

T0   No evidence of any primary tumour

Tis   Carcinoma *in situ* (Bowen's disease, high grade squamous intraepithelial lesions, anal intrathelial neoplasm)

T1   Tumour less than 2 cm

T2   Tumour larger than 2 cm but less than 5 cm

T3   Tumour larger than 5 cm

T4   Tumour of any size invading adjacent organs, e.g. vagina, urethra, bladder.

N staging

Nx   Regional lymph nodes cannot be assessed

N0   No regional lymph node metastasis

N1   Metastasis in perirectal lymph nodes

N2   Metastasis in unilateral internal iliac and/or inguinal lymph nodes

N3   Metastasis in perirectal and inguinal lymph nodes and/or bilateral internal iliac and/or inguinal lymph nodes

Spread of anal carcinoma: The distal anal carcinoma spread to inguinal lymph nodes but proximal anal canal tumours spread to perirectal nodes. From inguinal lymph nodes internal iliac lymph nodes are involved.

How will you investigate?

a. All patients should undergo examination under anesthesia and biopsy of suspicious lesion. The exact site of tumour should be noted to so that anal canal and anal margin tumours can be distinguished.

b. The inguinal lymph nodes should be palpated and FNAC or tru-cut biopsy should be performed if found to be enlarged.

c. CT of abdomen, pelvis, and thorax is performed to detect intra-abdominal metastasis or distant metastasis.

d. CT combined with PET appears to have greater sensitivity for detection of metastatic lymph nodes.

e. Endo-anal ultrasound is of use in staging of early anal tumours but it has limited ability in detection of nodal disease. However, MRI pelvis allows reliable local tumour and nodal staging of all patients with anal cancer. MRI should be employed with CT in staging of all patients with anal cancer.

Describe treatment.

Anal intraepithelial neoplasia (AIN)
- The grades 1 or 2 AIN can be observed and managed expectantly due to low rate of progression to invasive disease.
- Long-term follow is not required in these cases.
- Grade 3 AIN carries a high risk of conversion to invasive carcinoma. In these cases local excision can be carried out (involving less than one-third of circumference). Excision of wider areas is avoided due to risk of development of anal stenosis.
- These patients undergoing excision should have 6 monthly assessment of any residual lesion especially in HIV patients.
- Imiquimod, a topically applied immuno-modulator has been shown to cause regression of high grade dysplasia and can be considered in management of multifocal AIN 2.

Anal Verge Tumour
- Wide excision of tumour with a margin of 2.5 cm all around followed by RT to pelvic and inguinal lymph nodes in advanced cases. After RT patients undergo systemic chemotherapy.
- A combination of surgical excision followed by RT (external beam or brachy-therapy) is associated with 5 year loco regional control rate of 78 percent, sphincter preservation rate of 80 percent and overall survival of 55 percent at 5 years.
- Abdomino-perineal resection is necessary for patients with tumour involvement of the anal sphincter and in those who have not responded to initial therapy.

Anal Canal Tumour
- Chemoradiation forms the mainstay of the treatment (first described by Nigro and associates, Flowchart 18.1).
  External beam radiation to primary tumour and pelvic and inguinal lymph nodes is started on day one and given in 28 fractions over 5 and half weeks with dose of 51 Gy. Initially multi-field technique including lower pelvis and inguinal lymph nodes is used but later field is reduced to local tumour only.
  Systemic chemotherapy in the form of 5FU is started as continuous infusion in the dose of 1000 mg per sq meter for 24 hours and is given for four days starting from day one. The 5FU is again repeated on 28th day for 4 days. Mitomycin C is given as bolus dose of 15 mg per sq meter on day one.
- 2/3rd of all patients respond to chemoradiation alone.

Flowchart 18.1: Management of anal carcinoma

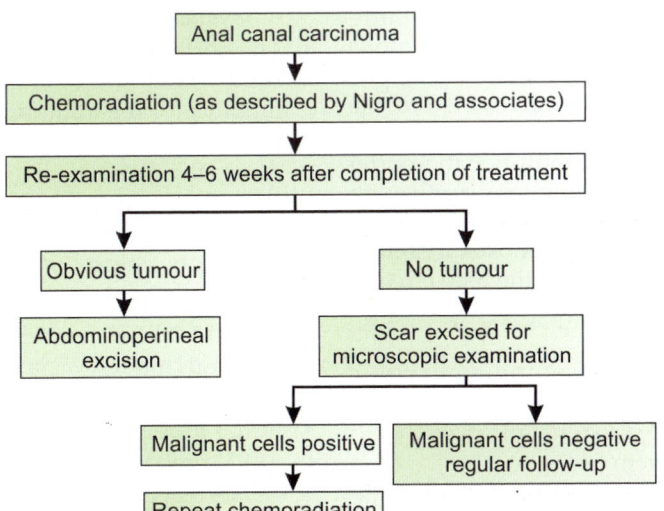

19

Portal Hypertension

Give a background of portal hypertension.

- "Porta" in Latin means gate or passage
- Portal pressure gradient (pressure difference between IVC and portal vein) 12 mmHg or more is known as portal hypertension
- Often associated with varices and ascites.
- Many conditions are associated with it, the most common being **cirrhosis** of the liver.

Describe embryology of development of portal vein.

The embryologic development of the portal circulation is from:

- Two vitelline veins, which bring blood from the yolk sac
- Two umbilical veins, which return blood from the placenta.
   The vitelline veins intercommunicate in the septum transversum from which the liver sinusoids develops. The extra-hepatic portal venous system develops primarily from the left vitelline vein. The right umbilical vein gives rise to the intra-hepatic right portal vein and the left umbilical vein forms the left intra-hepatic portal vein. The left vein also communicates directly with the sinus venosus, which connects to the inferior vena cava; through the ductus venosus therefore allowing blood to bypass most in the fetal circulation.
- Portal vein develops from
   - Post-duodenal plexuses of embryonic vitelline veins
- May form from pre-duodenal plexuses
   - Anterior portal vein
   - Associated with annular pancreas, malrotation and biliary tract anomalies

Describe anatomy of portal vein.

- 8 cm long, no valves, 8 mm diameter
- Begins at L2 behind neck of pancreas in front of IVC
- The superior mesenteric vein and splenic vein join behind the pancreas to form the portal vein.
- Portal vein drains blood from the small and large intestines, stomach, spleen, pancreas and gall bladder.
- Tributaries of portal vein
   - Splenic (short gastric, left gastro-epiploic, pancreatic, inferior mesenteric)
   - Superior mesenteric (jejunal, ileal, ileocolic, right colic, middle colic)
   - Left gastric
   - Right gastric
   - Para-umbilical
   - Cystic veins
- The portal trunk divides into 2 lobar veins, the right drains the cystic vein, the left receives umbilical and paraumbilical veins (that enlarge to form the caput medusae). The coronary vein drains the distal esophagus, which also enlarge in portal hypertension.

Describe physiology of portal circulation.

- Portal circulation
   - 1 to 1.2 litres per minute
   - 40 ml/min O_2 (72% of total O_2 supply)
   - 80% of total blood supply to liver
- Portal pressure gradient
   - PV pressure – IVC pressure
   - Normal 5 mmHg
   - 6–10 mmHg subclinical portal hypertension

– >10 mmHg esophageal varices
– >12 mmHg variceal bleeding/ascites

What is pathophysiology of portal hypertension?

The major theories in the pathophysiology of portal hypertension have been the 'backward' and the 'forward' flow theories:

- Backward theory postulates that all consequences of portal hypertension result from obstruction to portal venous flow.
- Forward flow theory postulates that increased inflow to the portal venous system (usually because of splenomegaly) causes the changes that lead to the clinical findings of portal hypertension.

Current evidence indicates that both theories contribute to the pathophysiology.

The stages in developing portal hypertension are summarised in the table given below.

Stages in the development of portal hypertension

- Increased resistance to portal venous flow
- Formation of portal systemic collaterals
- Dilatation of the splanchnic venous bed and increased splanchnic flow
- Expansion of the intravascular plasma volume
- Peripheral and splanchnic vasodilatation leading to development of a hyperkinetic systemic circulation

The initiating event is an increased resistance to portal venous flow which leads to the increased pressure on the splanchnic venous bed. Increased splanchnic pressure leads to the development of collaterals to bypass the blockage to flow. The compensatory increase in splanchnic inflow perpetuates and aggravates the portal hypertension. The major importance in clarifying this pathophysiology is that it has implications for clinical management, particularly in pharmacologic therapy.

- P=FR, where P is pressure gradient through the portal system, F is the volume of blood flowing through the system, R is the resistance to flow
- Changes in either F or R affect the pressure
- In most types of portal hypertension, both flow and resistance are altered.

Increase in Resistance

- Liver disease is responsible for a decrease in portal vascular radius, producing an increase in portal vascular resistance.

- In cirrhosis, the increase occurs at the microcirculation (sinusoidal).
- The resistance is also due to active myofibroblasts or vascular smooth muscle cells in the intra-hepatic veins.

Increase in Flow

- The increase in blood flow is caused by splanchnic arteriolar vasodilatation caused by release of endogenous vasodilators
- The increased flow aggravates the increase in portal pressure and contributes to portal hypertension despite the formation of portosystemic collaterals that divert as much as 80% of portal flow.

Manifestations of splanchnic vasodilatation are:
- Increased cardiac output
- Arterial hypotension
- Hypovolemia
- The above explains rationale for treating patients with low sodium diet and diuretics to attenuate the hyperkinetic state.

What is mortality/morbidity of portal hypertension?

- Variceal hemorrhage is the most common complication and cause of mortality and morbidity
- 90% with cirrhosis develop varices
- 30% of these bleed
- The first episode is estimated to carry a mortality of 30–50%

What are sites of collateral circulation?

- Lower end of oesophagus and fundus of stomach
- At the anus
- Around umbilicus
- Natural porto systemic shunts (NPSS) at following sites
  – Gastro-adrenrorenal
  – Lienorenal

NPSS is more common in extra-hepatic portal vein obstruction.

What is natural history of portal hypertension?

At the time of initial diagnosis of cirrhosis approximately 30% of patients have compensated disease and 60% with decompensated disease have varices. It is estimated that every year 8% of patients who have cirrhosis develop varices. Small varices slowly grow into large varices which have a higher risk of bleeding. All patients who are diagnosed with cirrhosis should have a screening endoscopy to look for varices and to determine the need to start therapy to reduce the risk of an initial bleed. The risk of the first variceal bleed is higher in following:

- Increased variceal size
- The presence of red color signs
- The portal pressure gradient greater than 12 mmHg (1.6 kPa)
- Poor liver function

An acute episode of variceal bleed has mortality of approximately 30% and majority of deaths occur among poorer risk patients having child score higher or equal to 8 points.

Early re-bleeding which occurs in 20–50% of patients in the first 7–10 days is a poor prognostic sign. After the first 6 weeks, the re-bleeding risk drops to approximately the same as before the initial bleed (i.e. about 30%). Overall, it is estimated that once there has been an initial bleed, the risk of re-bleeding is 75–80% within the first year. These natural history factors are **important** in making management decisions.

Describe clinical features of portal hypertension.

History

- Directed towards determining the cause and the presence of complications of portal hypertension
- Jaundice, transfusions, IV drug abuse, pruritis, hereditary liver disease
- Hematemesis, melena, mental status, abdominal girth, pain, fever, hematochezia

Physical Examination

- Signs of portosystemic collateral formation:
  - Dilated veins in abdominal wall
  - Caput medusa
  - Rectal hemorrhoids
  - Ascites
  - Umbilical hernia
- Signs of liver disease
  - Ascites
  - Jaundice
  - Palmar erythema
  - Asterixis

- Testicular atrophy, gynecomastia
- Muscle wasting, Dupuytren's contracture
- Splenomegaly

What is etiology of portal hypertension?

Portal hypertension can be classified into pre-sinusoidal, sinusoidal and post-sinusoidal causes. The clinical implication of this classification lies in separating patients who have normal hepatocellular function from those who have hepatocellular damage as this classification has important implications in outcome.

Prehepatic (Presinusoidal)

- Portal vein thrombosis
  - Neonatal umbilical sepsis
  - Hypercoagulable state in older patients such as polycythemia rubra vera or a myeloproliferative disorder.
  - Pancreatitis
  - Carcinoma head of pancreas
  - Metastatic nodes at hepatic hilum
- Banti syndrome—splenomegaly, normal liver, portal hypertension
- Increased portal flow
  - Arteriovenous fistula
  - Massive splenomegaly (primary hematologic disease)

Hepatic

- Pre-sinusoidal (affect terminal portal venule in pre-sinusoidal space) liver function is well preserved in pre-sinusoidal causes of portal hypertension and the main stay of treatment is to prevent variceal bleeding.
  - Schistosomiasis
  - Congenital hepatic fibrosis
  - Early stages of primary biliary cirrhosis
  - Hepatocellular carcinoma
  - Secondaries liver
  - *Toxins*: Vinyl chloride, arsenic, copper
  - Idiopathic portal hypertension

  Sinusoidal (in these cases sinusoidal anatomy is distorted, regenerative nodules form, fibrosis further obstructs portal venous flow and the normal metabolic processes are disrupted).
  - Hepatic cirrhosis: Alcoholic or post-viral
  - Noncirrhotic acute alcoholic hepatitis
  - Cytotoxic drugs

– Vitamin A intoxication
– Autoimmune liver disease
– Wilson's disease
– Hemochromatosis
– More advanced stages of primary biliary cirrhosis
– Sclerosing cholangitis
– Alpha one antitrypsin deficiency

The careful evaluation of liver function and an assessment of the activity of the underlying liver disease, its rate of progression and the hepatic reserve is needed in this group. The clinician has to evaluate whether the cirrhosis is compensated or decompensated as the prognosis depends upon this.

- Post-sinusoidal
  – Veno-occlusive disease

Post-hepatic

- Hepatic vein thrombosis (Budd-Chiari syndrome)
- Membranous obstruction of inferior vena cava
- Cardiac causes (e.g. constrictive pericarditis, restrictive cardiomyopathy).

Main Causes of Portal Hypertension in India

- Cirrhosis <50%
- Noncirrhotic portal fibrosis 10–25% (NCPF)
- Extra-hepatic portal vein obstruction 30–40% (EHPVO)
- Budd-Chiari syndrome 8–26%

What is non-cirrhotic portal fibrosis?

- NCPF occurs in northern and eastern part of India
- 30–50 years
- Peri-sinusoidal fibrosis takes place
- Obliteration of peripheral portal venule
- Normal sized liver
- Nodular type or non-nodular type
- Progressive loss of liver function

What is the natural course of portal hypertension?

- In cirrhotic patients progressive and early liver failure occurs
- In NCPF non-nodular variety liver failure occurs late
- Nodular type of NCPF leads to early liver failure
- In EHPVO liver perfusion is maintained.

What are the investigations to be done in portal hypertension?

Hematology

A complete blood count including hemoglobin concentration, hematocrit and white cell and platelet counts should be performed:

- The hematocrit can be low either secondary to chronic bleeding or as a result of the expanded plasma volume due to water retention
- The platelet count can be low and the white cell count less than $4000/mm^3$ because of increased break down due to hypersplenism.

Other useful blood test include prothrombin time and the plasma fibrinogen levels. Prothrombin time is used in calculating the Child-Pugh score. The prolongation of the international normalized ratio by more than 1.5 indicates moderate liver impairment.

A plasma fibrinogen level of less than 100 mg/dl is often seen in advanced liver disease due to poor synthetic hepatic function. The therapeutic implication of this is an increased risk of bleeding. The fresh frozen plasma should be transfused to these patients who are bleeding or require any interventional procedure.

Biochemistry

Serum electrolytes, blood urea nitrogen and serum creatinine provide valuable information during the management.

In portal hypertension total exchangeable body sodium is increased, but intravascular sodium is depleted, particularly following aggressive attempts at diuresis or due to dilution hyponatermia.

A low blood urea nitrogen at presentation is indicative of poor liver function because liver is the sole site for urea production, whereas an elevated blood urea nitrogen in such a patient indicates more severe renal insufficiency than suspected. Patients with advanced liver disease have a decreased lean body mass, so an elevated serum creatinine indicates more severe renal insufficiency than in a normal subject.

Other biochemical parameters of importance in investigating patients who have liver disease are:

↑serum bilirubin
↓albumin
↑aminotransferases
↑alkaline phosphatase
↑γ-glutamyltranspeptidase

These parameters are used to assess the severity and activity of the underlying liver disease:

- Serum bilirubin and albumin are used to calculate the Child-Pugh score.
- Aminotransferases are elevated as a result of acute hepatocellular injury and are used as an index of ongoing 'hepatitis', but do not help in differentiating the aetiology of the hepatitis.
- Increases in alkaline phosphatase and γ-glutamyltranspeptidase are indicative of cholestasis either at large duct or canalicular levels.

Serology

Hepatitis A, B and C serologies should be carried out routinely and for those who are positive for hepatitis B or C, a more detailed analysis for evidence of active viral replication by testing for hepatitis B DNA or hepatitis C RNA titres should be performed.

- Antimitochondrial antibody (primary biliary cirrhosis);
- Antinuclear antibody (for evidence of auto-immune hepatitis);
- Ceruloplasmin for Wilson's disease
- Alpha 1-antitrypsin deficiency

What is the role of imaging studies?

Endoscopy

All patients of cirrhosis suspected or confirmed should have a upper gastrointestinal endoscopy to define a bleeding risk if varices are present. If varices are identified at first endoscopy, patients should be started on appropriate prophylactic pharmacologic therapy to reduce the risk of an initial bleed.

The major aims at the time of endoscopy are:

a. To find out whether the patient has esophageal and/or gastric varices.
b. To establish whether there is portal hypertensive gastropathy.
c. Other pathologies such as peptic ulcer disease, gastric antral vascular ectasia or malignancies should be excluded.
d. The grading of the severity of portal hypertensive changes can done using Japanese and European workers classification. Another classification which is more commonly used is Sarin's classification.

Radiologic Imaging

The initial imaging study is Doppler ultrasound evaluation of the major vessels. An ultrasound scan of the liver should inspect overall morphology including any focal intra-hepatic lesions that may suggest hepatocellular carcinoma.

The Doppler imaging focuses on the main portal vein, the splenic vein, hepatic veins and the infra- and intrahepatic inferior vena cava. The aim of this study is to evaluate portal vein patency and directional flow. It identifies most of the extra-hepatic causes of portal hypertension. The value of portal vein size measurement and flow velocities as measures of the severity of portal hypertension has not been fully established.

Angiography

Angiography which is a gold standard for abdominal vascular imaging in patients with portal hypertension is done through a transvenous or a transarterial approach.

The hepatic arterial phase imaging has benefit of detecting small vascular lesions suggestive of hepatocellular carcinoma.

The venous phase imaging of arterial injection is used to delineate the portal venous anatomy in patients being considered for decompressive shunt surgery. Splenic artery injection followed through the venous phase gives the best imaging of the splenic vein and its tributaries. Superior mesenteric artery injection through the venous phase is the preferred method of imaging for the superior mesenteric and portal vein. Identification of the site, size and flow parameters of the major collaterals such as the left gastric and inferior mesenteric vein is best defined on arteriography.

Venography

This is used to assess the hepatic veins, the inferior vena cava and the left renal vein and may be carried out by either a transfemoral or a transjugular approach.

Hepatic venography combines both pressure measurements and imaging.

Pressures are measured in the hepatic vein in both the occluded and free vein, using the same principle as pulmonary pressure measurement with a Swan-Ganz catheter. The occluded pressure is an indirect measurement of hepatic sinusoidal pressure. The difference between the occluded and free pressure—the hepatic venous pressure gradient (HVPG) is used as a clinical measurement of portal hypertension.

If a catheter is placed in the wedged position in a hepatic vein and contrast is injected, the contrast refluxes into the hepatic sinusoids and, in patients who have sluggish portal venous flow, into the main portal vein and/or its feeding tributaries . This can serve as an excellent imaging modality for portal vein patency. Imaging and pressure measurements within the inferior vena cava and left renal vein may be important in making decisions for surgical intervention. The vena cava may be compressed by an enlarged and cirrhotic liver with distortion or pressure gradient. The left renal vein has anomalies in 20% of the population, with a circum-aortic vein present in 16% and a totally retro-aortic left renal vein in 4%.

The trans-jugular route of venous access has become the preferred method because it allows easier intervention for liver biopsy and is the route for a trans-jugular intra-hepatic portal systemic shunt (TIPS) if indicated.

What is the role of liver biopsy?

A histologic diagnosis is needed before initiating therapy, for patients who have hemochromatosis before phlebotomy or patients who have Wilson's disease before copper chelation. For all types of cirrhosis, the morphologic findings of acute cellular injury and the extent of fibrosis are parameters that help in assessing the degree of underlying liver disease and dictate therapy. Finally, image-guided biopsy may be required for focal lesions.

There are three techniques for liver biopsy.

a. *Percutaneous*
   1. 'Blind' percutaneous biopsy
   2. Used to evaluate diffuse liver disease, but is inadequate if focal changes are suspected
   3. The most serious complication of percutaneous biopsy is bleeding, which occurs in 0.1–0.2% of patients
   4. Performed using either a suction-type Menghini needle or a tru-cut biopsy needle
   5. Can be done under CT or ultrasound guidance

b. *Transjugular*
   1. May be combined with angiographic images
   2. Used in patients when percutaneous biopsy contraindicated as in massive ascites or severe coagulopathy.
   3. A catheter is advanced into major hepatic vein through jugular vein and biosy taken by biopsy forceps or needle.

c. *Laparoscopic*:
   1. For directed biopsies of focal lesions when direct visualisation during laparoscopy can combined with ultrasonography.
   2. In Budd-Chiari syndrome.

What is quantitative liver function testing?

Quantitative tests can be broadly divided into those:

- Which assess hepatocyte function
- Which are dependent upon liver blood flow.

Substances such as galactose, indocyanine green, antipyrine or lidocaine (lignocaine)have been most widely used for quantitative testing. Recently, monoethylglycinexylidide (MEGX) formation from lidocaine has received attention.

Other methods used to quantitate liver function include rates of urea synthesis and high first-pass clearance methods to estimate liver blood flow, such as sorbital and galactose.

What are the treatment strategies for esophagastric varices?

Treatment strategies include:
Pharmacologic therapy
Endoscopic therapy
Tamponade
Decompression—radiologic, surgical
Devascularization operation
Liver transplantation

Medical Treatment

Different points of time in the treatment of esophagogastric varices
To prevent the initial bleed
Treatment of acute variceal bleeding
Treatment to prevent recurrent variceal bleeding
- First-line treatment
- Second-line treatment
Treatment of end-stage liver disease
Treatment is directed at cause:
- Emergent treatment
- Primary prophylaxis
- Elective treatment

Emergent Treatment

- Bleeding from varices ceases spontaneously in 40%. They rebleed in 40% within 6 weeks
- Following resuscitation, treatment includes control of bleeding, prevention of recurrence, blood replacement, avoiding over expansion of volume status
- Diagnose source of bleed, specific treatment of bleeding lesion
- All patients with cirrhosis and upper GI bleed are at risk for severe bacterial infections, which are associated with early rebleed
- Use of antibiotics has been shown to increase survival, decrease rate of infection, thus prophylactic use of antibiotics in acute bleeding is recommended

Pharmacologic Therapy

- Somatostatin—decreases portal flow and causes, splanchnic vasoconstriction
- Octreotide—50 mcg/h has been shown to reduce complications of bleeding after sclerotherapy
- Vasopressin—reduces blood flow to all splanchnic organs, decreases portal pressure and venous blood flow.

Endoscopic Therapy—Endoscopic Sclerotherapy and Variceal Ligation (EST, EVL)

- No more than 2 sessions should be given before deciding on TIPS or surgery
- Complications include fever, stricture, perforation, mediastinitis, ulceration, pleural effusion
- EVL and EST are comparable in control of bleeding
- EST is associated with more complications

Minnesota Tube

- Balloon tamponade is used only in massive bleeding as a temporizing measure
- Complications—esophageal rupture, rebleed, mediastinitis
- Has 4 lumens—1 for gastric aspiration, 2 lumens to inflate the balloons, 1 lumen above the esophageal balloon to prevent aspiration
- Usually only need to inflate gastric balloon

Prophylaxis

- Beta-blockers (propanolol, nadolol) are non-cardio-selective; reduce portal and collateral blood flow. Also reduces cardiac output, and splanchnic vasoconstriction with significant reduction of bleeding rates.
- No role for sclerotherapy in primary prophylaxis
- EVL is more effective than no treatment to prevent first bleed. Similar efficacy to beta-blockers, with more adverse effects.
- EVL not recommended for primary prophylaxis except perhaps in patients with very large varices.

Elective Treatment

- This is for prevention of rebleeding (2 years recurrence rate of 80%)
- Propanolol and nadolol, reduce rebleed, and increase survival
- Beta-blockers vs sclerotherapy have comparable rates of prevention
- EVL is considered treatment of choice in prevention of rebleeding, may be combined with drugs
- Methods of decompression for portal hypertension and gastroesophageal varices
  - a. TIPS: Nonoperative, radiologic
  - b. Portosystemic surgical shunts
    - Total portacaval (using portal vein)
    - Mesocaval, mesorenal, mesoatrial (using superior mesenteric vein)
    - Partial portacaval or mesocaval (interposition graft of restricted diameter to allow some prograde portal flow)
    - Selective variceal decompression
    - Distal splenorenal shunt.

Surgical Treatment (Shunts)

- Total portosystemic shunts include any shunt larger than 10 mm between portal vein and IVC. Includes Eck (end to side) and side to side portocaval shunts.
  - Eck fistula controls bleeding, but ascites unrelieved.
  - Side to side controls bleeding and ascites, but encephalopathy is a problem (40–50%).
- Partial portal systemic shunts reduce the size to 8 mm in diameter.
  - Use an interposition graft between portal vein and IVC.
  - 90% control of bleeding, decreased incidence of encephalopathy and liver failure.

- Selective shunts aim to decompress varices whilst maintaining portal hypertension to maintain portal flow to liver.
  - Warren distal splenorenal shunt is the most commonly used for patients with refractory bleeding and good liver function. Decompresses gatroesophageal varices through short gastrics, spleen, splenic vein to left renal vein. Lower incidence of encephalopathy (15%), preserves some liver function. It produces ascites.

Types based on anatomy:

- Direct bypass
  - Porto-caval
  - Distal spleno-renal
  - Proximal spleno-renal
- H type bypass
  - Porto-caval
  - Meso-caval
  - Splenorenal
- *Risks*:
  - Shunt thrombosis—risk is low. If the shunt thromboses, then portal hypertension recurs.
  - Liver failure—creation of a shunt reroutes the blood away from the liver and deprives partly the liver of the portal flow and this can lead to liver failure mostly in patient with advanced cirrhosis. This is avoided by adequate selection of the candidates.
  - Encephalopathy—re-routing the blood flow directly to the heart also carries some risk of encephalopathy and other problems at long term.
- *Indications*:
  - Well compensated cirrhosis
    - Bleeding ectopic varices
    - Unsuccessful sclerotherapy/banding
    - Untractable ascites
  - Non-cirrhotic portal hypertension
    - Inadequate local medical support
    - Refractory/recurrent bleeding

Devascularization Procedures

- Include splenectomy, gastroesophageal devascularization, and esophageal transection.
- Incidence of encephalopathy is low, because of maintenance of portal flow.

- Used in patients who are not candidates for decompression in whom 1st line therapy has failed. This includes patients with splenic or portal vein thrombosis in addition to cirrhosis.
- Splenectomy—the spleen is a major inflow path to GE varices. Splenectomy gives better access to fundus and distal esophagus to complete the devascularization.
- Complicated by portal vein thrombosis and ascites.
- Sugiura procedure—devascularizes whole greater curve from pylorus to esophagus, upper two-thirds of lesser curve. The esophagus is devascularized by a minimum of 7 cm.

Liver Transplant

- The ultimate choice as it relieves portal hypertension, prevents bleeding, manages ascites and encephalopathy by restoring liver function.

Class C	Class B	Class A	The child classification
Moderate	Slight	None	Ascites
III and IV	I and II	None	Encephalopathy
28–35	>35	<28	Albumin (g/L)
>3	2–3	<2	Bilirubin (mg/dl)
>6	4–6	1–4	PT (INR)

- Child class A: Shunt surgery
- Child class B: Shunt or TIPS
- Child class C: TIPS or liver transplant

What is Transjugular Intrahepatic Portosystemic Shunt (TIPS)?

- For continued bleeding despite medical and endoscopic treatment in patients with Child C disease and selected Child B disease, TIPS is the management of choice.
- It is only useful in portal hypertension of hepatic origin.
- Shunt is created from internal jugular to hepatic vein through hepatic parenchyma to portal vein. Tract is dilated and stented.
- *Accepted indications*:
  - Active bleeding despite endoscopic or pharmacologic treatment
  - Recurrent variceal bleeding despite adequate endoscopic treatment.
  - Bleeding gastric fundic varices, refractory ascites
  - Preparation to transplant

- *Complications of TIPS*:
  - Hematoma, cardiac arrhythmias, bacteraemia
  - Perihepatic hematoma, rupture of liver capsule
  - Extrahepatic puncture of portal vein
  - Arterioportal fistula, portobiliary fistula
  - Encephalopathy (30%)
  - Liver failure

What are the Guidelines for Management of Portal Hypertension?

- Wait and see
  - Compensated liver disease
  - No complications yet
  - Minor/moderate risk of bleeding

- Medical treatment
- β-blockers
- Diuretics
- ? TIPS
- ? Shunt surgery
  - Compensated liver disease
  - Previous bleeding, banding
  - Ascites

- Transplant
  - End-stage liver disease
  - Recurrent varices and bleeding
  - Refractory ascites

Gastro-intestinal Bleeding

Emergency Therapy of Variceal Hemorrhage

- Fluid resuscitation
- Platelet transfusion (if platelet count <50,000/mm^3)
- Vit. K/fresh frozen plasma
- Esogastroscopy (diagnostic + variceal obliteration)
- *Pharmacologic intervention*:
  - Somatostatin
  - Vasopressin
- *Rescue therapy*:
  - Balloon compression
  - TIPS
  - Shunt surgery

Sclerotherapy/Banding

- *Limits*:
  - Ectopic varices
  - Recurrence
- *Complications of sclerotherapy*:
  - Ulcer
  - Stricture
  - Mediastinitis
  - Esophageal dysmotility
  - Gastroesophageal reflux.

Urinary System

Section 4

20

Suprarenal or Adrenal Mass

What are the important differentials to consider in a patient presenting with suprarenal mass?

Differential diagnosis of suprarenal mass or adrenal mass includes the following:

In children

- Neuroblastoma
- Extralobar pulmonary sequestration/broncho-genic cyst
- Congenital adrenal hyperplasia
- Partial multicystic dysplastic kidney
- Renal duplication
- Gastric duplication cyst or right side
- Splenic cyst/splenunculi or left side

In adults

- Kidneys, spleen, pancreas, lymph nodes masses
- Adrenal cortical hyperplasia
- Adrenal cortical neoplasms
- Infiltrative diseases, e.g. amyloidosis
- Medullary neoplasms
- Metastatic disease
- Adrenal pseudocyst
- Adrenal myelolipomas
- Lymphoma

How does one work up a patient with adrenal mass?

Evaluation of adrenal masses is focused at determining the organ of origin in the first place. Surrounding organs may present as a suprarenal mass and renal tumours are especially confused with till the end. It is necessary to look for congenital anomalies if the patient is a newborn or child and keep the possibility of non-adrenal origin of the mass. Looking for features of virilization may be suggestive of functional lesions or congenital adrenal hyperplasia which is a urological emergency and requires electrolyte correction so that the child can survive. External genitalia must be examined and history of maternal use of steroids must be taken.

In adult patients it is important to discern the functional status of the mass. Depending on the tissue of origin of the lesion different types of hormones could be produced like catecholamines, glucocorticoids, mineralocorticoids and sex steroids. Directed history should be taken for excess production of each of these. Clinical features have been described in detail separately in the chapter. Functional masses are dealt with suspicion as they are likely to be malignant. The various functional tests that must be performed as described in detail within the chapter.

General examination should focus of general features of hypercortisolism and virilization. A detailed cardiovascular examination is important due to hypertension and its sequel. Blood pressure must be taken in both the arms in different positions. Abdominal examination to look for any palpable lump and examination of other systems to rule out any metastasis from undetected primary must also be performed.

What are the findings suggestive of benign adrenal mass?

Some of the important clues that point to the benign nature of adrenal mass include:

- No history of other malignancy (lowers risk to 0.3% chance of cancer)

- Imaging findings suggestive of benign mass:
  - Size <4 cm with smooth borders
  - Fat containing lesions
  - CT with low attenuation value (<10 Hounsfield units) homogeneous mass (Fig. 20.1)
  - MRI with signal loss on out-of-phase imaging
  - Rapid contrast washout

What is an incidentaloma?

An adrenal "incidentaloma" is an adrenal mass, generally 1 cm or larger, discovered incidentally during a radiologic examination performed for indications other than an evaluation for adrenal disease. The incidence of an incidentaloma is about 4–6% being uncommon in the younger age (0.2–1%) and incidence rising to as much as 7% at an age of 70 years. Incidental adrenal mass may be found on up to 3–4% of abdominal CTs or MRIs and 20% of the autopsies. Most of these lesions are histologically benign and turn out to be adrenocortical adenomas. The nature of these masses has to be diagnosed and in the presence of growth >1 cm or secretion of hormones they have to be removed surgically.

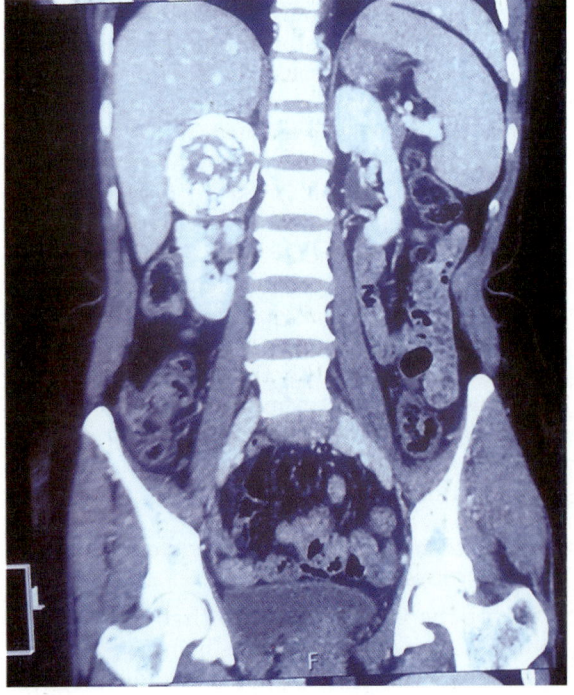

Fig. 20.1: CT scan showing calcified suprarenal mass

Differential diagnosis of incidental adrenal mass includes:

1. Adrenal adenoma (50%)
2. Non-functioning adenoma
3. Functioning adenoma
   a. Cushing's syndrome
   b. Pheochromocytoma
   c. Hyperaldosteronism
   Metastatic cancer (30%)
   Bronchogenic carcinoma
   Renal cell carcinoma
   Melanoma
   Adrenal carcinoma (1–4%)
   Adrenal cyst (4%)
   Adrenal hyperplasia (2%)
   Lipoma (2%)
   Myelolipoma (2%)

How are incidentalomas worked up and managed?

All incidentally detected adrenal masses are subjected to CT scan.

Adrenal mass on CT scan <1 cm in greatest diameter require no further evaluation where adrenal mass on CT Scan >4 cm in greatest diameter need endocrine evaluation especially to rule out pheochromocytoma. Such tumours have to be removed surgically owing to high incidence of malignancy. Adrenal mass between 1 and 4 cm and lipid containing lesion on initial imaging should be evaluated for function and repeat unenhanced CT abdomen should be performed in 12 months to confirm no change. Adrenal mass 1–4 cm which is not a lipid containing lesion should be further evaluated using endocrine assays along with CT abdomen with IV contrast and delayed phase (or MRI as alternative). If CT or MRI is non-diagnostic, FDG-PET may also be used. If there is any suspicion of malignancy, early surgery should be considered.

What is the metabolism of adrenal hormones?

Adrenal hormones are derived from L tyrosine which is converted to norepinephrine and epinephrine as explained in the flowchart (Fig. 20.2).

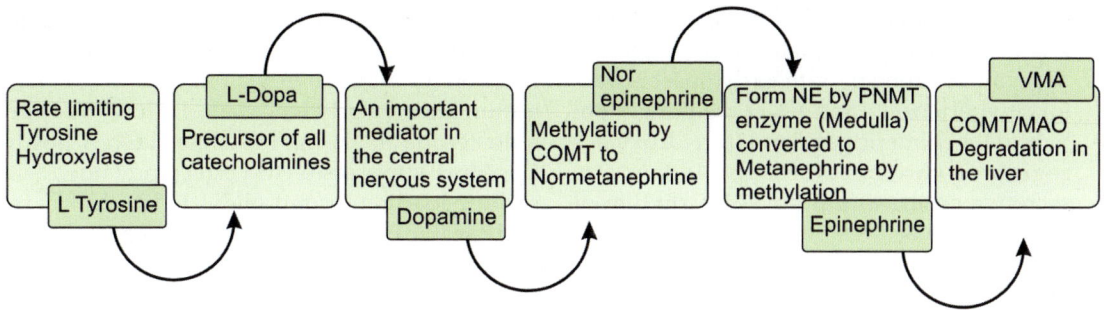

Fig. 20.2: Steps in the synthesis and degradation of adrenal hormones

What are the causes of Cushing's syndrome?

The etiology of Cushing syndrome has been summarized in Fig. 20.3.

What is Conn's syndrome?

Conn's syndrome or primary aldosteronism occurs as a result of aldosterone secretion independent of renin angiotensin aldosterone secretion. In contrast to secondary hyperaldosteronism where high plasma rennin levels are the cause of increased aldosterone production, plasma rennin levels are suppressed in primary aldosteronism.

Increased aldosterone leads to sodium and water reabsorption along with potassium loss leading to increased volume of fluid within the body.

What are the common causes of Conn's syndrome?

The common causes leading to Conn's syndrome include:

- *Bilateral hyperplasia*: It is the most common causes in more than half of the patients and is usually idiopathic.
- *Adenoma*: A secreting adenoma is the second most commonly found etiology. It is associated with a more severe hypertension and potassium loss.
- Unilateral hyperplasia.
- Carcinoma <1% (represents 2–5% of adrenal cortical carcinoma).
- Ectopic tumour producing aldosterone (<1%).
- *Familial hyperaldosteronism*: There are two variants of familial hyperaldosteronism both of which are autosomal dominant.

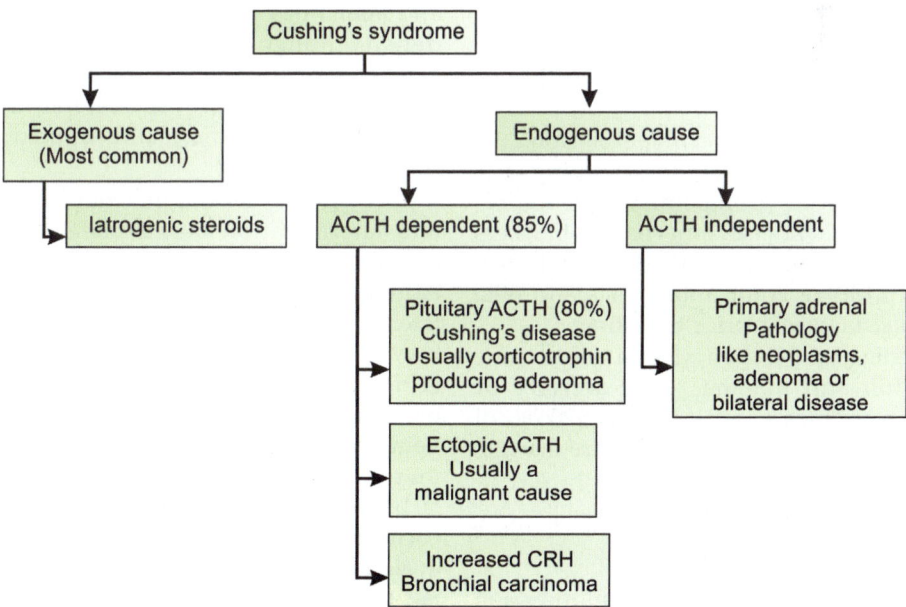

Fig. 20.3: Etiology of Cushing's syndrome

- *Familial hyperaldosteronism type 1:* It is a glucocorticoid remediable form of familial hyperaldosteronism with early onset refractory hypertension and CKD resulting from hybrid for chimeric gene on 11β-hydroxylase region of chromosome 8q. Aldosterone secretion occurs as per circadian rhythm of ACTH.
- *Familial hyperaldosteronism type 2:* It is heterogeneous variant of familial hyperaldosteronism. Aldosterone producing adenomas may be found on imaging.

What is the clinical feature of Conn's syndrome?

Conn's syndrome is seen in 3rd–6th decade and most commonly patients are normokalemic and normonatremic at presentation (up to 90%). A smaller percentage has hypertension, cardiovascular, renal and end organ damage.

Who should be screened for Conn's syndrome and how is screening performed?

The following patients should undergo screening for hyperaldostronism:
- Hypertension with hypokalemia
- Uncontrolled and refractory hypertension for >3 days
- Detection of incidentaloma with hypertension
- Early onset hypertension at age <20 yrs
- Severe hypertension (160/110) refractory to a combination of anti-hypertensives
- Unexplained hypokalemia
- End organ damage in excess of degree and duration of hypertension
- Consideration of secondary hypertension

Before subjecting patients to screening it is essential to correct hypokalemia, shift hypertensives to α_1 blocker or calcium channel blockers (ACE inhibitors can be continued) and stop mineralocorticoid receptor antagonists and beta blockers at least 6 weeks prior to testing.

For screening an 8–10 am plasma aldosterone concentration and plasma renin activity or concentration are measured. If PAC is >20 ng/dl and aldosterone to rennin ratios are more than 30, confirmatory testing must be performed.

What are the confirmatory tests for Conn's syndrome?

Confirmatory testing is done using suppression tests. These tests are positive in about half of the cases who have a positive screening test. In fludrocortisone suppression test, fludrocortisone in a dose of 0.1 mg 6 hrly along with 2 gm NaCl is administered 8 hrly for 4 days. Failure to suppress aldosterone to <6 ng/ml is considered positive. Captopril suppression test is recommended where sodium loading is contraindicated such as in renal and cardiac patients. 25–50 mg of captopril is used and a plasma aldosterone concentration of >15 ng/dl is considered as a positive test.

When sodium is administered exogenously such that a high serum level is achieved, no further aldosterone rise is observed. High salt diet (>12.8) is administered for 3 days such that 24 hr urinary sodium is >200 mmol. A 24 hr aldosterone >12 mcg/day is considered as a positive test. Suppression can also be achieved using intravenous saline infusion wherein 2 litre of normal saline is administered intravenously over 4 hrs. Plasma aldosterone concentration >5 ng/dl is considered as positive (s/o adenoma if >10 ng/dl).

5% of newly diagnosed hypertensives may harbor aldosteronoma and genetic testing is indicated in patients with a positive family history, Early onset hypertension <20 yrs and family history of CVA at a young age. Aldosterone renin ratio of 20 with aldosterone concentration >15 ng/ml are indicative of Conn syndrome.

Imaging is used to supplement the biochemical findings. CT scan is the initial modality of choice and adenomas usually present as unilateral low density nonenhancing lesions <10 HU with average size of 1.6–1.8 cm. Adrenal hyperplasia is associated with multiple bilateral nodules with enlargement and the glands appear essentially normal.

Occasionally lesions may not be readily visible and lateralization may be needed so that the affected gland can be identified and removed. Adrenal vein sampling is an important method of lateralization. Without this test 20% of the patients may be under treated and 25% may be overtreated. Aldosterone and cortisol concentration are measured in the right adrenal vein, left adrenal vein and inferior vena cava. Nuclear scintigraphy may be performed if vein sampling is inconclusive. [131]I-6β-iodomethylnorcholestrol (*NP59*) is a cortical analogue which is injected 4 days prior to evaluation. Unilateral uptake earlier than 5 days is suggestive of an adenoma while bilateral uptake suggests idiopathic hyperplasia. 18 hydroxy cortisone measurement may also be done. 18 hydroxy cortisone is an immediate precursor of aldosterone and value >100 ng/dl suggests aldosterone producing adenoma while value <100 ng/dl is suggestive of idiopathic hyperplasia.

What are the treatment options for Conn's syndrome?

Adrenalectomy is the mainstay of therapy for surgically correctable primary hyperaldosteronism that may be seen in conditions like aldosterone-producing adenoma, primary unilateral adrenal hyperplasia, ovarian aldosterone-secreting tumour and functional adrenal carcinoma but conditions like familial hyperaldosteronism and bilateral hyperplasia require medical management. Spironolactone and eplerenone (25–100 ng) are the agents of choice for hyperaldosteronism that is not amenable to surgical management. It is essential to maintain high sodium diet and monitor hyperkalemia following treatment (25–400 ng). Familial hyperaldosteronism I can be managed with glucocorticoids.

What is Pheochromocytoma?

Pheochromocytoma is an endocrine neoplasm that secretes metanephrines resulting in tachycardia, sweating and hypertension. Pheochromocytomas are often called the 10% tumour as roughly 10% are bilateral, 10% occurs in pediatric population, 10% are asymptomatic, 10% occur in extra-adrenal tissues and 10% are malignant. Pheochromocytomas are responsible for 0.5% of all causes of hypertension and 5% of incidentalomas. Epinephrine secreting tumours generally lead to syncope or hypotensive spells while norepinephrine secreting tumours present with HTN and sweating. Most familial cases present in the 2nd and 3rd decades of life, whereas sporadic cases present in the 4th or 5th decade.

What are the biochemical and radiological investigations needed in a case of pheochromocytoma?

Testing for catecholamines and their byproducts is the first step in proving a suspected diagnosis of pheochromocytoma. Serum levels of catecholamines like dopamine, epinephrine and NE released paroxysmally can be measured. Urinary levels are now preferred.

Catecholamines are converted to metanephrines and normetanephrines by the enzyme catechol O-methyltransferase, which can be measured in the serum. Plasma free metanephrines and 24 hours fractionated urinary metanephrines are used to make a diagnosis of pheochromocytoma. Before testing drugs like tricyclic antidepressants and phenoxybenzamine should be stopped. To measure plasma-free metanephrine samples should be taken in the supine position. Acetaminophen which can interfere with these levels should also be stopped at least 5 days prior. Before measuring 24 hr fractionated urinary metanephrines, it is essential to verify that renal function is normal.

VMA testing also has high specificity in especially in non-familial cases of pheochromocytoma. It has a less dramatic rise and low sensitivity. Certain drugs can suppress normal catecholamine secretion in the body but cannot suppress norepinephrine secretion by pheochromocytoma. Clonidine is an α_2 agonist that suppresses sympathetic norepinephrine and comparison of levels before and after clonidine suppression can be used to evaluate pheochromocytoma.

Cross-sectional imaging in the form of a computerized tomography scan or magnetic resonance imaging scan may be performed to delineate the lesion prior to surgery. On the CT scan pheochromocytoma appears as a well circumscribed, richly vascular, low lipid containing mass with HU >10 (mean 35) with a slow contrast washout. On MRI bright intensity on T2 weighted image "light bulb sign" is appreciated with no signal dropout (unlike lipid rich adenoma) on out of phase sequences. Pheochromocytoma can be best appreciated on fat suppression sequences.

Functional imaging in the form of MIBG scan can be used to locate the side of catecholamine production. It is of importance when no lesion can be delineated on cross-sectional imaging such as in extra-adrenal pheochromocytomas. MIBG scan is considered an integral part of workup for recurrent, extra-adrenal, metastatic pheochromocytomas, and masses exclusively secreting norepinephrine (associated with malignancy). Its normal uptake can be seen in liver, thyroid, salivary gland and bladder. Metaiodobenzylguanidine is an analogue of norepinephrine that is taken up by pheochromocytoma. However, pheochromocytomas associated with VHL and

SDHB gene may have cold MIBG scans and certain aggressive metastatic lesions may not accumulate MIBG. In such situations somatostatin and $_{18}$F dopamine PET may be useful.

How is pheochromocytoma managed?

Pheochromocytomas are best served by surgical excision or adrenalectomy. Laparoscopic adrenalectomy is the gold standard. Hereditary pheochromocytoma with MEN 2 and VHL may require cortical sparing adrenalectomy. Since these patients usually are hypertensive cardiac evaluation and preanesthetic considerations must be given importance. Echocardiogram should be performed preoperatively to assess the effects of hypertension and cardiac performance status. Pre-operative catecholamine blockade should be given in all patients. For alpha blockade, phenoxybenzamine is the most common agent used. The agent is started 7–14 days prior in a dose of 1 mg/kg to provide irreversible blockade. BP is maintained in the normotensive range. Beta Blockade is started after alpha blockers have been given to prevent reflex tachycardia and arrhythmias to avoid unopposed alpha agonism. Selective β1 blockade is preferred with atenolol or metoprolol. In refractory patients metyrosine may be added to an alpha blocker or in refractory/metastatic cases due to CNS and extrapyramidal side effects. Calcium channel blockade like nicardipine can also be used in refractory cases. Fluid loading and salt loading increases the intravascular volume to prevent postural hypotension which is a sign of adequate blockade.

What is the prognosis and follow up of patient with pheochromocytoma?

Once tumour has been successfully removed repeat metabolic testing should be done at 2 weeks to confirm the absence of tumour at any other site and achieve a baseline level. Lifelong screening is recommended for monitoring of recurrence in the form of annual biochemical testing. Up to 20% of patients may develop recurrence within a decade and a large number of these tumours are malignant (up to 50%).

How are metastatic malignant pheochromocytomas managed?

Treatment of metastatic disease is largely palliative and surgical removal is the standard of care.

Systemic treatment of metastatic patients can be done with ^{131}I MIBG and up to half of these patients demonstrate reduction in tumour volume. Chemotherapy in the form of cyclophosphamide, vincristine, dacarbazine may be useful for failed MIBG therapy or poor MIBG uptake pheochromocytomas.

What are the features of adrenal carcinoma?

Adrenal carcinomas present either as functional masses (60–80%) or are incidentally detected. Most commonly they secrete cortisol in an ACTH independent fashion, but many tumours secrete more than one hormone. 90% of pediatric adrenal cancers are functional and lead to virilization by increased DHEA and 17 keto steroid secretion. Adrenal carcinomas have a bimodal distribution with children presenting with lower stage functional tumour with increased survival. Most cases are sporadic and unilateral. Adrenal cancers grow rapidly and more than 90% of these tumours are greater than 5 cm in size at presentation.

What are the distinguishing features of adrenal carcinoma on imaging?

Computerized tomography is the imaging of choice. Carcinomas are suspected based on the following features:

1. Irregular borders
2. Irregular enhancement
3. Calcifications
4. Necrotic areas with cystic degeneration
5. Higher mean attenuation 40 HU

Carcinomas show marked contrast uptake on gadolinium enhanced MRI.

What is Weiss criteria?

Based on tumour structure, cytology and invasion malignant potential of tumours can be defined using the Weiss criteria. Presence of 3 or more of these features is suggestive of malignancy.

- *Nuclear grade*: Nuclear grade III and IV based on criteria of Führman
- *Mitotic rate*: Greater than 5/50 HPF (×40 objective)
- Atypical mitotic figures
- *Cytoplasm*: Presence of less than or equal to 25% clear or vacuolated cells resembling the normal zona fasciculata

- *Diffuse architecture*: If greater than one-third of the tumour formed patternless sheets of cells
- Necrosis
- Venous invasion
- Sinusoid invasion
- Invasion of tumour capsule

What is the staging for adrenal carcinoma?

Stage 1: Confined <5 cm (wt <200 gm)

Stage 2: Confined >5 cm

Stage 3: Extension to adjacent adipose tissue, regional LN involved

Stage 4: Adjacent organ invasion, distant metastasis

How are adrenal carcinomas managed?

For locally confined disease surgery is the main-stay of treatment but despite radical surgery up to 60–80% of these tumours recur. Cytoreductive surgery should be offered only if >90% of the tumour can be removed. For metastatic disease radiotherapy is the treatment of choice. Adjuvant therapy with mitotane can also be offered and the drug can be combined with streptozocin, etoposide, cisplatin or duanorubicin. Adjuvant treatment or enrolment into clinical trial must be considered due to high recurrence and metastatic progression.

What are the adverse prognostic variables for adrenal carcinoma?

Adverse prognostic variables for adrenal carcinoma include:
- Size >12 cm (10.5 in pediatric/>40 yr)
- High mitotic rate
- Tumour necrosis
- Atypical mitotic figures
- High Ki-67 staining

What are the indications of adrenalectomy?

Adrenalectomy is indicated in patients with:
- Functional adrenal mass
- Mass >4 cm except myelolipoma
- Imaging s/o malignancy—lipid poor, hetero-genous, invasion, irregular
- Incidentaloma with growth >1 cm
- Large >10 cm or symptomatic myelolipoma
- Isolated adrenal metastasis
- Failed neurosurgical treatment of Cushing
- Patient with ectopic ACTH syndrome with non-localized primary
- During radical nephrectomy if adrenal abnormal on imaging
- Large ≥7 cm upper pole mass
- Vein thrombus up to the level of adrenal vein.

21

Renal Lump

What are the common differentials of a mass in the lumbar region?

- Renal mass
- Colonic mass
- Liver mass on right side
- Retroperitoneal mass
- Splenic enlargement
- Pancreatic pathology arising from tail or body of pancreas

What are the clinical features of renal mass?

- Renal swelling is located in the loin or can be moved back into the loin.
- Usually maintains the original reni-form or bean shape.
- It just moves with respiration.
- *Ballottement*: It is felt bimanually and can be balloted with 2 hands. Short, quick forward thrusts are made by the posterior hand lead to a bouncing sensation to the anterior hand.
- There may be a band of colonic resonance anteriorly.
- It is dull posteriorly with oblitration or bullness of renal angle.

What are the common differentials of a renal mass (Fig. 21.1)?

Inflammatory conditions: Renal abscess, perinephric abscess, pyonephrosis or infected hydronephrosis, emphysematous pyelonephritis, xanthogranulo-matous pyelonephritis.

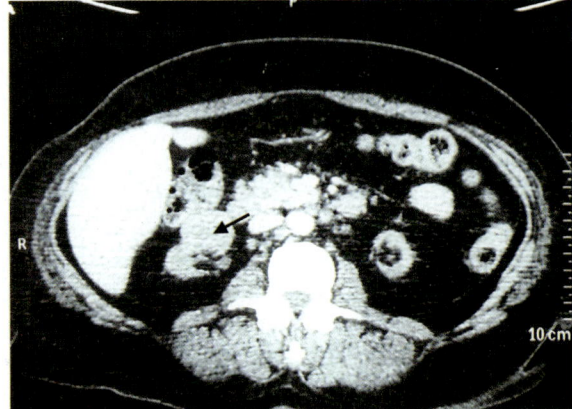

Fig. 21.1: Computerized tomogram showing a right upper polar renal mass

Clinical Features of Pyonephrosis

- Unilateral mass of moderate size.
- May not maintain reniform shape.
- Irregular, ill-defined border with irregular surface.
- Tender and may be fixed due to perinephritis.
- Firm consistency.
- Patient looks toxic.

Hydronephrosis

Clinical Features of Hydronephrosis (Fig. 21.2)

- Unilateral, large, bean-shaped, mobile mass.
- Well-defined border with rounded lower pole.
- Not tender unless infected.
- Boggy in consistency, i.e. like a half-full cyst, and becomes tensely cystic if infected

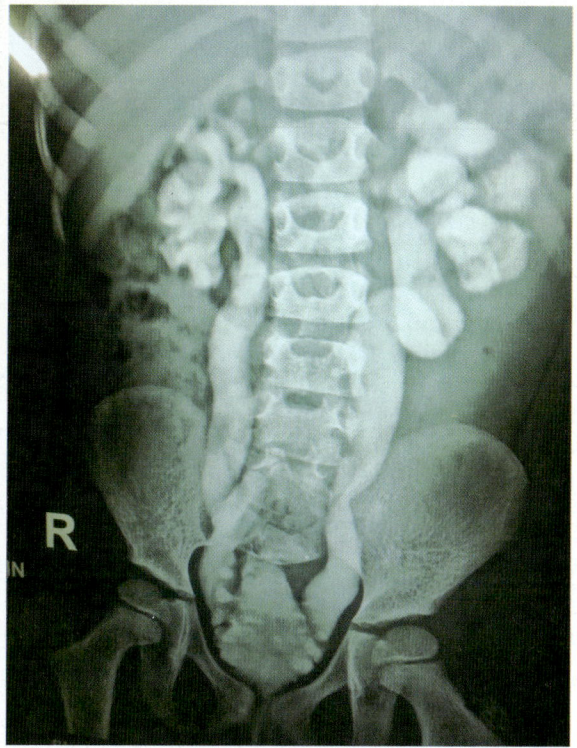

Fig. 21.2: IVU showing with bilateral hydroureteronephrosis due to back pressure changes

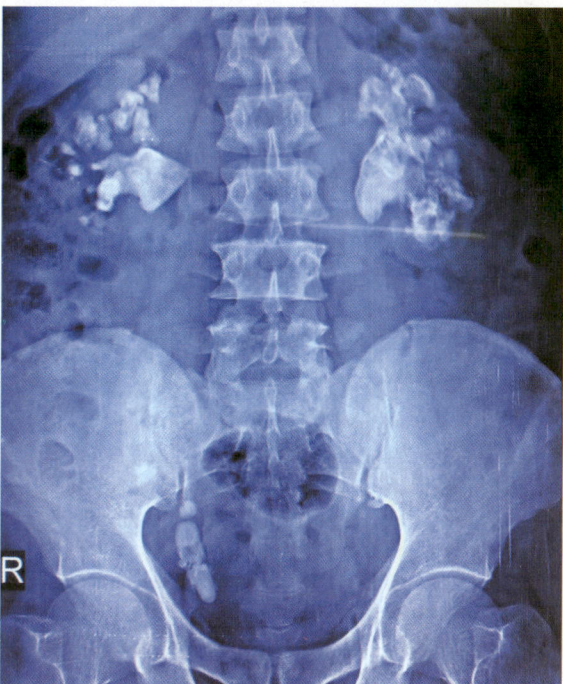

Fig. 21.3: Plain X-ray of the kidney ureter and bladder region showing bilateral renal calculi and ureteric calculi

It is caused by the obstruction to flow of urine. It can be caused by stone (Fig. 21.3), pelvi ureteric junction obstruction (Fig. 21.4)or malignancy causing obstruction to the outflow. Causes of obstruction may be present within the kidney, ureter, bladder or urethra. The causes may be intra-luminal, intramural or extramural.

Polycystic Kidney Disease

Clinical Features of Polycystic Kidney Disease

- Bilateral, large, mobile masses.
- The mass is irregular with beaded nodular surface.
- Non tender except in cases of hemorrhage and infection.
- Firm in consistency.
- Patient usually has features of uremia.
- Hypertension is seen in two-thirds of cases.

Both acquired and congenital polycystic kidney disorders may present as a renal mass. The congenital conditions include autosomal recessive polycystic kidney disease and autosomal dominant polycystic kidney diseases.

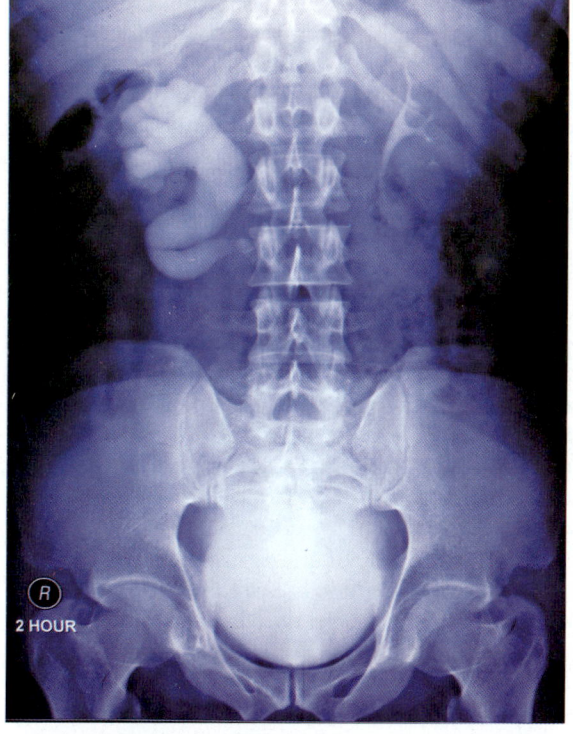

Fig. 21.4: Plain X-ray of the kidney ureter and bladder region showing pelvi ureteric obstruction

Simple renal cyst and acquired renal cystic disease are some of the most common acquired causes of cystic and enlarged kidneys in adults.

Benign renal tumours: These include angio-myolipoma, oncocytoma, myelolipomas, fibromas, lipomas and other benign tumours.

Malignant renal tumour: Malignant tumours may arise from various parts of the kidneys like nephrons (renal cell carcinoma), urothelium/collecting system (transitional cell carcinoma), lymphoid tissue (lymphoma), soft tissue (sarcoma) and Wilms' tumour.

What are the common presentations of a Renal Cell Carcinoma (RCC)?

RCC comprises 2–3% of all malignancies. The median age at diagnosis is about 65 years. A renal mass may cause patients to present with pain, fullness, urinary symptoms like hematuria, pyuria, dysuria and other systemic manifestations arising from dissemination of malignancy or uremia arising out of renal failure (in bilateral conditions or solitary kidneys). Pain arising from acute obstruction may mimic a colicky pain but more commonly, obstruction located in the kidneys causes a dull ache. Ureteric obstruction may lead to a colicky pain which has a waxing and waning phase. Heaviness due to the mass may also lead to a vague heaviness or fullness which causes a constant dull ache. More commonly renal pain is a dull continuous pain with episodes of acute colic.

Association with urinary symptoms is an important pointer to the pain being from the genitourinary system. These symptoms may include dysuria or burning micturition, hematuria or the presence of blood in urine, pyuria or presence of turbid urine containing pus, chyluria arising from presence of chyle in urine that gives urine a milky white appearance, passage of fragments of stones in urine or lithuria and occasionally lower urinary tracts symptoms (described in detail in the Chapter on *Bladder Outlet Obstruction*).

Dissemination of malignancy may lead to anorexia and weight loss. Spread of inflammation which is renal in origin may lead to symptoms of septicemia. Poor renal function arising from loss of functioning nephrons leads to uremia the symptoms of which include: Nausea, vomiting, fatigue, anorexia, and weight loss, muscle cramps, pruritus, mental status changes, visual disturbances and increased thirst apart from affecting all the major organ systems of the body.

History taking with special reference to the Kidneys and Genito-urinary System

Pain and all its characteristics must be enquired about as already described. Ask if relief in pain is associated with diuresis as in pelvi-ureteric junction obstruction. It is also important to ask about the radiation of pain to the lower abdomen, genitilia or inner thigh which is quite typical of a ureteric calculus. It is important to know the duration of such episodes and how bothersome they are to the patient. Enquire whether the pain is associated with any urinary symptoms as described previously or lower urinary tract symptoms.

Hematuria and weight loss are suggestive of renal malignancy. Elicit if the patient has recently developed hypertension that is poorly controlled with medication. Persistant cough, bone pain, cervical lymphadenopathy and constitutional symptoms like significant unintentional weight loss, malaise and anorexia may point towards a disseminated malignancy.

The daily water intake must also been asked from the patient.

Symptoms of uremia must be asked about especially if bilateral disease is in question. Also, it is not possible to rule out congenital solitary kidney by mere history taking unless the patient has that information based on prior investigations as a part of routine health checkups.

History of smoking which is another recognized risk factor for renal cancer must be asked. Performance status of the patient must be calculated based on questions about daily living.

History of fever may suggest infective origin of the mass.

How do we perform examination of the Patient with Renal Mass?

Blood pressure may be raised in a patient with uremia and chronic kidney disease apart from renal carcinoma. The general examination lays special emphasis on body mass index. Obesity is a risk factor of renal cell cancer and also for stone disease. Anaemia is a common paraneoplastic syndrome associated with renal cancer. Look for stigmata of gout such as joint pain and inflammation. Tophi are classically located along the helix of the ear, but they can be found in multiple locations, including the fingers, the toes, the prepatellar bursa, and along the olecranon, where they can resemble rheumatoid nodules.

Edema especially in the periorbital and sacral region is an important clue to uremia. The skin may be dry and scaly and there is sallow coloration of skin due to urochrome and eventually melanosis as uremia progresses. Unilateral limb edema and varicocele that has developed recently and suddenly are indicative of compression of pelvic veins and venous invasion by renal tumours.

On examination of the abdomen, there may be fullness of the renal angle or the lumbar region and occasionally the hypochondrium. There may be restricted movement of the occupied quadrants. Initially the swelling may be appreciable only on palpation but as the mass progresses a bulge may become apparent. Examination of the back is of utmost importance in these cases.

Palpation reveals the extent and nature of the mass. It is important to note the various characteristics of the mass as explained earlier to narrow down the diagnosis. Compared to the splenic mass it is possible to insinuate ones fingers between the subcostal margin and the mass of renal origin. The inferior borders are not sharp but round with the absence of the characteristic splenic notch. Renal masses may be covered by the colon anteriorly which provides a band of resonance to renal masses until they grow large enough to push the colon to the side.

In contrast to a retroperitoneal swelling the renal mass is mobile owing to its continuity with the diaphragm and has a relatively well-defined inferior border. Unlike retroperitoneal masses which arise in or have a propensity to cross the midline renal masses rarely if ever cross the midline. Being attached to a central pedicle renal masses are often ballotable if not large enough to be bimanually palpable. They often have a reniform shape conferring to the kidney and the colonic band of resonance.

Investigations Pertaining to Diagnosis of a Lumbar/Renal Mass

Basic hemogram depicts anaemia and occasionally polycythemia (a systemic syndrome associated with renal cell carcinoma). Infective renal conditions may reveal leukocytosis or neutrophilia. Kidney function may be deranged when the renal mass is associated with parenchymal loss. It must be remembered that both the kidneys must be diseased to result in an abnormal kidney function or the disease must involve a solitary kidney. Abnormal liver function may be sign of Stauffer's syndrome which is an idiopathic liver involvement in renal cell carcinoma. Alkaline phosphatase may be raised in skeletal related events like metastasis from a renal or retroperitoneal tumour.

Hypercalcaemia is also an important paraneoplastic syndrome of renal tumour. Patients with uremia, on the other hand, manifest with hyperkalaemia, hyperphosphatemia and hypocalcaemia.

Routine urine investigations may reveal red blood cells which are often helpful in delineating the source of haematuria. Dysmorphic RBCs are indicative of glomerular origin of blood while intact RBCs indicate that the source is non-glomerular and may be from the tubules, ducts or the pelvicalyceal system. Non-dysmorphic or intact RBCs also indicate that the blood may have a non-renal origin that is from the ureters, bladder or the urethra and accessory glands. Dysmorphic RBCs and RBCs of tubular origin may be associated with protienuria and casts which again indicate a renal cause of haematuria. Pus cell and crystals may point towards stones and infection as the cause of the renal mass.

The first investigation that is preferred to make a diagnosis is an ultrasound of the abdomen which reveals the organ of origin, possible pathology, the extent of the disease and evidence of metastasis in the form of liver involvement and ascites. A chest X-ray can reveal pulmonary metastasis which is often seen as rounded opacities called cannon ball metastasis (Fig. 21.5).

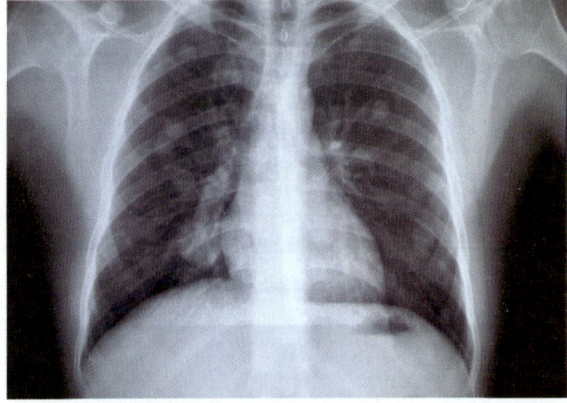

Fig. 21.5: Plain chest skiagram showing multiple cannon ball metastases in a case of renal cell carcinoma

A contrast enhanced computerized tomography is the best investigation to evaluate renal masses and differentiate them from other possible disease conditions. A computerized tomogram has very high detection rate for calculi and the presence of enhancement in renal masses is virtually diagnostic of renal cancer. It also gives information about the involvement of renal vein and inferior vena cava, involvement of surrounding organs like the adrenals and the presence of distant metastasis.

In patients with renal insufficiency, magnetic resonance imaging may be a useful diagnostic tool. It also shows enhancement of renal cancer and can better delineate the involvement of the wall of inferior vena cava by renal tumour than the CECT scan.

PET CT scan does not have an established role in the diagnosis or management of renal tumour. In doubtful cases a renal angiogram may be helpful in differentiation of benign tumours from malignant ones.

Renal cysts are difficult to differentiate from renal cancer and it is essential to detect if these cysts are harboring renal tumour. Based on their appearance, renal cysts have been classified by Bosnaik as given in Table 21.1.

Renal cell carcinoma shows enhancement of more than 15 Hounsfield units while a negative enhancement of –20 HU or more is indicative of fat containing benign tumours like angiomyolipoma, an important differential of a renal mass. In up to 10–20% masses the CT scan may be inconclusive and such tumours require further testing.

Renal biopsy for detection of renal cancer is plagued by unacceptably high false negative rates (about 15–18%), and thus is not used for diagnosis. Although these rates have been declining, the overall accuracy is in the order of 80%. Biopsy is thus presently indicated when there is a suspicion of renal abscess, metastasis or renal lymphoma.

What is Renal Cell Carcinoma?

Renal cell carcinoma is an adenocarcinoma that arises from the proximal convoluted tubules. Certain subtypes of renal cancer like chromophobe and collecting duct cancer are derived from the distal nephron. Renal cell carcinoma accounts for 2–3% of all malignant neoplasms in adults with a slight male predominance (3:2). The disease presents in the elderly usually in the 6th to 7th decade and most cases are sporadic with only 2–3% being familial.

Risk Factor for Renal Cell Carcinoma

- Smoking/tobacco
- Hypertension
- Obesity
- Occupational exposure
    - Lead, cadmium, asbestos, aromatic hydrocarbons, trichloroethylene, thorotrast
    - Radiation

Presentation of Renal Cell Carcinoma

Almost half of the cases of renal cell carcinoma are incidentally detected during routine investigations for other causes or annual health checkups. The classical triad of presentation consists of gross hematuria, flank pain and abdominal mass. However, this triad is found late in the course of disease and presently only 4–10% patients present with this "Too Late Triad". Bleeding may lead to clot colic and flank pain associated with hematuria. Extensive growth of the mass may cause stretching of the renal capsule and also result in flank pain. Renal cancer exhibits venotropism and as it grows,

Classification	Features of contrast enhanced CT	Malignancy risk	Management
I	Homogeneous, uncomplicated benign cysts	None	None
II	Thin hairline septa with fine calcifications	0–5%	None
IIF	Hyperdense cyst, with multiple hairline septa and minimal smooth wall thickening		Periodic surveillance
	Thick and nodular calcification without enhancement	5–10%	
III	Indeterminate cyst with thickened irregular or smooth wall septa with enhancement	50%	Excision
IV	Enhancing soft tissue components present	75–90%	Excision

Table 21.1: Bosnaik's classification of renal cysts

it invades the renal vein and inferior vena cava. This presents as edema of the lower limbs and a suddenly developing non-reducing right sided varicocele. Renal cancer may give rise to various paraneoplastic syndromes like anaemia, polycythemia, hypertension and hyperkalaemia. Idiopathic derangement of liver function has also been found to be associated with renal cancer (Stauffer's syndrome). If the disease has metastasized to the lungs, it may lead to persistent cough and dyspnoea. Bony metastasis causes bony pain, and spread to other organs may cause constitutional symptoms like fever, malaise and weight loss. Cervical lymphadenopathy may also be present. Presence of weight loss, fever and nights sweats indicates advanced disease. Rarely renal cell cancer may present as peri-renal haematoma.

Subtypes of Renal Cell Carcinoma (see Table 21.2)

Staging of RCC

T: Primary tumour

TX: Primary tumour cannot be assessed

T0: No evidence of primary tumour

T1: Tumour <7.0 cm and confined to the kidney

- T1a: Tumour ≤4.0 cm and confined to the kidney
- T1b: Tumour >4.0 cm and ≤7.0 cm and confined to the kidney

T2: Tumour >7.0 cm and confined to the kidney

- T2a: Tumour >7.0 cm and ≤10.0 cm and confined to the kidney
- T2b: Tumour >10.0 cm and confined to the kidney

T3: Tumour extends into major veins or perinephric tissues but not into the ipsilateral adrenal gland and not beyond the Gerota fascia

- T3a: Tumour grossly extends into the renal vein or its segmental (muscle containing) branches or tumour invades perirenal and/or renal sinus fat but not beyond the gerota fascia
- T3b: Tumour grossly extends into the vena cava below the diaphragm
- T3c: Tumour grossly extends into the vena cava above the diaphragm or invades the wall of the vena cava

T4: Tumour invades beyond the gerota fascia (including contiguous extension into the ipsilateral adrenal gland)

N: Regional Lymph Nodes

- NX: Regional lymph nodes cannot be assessed
- N0: No regional lymph nodes metastasis
- N1: Metastasis in regional lymph node(s)

M: Distant Metastases

- MX: Distant metastasis cannot be assessed
- M0: No distant metastasis
- M1: Distant metastasis present

Stage Grouping

- Stage I: T1 N0 M0
- Stage II: T2 N0 M0
- Stage III: T1 or T2 N1 M0
  - T3 Any N M0
- Stage IV: T4 Any N M0
  - Any T Any N M1

Table 21.2: Subtypes of RCC		
Subtype	Defect	Presentation and Peculiarities
Clear cell RCC (70–80%)	3p deletions	Most common type of RCC Exhibit venotropism Responsive to immunotherapy
Papillary RCC (10–15%)	Trisomy of chromosome 7 and 17; loss of Y	Hypovascular tumours Multicentric tumours Associated with acquired renal disease
Chromophobe RCC (2–5%)	Fumarate hydratase gene 1q mutation	Well circumscribed with good prognosis Originate from collecting duct
Collecting duct cancer	Multiple chromosomal defects	Poor prognosis Originate from collecting duct Chemo responsive
Medullary carcinoma	Multiple chromosomal defects	Poor prognosis Originate from collecting duct Associated with sickle cell disease

What are the guidelines for management of RCC?

The management of renal cell carcinoma is essentially restricted to the surgical domain in the present time. All incidentally detected and localized renal cancers are subjected to radical nephrectomy which include typically, the removal of the kidney along with upper 1/3rd of the ureter, the ipsilateral adrenal, Gerota's fascia, and the lymph nodes from crus of diaphragm to bifurcation of aorta. With due course it has been realized that we can be more conservative during the surgery for renal masses. The advantage of lymphadenectomy is not clear and the fact that it increases the surgical morbidity makes it underutilized. Routine lymphadenectomy is no longer recommended and enlarged lymph nodes if encountered can be selectively removed. Ipsilateral adrenal gland can also be spared if the tumour is not in close vicinity of the adrenal, well confined locally and there is no radiological evidence of invasion.

For all T1 tumours and some T2 tumours partial nephrectomy has become the norm. In partial nephrectomy only the affected part of the tumour is removed with a 2–3 cm margin of healthy renal parenchyma after achieving/vascular control. The collecting system is repaired and the capsule is closed using interrupted absorbable sutures. Patients subjected to partial nephrectomy require a more stringent follow up but the overall survival is comparable to radical nephrectomy. For larger and locally advanced tumours radical nephrectomy is the gold standard whether performed using the open route, laparoscopic means or assisted by a robot.

Patients with tumour thrombus invading the vein require more extensive surgery and venotomy is done after taking distal, contralateral and proximal control with vascular clamps. For tumours reaching up to the atrium, cardiopulmonary bypass may have to be used to remove the tumour in its entirety.

What is the role of Minimally Invasive Therapies for Renal Cell Cancer?

Renal cryoablation and radiofrequency ablation are minimally invasive therapies available for renal tumour ablation. These can be used in patients with multifocal tumours, or tumours in solitary kidneys where ischemia may lead to dialysis dependence. Patients' choice may also guide treatment towards ablative therapy. In cryoablation the cryoprobe is used to first passively freeze and then actively thaw the tumour. A temperature of –40°C is achieved which causes direct cellular damage followed by reperfusion injury during active thawing. Argon is used to form an ice ball which is monitored laparoscopically or using the ultrasound and helium is used to thaw the tumour. In radiofrequency ablation, the ablation probe is guided into the lesion and continuous monopolar radiofrequency current is use to achieve temperatures above 60°C which leads to necrosis of tumour tissue. 2–3 cycles of 5–10 minutes are used to ablate the tumour. Patients are followed up with imaging where loss of enhancement and decrease in size are predictors of successful ablation. Even though no significant differences in overall survival have been observed these modalities still need to pass the test of time.

How do we manage a patient of metastatic RCC?

Up to one-third of patients with renal cell carcinoma develop metastatic spread. Common sites of metastasis include lung, liver, bone and the brain. It is the most important feature in the selection of appropriate therapy. Shorter interval between surgery and development of metastatic is one of the poor prognostic factors. Patients with metastatic RCC were believed to have a dismal prognosis. Often there is involvement of more than one organ system. 20–50% patients may develop metastasis post-nephrectomy.

Clinical signs do not develop early due to the location of the tumour, consequently the overall five-year survival is as low as 20–25%. Last decade has seen a major improvement in management of metastatic RCC. Better knowledge about the renal cancer biology has led to development of new targeted molecules for treatment of mRCC.

In patients with potentially resectable solitary metastatic site, nephrectomy and surgical metastatectomy is the recommended treatment. If only the primary tumour is potentially resectable then cytoreductive nephrectomy should be done prior to systemic therapy. The patients with metastatic RCC are divided into various risks based on the number of risk factors. The various adverse prognostic factors are:

- Haemoglobin less than the lower limit of normal (LLN)

- Corrected calcium greater than the upper limit of normal (ULN).
- Karnofsky performance score of less than 80.
- A time from diagnosis to treatment initiation of less than 1 year.
- Absolute neutrophil count greater than ULN.
- Platelets greater than ULN.

Patients with no risk factors are good risk metastatic patients, patients with 1–2 risk factors are categorized as intermediate risk and patients with 3–6 risk factors are poor risk patients.

Optimal IL-2 regimen is not clear, but long-term (>10 years) complete responses have been achieved with high-dose bolus IL-2 in a randomized phase III study. Response rates range from 7 to 27% but the toxicity of IL-2 is substantially greater than IFN-α. The positive effect of IFN-α is particularly apparent in mRCC patients with clear cell histology.

Only selected patients with mRCC with good risk profile and clear cell subtype histology show clinical benefit from immunotherapy with IL-2. Monotherapy with IFN-α or high-dose bolus IL-2 can only be recommended as a first-line treatment for mRCC in selected patients with clear cell histology and good prognostic factors. Bevacizumab + IFN-α is recommended as first-line therapy in low-risk and intermediate-risk patients. Alternatively targeted therapy using Tyrosine Kinase Inhibitors (TKIs) has been widely accepted as first line therapy in mRCC and till date seven agents have been approved by FDA for treatment of advanced and mRCC:

- Sunitinib
- Sorafenib
- Pazopanib
- Axitinib
- Temsirolimus
- Everolimus
- Bevacizumab in combination with interferon

There is a lack of clear consensus on drugs useful in systemic therapy for non-clear cell mRCC. Enrollment in clinical trials is the preferred strategy for such patients.

Follow up of Patients with RCC

After partial nephrectomy patients are more aggressively followed up with yearly clinical examination and blood tests like urea, creatinine electrolytes, calcium and liver function for tumours less than 4 cm (T1a). For higher stage tumours up to 10 cm (T2b) yearly clinical examination, test and chest X ray are performed along with an abdominal CT scan 2 yearly. CT scan can be avoided if radical nephrectomy has been done. For T3 tumours these investigations are done 6 monthly. After radical nephrectomy, the follow-up protocols are essentially similar but abdominal CT is done on a 2 yearly basis for T2 tumours and yearly for T3–4 tumours and 6 monthly for node positive disease.

What are the Familial Syndromes Associated with Renal Cell Carcinoma? (*see* Table 21.3)

What are the various Subtypes of von Hippel-Lindau Syndrome? (*see* Table 21.4)

Table 21.3: Various familial syndromes associated with renal cell carcinoma		
von Hippel-Lindau syndrome	Affects the VHL gene on chromosome 3	Clear cell renal cell cancer (in 50% patients) CNS hemangioblastomas Retinal angiomas Pheochromocytomas Pencreatic islet cell tumours Renal and pancreatic cysts Cystadenoma of epididymis Endolymphatic sac tumour
Hereditary papillary renal cell carcinoma	Affects the cMET proto-oncogene on Ch. 7 and other chromosomes like Ch. 17	Type 1 papillary renal cell cancer
Familial leiomyomatosis and renal cell carcinoma	Fumarate hydratase chromosome 1	Type 2 papillary renal cell cancer: Uterine and cutaneous leiomyomas
Birt-Hogg-Dubé syndrome	BHD1 gene on Ch. 17	Cutaneous fibrofolliculomas, lung cysts, spontaneous pneumothoraces, renal tumours primarily derived from the distal nephron (chromophobe RCC, oncocytomas, and hybrid or transitional tumours)

Table 21.4: Subtypes of von Hippel-Lindau syndrome		
Type 1	RCC with other manifestations	Full and partial deletions of the genes
Type 2A	Pheochromocytomas with other manifestations	Missense mutations
Type 2B	RCC along with pheochromocytomas and other manifestations	Missense and nonsense mutations with partial deletions
Type 2C	Pheochromocytomas	Missense mutations

RENAL SARCOMA

Renal sarcomas present in a manner very similar to renal cell cancer with abdominal mass, hematuria and flank pain in a similar age bracket. The tumours arise from perirenal tissues and do not invade but displace the renal tissue. These tumours are rapidly growing and are less vascular compared to renal cancer and despite of their large size lymph nodes are rarely involved. Based on the source of origin, fat, bones and other tissues may be found on imaging which may be useful in differentiating these lesions from renal cell cancer. These tumours are best managed by nephrectomy and en bloc excision of surrounding organs. Adjuvant chemotherapy and radiotherapy can be given but have a poor response rate. Margin status and tumour grade are the most important factors predicting prognosis and surgery performed with wide local excision gives the best chance of cure. Leiomyosarcomas are the most common renal sarcomas followed by liposarcomas.

RENAL LYMPHOMA

Renal involvement in non-Hodgkin lymphoma may been seen in up to 30% of patients. Compared to Hodgkin's lymphoma which remains confined to the nodes, tumour spread to organs and extranodal sites is frequent in non-Hodgkin's lymphoma. About half of the patients present as multiple renal masses and presence of lymphadenopathy and splenomegaly are useful pointers for lymphoma rather than renal cell carcinoma. Isolated renal involvement or primary renal lymphomas are rare. These tumours are managed with chemotherapy (CHOP regime, see chapter on Generalized Lymphadenopathy for details) and surgery is avoided unless there is massive refractory hematuria. Renal biopsy is indicated in patients with suspected renal lymphoma.

WILMS' TUMOUR

Wilms' tumour is the most common renal malignancy in children occurring slightly more commonly in females (especially bilateral disease). Most cases are sporadic and unilateral and present with an abdominal mass discovered by the parents along with abdominal pain, hematuria and hypertension. The mass is usually firm and non-tender and does not cross the midline. Approximately 10% of these tumours are bilateral and/or multifocal.

Tumour has a triphasic nature and can contain a mixture of blastemal cells, stromal cells and epithelial cells. Histology has prognostic implication and high degree of anaplasia is associated with poor outcomes. Most tumours have high levels of WT1 expression but 10–15% of sporadic have been found to have WT1 inactivation.

What are the various syndromes associated with Wilms' tumour?

Syndrome that are associated with mutations or deletions in WT1/FWT1/FWT2/p53 genes include Wilms' tumour as one of the components. These include:

- *Beckwith-Wiedemann syndrome*: It consists of macrosomia, macroglossia, omphalocele, large kidneys, hemihypertrophy with Wilms' tumour
- *WAGR syndrome*: It consists of Wilms' tumour, aniridia, GU anomalies, mental retardation
- *Denys-Drash syndrome*: Male pseudohermaphroditism with renal disease.

How is Wilms' Tumour Staged?

Stage I: Contained within one kidney that can be completely removed by surgery with intact capsule. No local tumour extension, no prior biopsy.

Stage II: Grown beyond the kidney, either into nearby fatty tissue or into blood vessels in or near the kidney but completely removed by surgery. Negative nodes and no prior biopsy.

Stage III: Incompletely removed tumour confined to abdomen with:

- Lymph node involvement of abdomen and pelvis
- Invasion to surrounding organs

- Peritoneal seeding
- Positive margins
- Intraoperative spillage
- Piecemeal removal
- Prior biopsy

Stage IV: Metastatic tumour

Stage V: Bilateral involvement

How is Wilms' Tumour Managed?

Resection of the tumour is the mainstay of treatment. This is followed by management as per any of the two commonly used protocols.

Based on the National Wilms' Tumour Study Group **(NWTSG) Protocol,** the management of Wilms' tumour based on stage is as under:

- *Stage I favourable/unfavourable histology*: 18 weeks of dactinomycin/vincristine
- *Stage II favourable histology*: 18 weeks of dactinomycin/vincristine
- *Stage III+IV favourable histology*: 24 weeks of dactinomycin/vincristine/doxorubicin with radiotherapy to tumour bed and involved sites
- *Stage II–IV unfavourable histology*: 24 weeks of dactinomycin/vincristine/doxorubicin/cyclophosphomide/etoposide with radiotherapy to tumour bed and involved sites.

Regime of post-operative therapy as per Societe Internationale D'oncologie Pediatrique **(SIOP) Protocol** is as follows:

Localized

- *Stage I*: No treatment apart from surgical excision
- *Stage I (intermediate grade/anaplasia)*: 18 weeks of dactinomycin/vincristine
- *Stage II (no lymph nodes)*: 28 weeks of dactinomycin/vincristine/epirubicin
- *Stage II with nodes/III*: 28 weeks of dactinomycin/vincristine/epirubicin with radiotherapy to tumour bed
  High grade: 34 weeks of epirubicin/ifosfamide/VP16/carboplatin with radiotherapy to tumour bed.

Metastatic

- Stage IV: As per local stage of tumour with treatment of metastases with radiotherapy and/or excision.

Prognosis of Wilms' Tumour

Response rates of up to 90% can be achieved with chemotherapy and resection. The best prognostic factors are favorable histology with age under 2 years and stage 1 disease. The recurrence rate for favorable histology is nearly 15% but almost half of the cases recur if anaplasia is present.

Metastatic Tumours to the Kidneys

Lung, breast, and intestinal tumours, malignant melanoma and leukemia and lymphomas are the most frequent malignancies that metastasize to the kidneys. There tumours are multifocal (except for lung, breast and colon which may be large and solitary) and history of another concomitant malignancy is a useful pointer. Diagnosis is confirmed on biopsy. Management is by systemic therapy of the primary tumour. Only in cases of haematuria nephrectomy is indicated.

Benign Renal Tumours (*see* Table 21.5)

Transitional Cell Tumours of the Kidney (TCC)

Transitional cell tumours comprise 5% of all renal tumours. They arise from the transitional epithelium that lines the collecting system and ureters and not the renal parenchyma or glomerulus. These tumours thus have a different prognosis than RCC. TCCs are rarely bilateral (less than 2%) and are usually symptomatic as they cause hematuria early due to their location within the urine channel. The tumours are more likely to occur in the lower ureter due to downstream implantation and may lead to bladder cancer in 15–75% within 5 years. These tumours affect older individuals compared to RCC (Age: Elderly 75 to 80 years. Mean age 65 years) and are more predominant among males.

What are the Etiological Factors for TCC?

- Bladder cancer increases risk for TCC. The risk is higher with carcinoma *in situ* than invasive cancer and high-grade lesions.
- Balkan degenerative interstitial nephropathy (mediated by aristocholic acid)
- Smoking (up to 7 times increased risk)
- Coffee (up to 2 times increased risk)
- Analgesic abuse: Renal papillary necrosis (7 × risk) and phenacitin (4 × risk) or both (20 × risk)

Table 21.5: Benign renal tumour	
Oncocytoma	Most common benign renal tumours that take origin from distal part of nephron. Cells are eosinophilic because of abundance of mitochondria. On angiography a typical spoke wheel pattern is seen. It is very difficult to differentiate between oncocytomas and eosinophilic RCCs and tumours are managed on lines similar to RCC. When suspected a nephron sparing surgery is performed.
Angiomyolipoma	Angiomyolipomas arise from the neural crest and are closely associated with tuberous sclerosis (adenoma sebaceum, mental retardation and epilepsy). These can be reliably differentiated from renal cancer on CT scan due to the presence of fat. Angiomyolipomas may undergo spontaneous haemorrhage and tumours more than 4 cm in size should be excised due to high chances of spontaneous haemorrhage (Wunderlich's syndrome characterized by Lenk's triad; acute flank pain, increasing flank mass and hypovolaemic shock). Pregnancy may also be associated with higher chances of spontaneous haemorrhage and in such situations of life threatening haemorrhage embolization is the first choice of treatment.
Metanephric adenoma	Consists of small basophilic epithelial cells with an acellular stromas that may represent the epithelial version of the Wilms' tumour. Very hard to differentiate form renal cell cancer and biopsy is the only way to diagnose it pre-operatively. Expression of S100 and WT1 may give a clue on histopathology.
Cystic nephromas	Cystic nephromas consist of cystic masses with intervening stroma that closely resemble cystic RCC and Wilms' tumour. They present in a younger age group and are conventionally managed by radical nephrectomy.
Mixed epithelial and stromal tumours	MEST are an important differential of RCC usually appearing as complicated renal cysts on imaging. This affects perimenopausal women on hormonal replacement therapy.
Leiomyoma	Leiomyomas present as well circumscribed and often exophytic renal masses that may show enhancement and thus become difficult to differentiate from an RCC. Management is often in the form of radical nephrectomy.
Reninoma	Reninomas are tumours arising from the juxtaglomerular apparatus found in the younger age group. Renin secretion by these tumours is associated with hypertension, polyuria, hypokalemia and myalgia. Plasma renin levels may be raised and these tumours are managed by surgical excision.
Others	Fibromas, lipomas, lymphangiomas, and haemangiomas.

- Excess inorganic arsenic
- Occupation in petroleum chemical plants
- Chronic bacterial infection with stones and obstruction
- Cyclophosphamide
- Familial syndromes like lynch 2 syndrome

How are TCCs Staged?

Tx   Primary tumour cannot be assessed.

T0   No evidence of primary tumour.

Ta   Papillary noninvasive carcinoma.

Tis   Carcinoma *in situ*.

T1   Tumour invades subepithelial connective tissue.

T2   Tumour invades the muscularis (renal pelvis).

T3   Tumour invades beyond muscularis into peripelvic fat or the renal parenchyma.

T3   (Ureter) tumour invades beyond muscularis into periureteric fat.

T4   Tumour invades adjacent organs, or through the kidney into the perinephric fat.

NX   Regional lymph nodes cannot be assessed.

N0   No regional lymph node metastasis.

N1   Metastasis in a single lymph node, ≤2 cm in greatest dimension.

N2   Metastasis in a single lymph node, >2 cm but not >5 cm in greatest dimension; or multiple lymph nodes, none >5 cm in greatest dimension.

N3   Metastasis in a lymph node, >5 cm in greatest dimension.

M0   No distant metastasis.

M1   Distant metastasis.

Staging

0a	Ta	N0	M0
0is	Tis	N0	M0
I	T1	N0	M0
II	T2	N0	M0
III	T3	N0	M0
IV	T4	N0	M0
Any T	N1	M0	
Any T	N2	M0	
Any T	N3	M0	
Any T	Any N	M1	

Management of Transitional Cell Tumours

The gold standard for management of transitional cell tumours of the ureters and renal pelvis is radical nephroureterectomy in which apart from the kidney and upper part of ureter, the entire length of ureter is removed along with excision of bladder cuff. This is done so because transitional cell tumours result from a field change as a result of risk factors and tumours may be present elsewhere in the urothelium which may recur if the urothelium is not completely removed. Regional lymphadenectomy is also performed as it has a prognostic significance and adds a little to the morbidity.

Nephron sparing surgery can be performed in solitary kidneys, multiple tumours and patients with Balkan nephropathy but radical nephro-ureterectomy offers the best chances of cure. Very small tumours Tis/T1 may be subjected to endoscopic resection if the patient can be followed up on a regular basis. Uretertectomy and uretero-ureterostomy involves excision of the involved ureteric segment. This can be performed in patients with low grade tumours which cannot be removed endoscopically.

Prognosis and Follow up of Transitional Cell Tumours of the Kidneys

Mortality rates are low if treated in a timely fashion and overall 5 year survival is 75 percent. For early and *in situ* tumours the survival is 95 percent but it decreases as disease advances. For disease with distant involvement the survival is only 15%. Mortality is greater in blacks and women.

Follow up of these patients after definitive treatment is by clinical examination, liver function tests (alkaline phosphatase) and urine cytology, annual intravenous pyelography, endoscopy and CT scan. Bone scan can be done if there is bone pain or an elevated alkaline phosphatase.

22

Bladder Outlet Obstruction

Bladder outlet obstruction (BOO) is an urodynamic concept characterized by high intravesical pressure, i.e. up to 80 cm of water (normal filling intravesical pressure is 30–50 cm of water) with low peak flow rate (less than 10 ml per second). If there is low peak flow rate with low intravesical pressure, it indicates neurogenic bladder. Common presentation in older men arises from benign prostatic hyperplasia or prostatic carcinoma, however, even in younger men bladder outlet obstruction may arise due to stricture of the urethra.

What is the differential diagnosis for bladder outlet obstruction?

Etiology of BOO can be:
- Urethral stricture (Fig. 22.1)
- BPH
- Urethral calculus (Fig. 22.2)
- Ca prostate

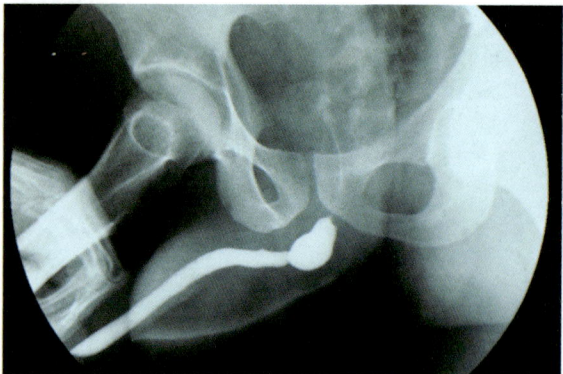

Fig. 22.1: Retrograde urethrogram showing midbulbar partial stricture of the urethra

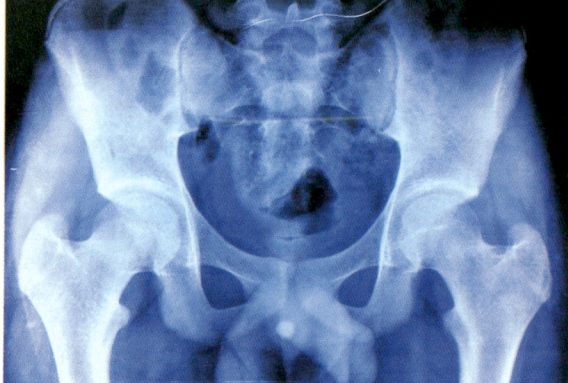

Fig. 22.2: Plain skiagram showing urethral calculus causing bladder outlet obstruction

- Vesical calculus impacted at neck (Fig. 22.3)
- Carcinoma at the base of urinary bladder
- Large ureterocele encroaching upon bladder neck
- Large cystocele
- Urethral caruncle
- Urethral leiomyoma
- Posterior urethral valve
- Paraurethral mass/abscess (Fig. 22.4)
- Urethral diverticulum
- Uterine fibroid
- Sacrococcygeal teratoma

How will you work up a patient with suspected bladder outlet obstruction?

Patients with bladder outlet obstruction present usually with lower urinary tract symptoms (LUTS) which could include storage, voiding and post-voiding symptoms.

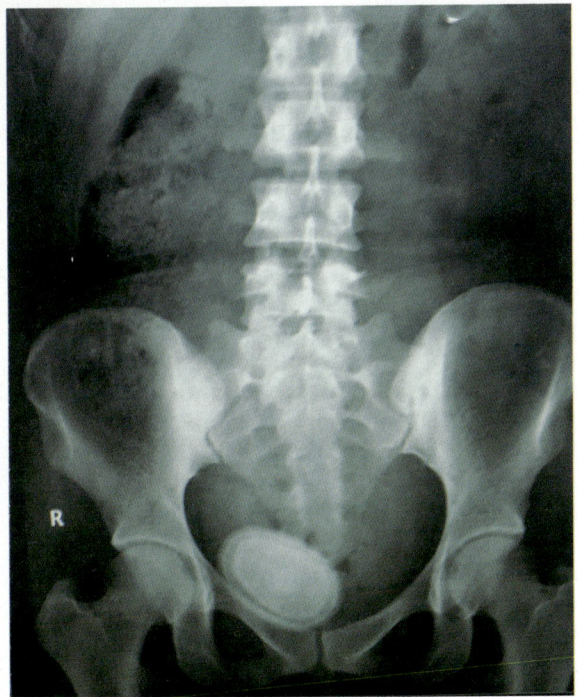

Fig. 22.3: Plain skiagram showing vesical calculus causing bladder outlet obstruction

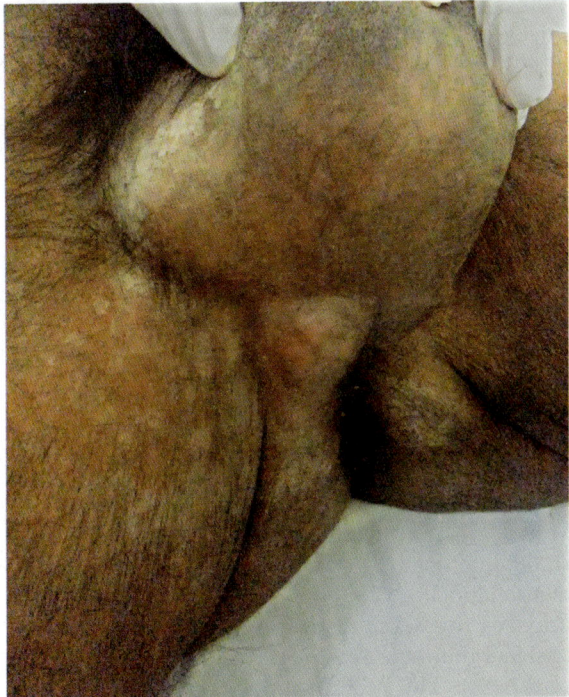

Fig. 22.4: Periurethral abscess in case of complicated stricture urethra

Storage symptoms include frequency, urgency, nocturia and urge incontinence. They can be remembered by mnemonic FUNI. The frequency occurs due to reduced functional bladder capacity.

Voiding symptoms include stream related symptoms, hesitancy, straining to void, poor urinary stream, intermittency, urinary retention and duplication of stream.

Post-void symptoms include feeling of incomplete voiding and post-void dribbling.

Thorough history and calculation of the AUA IPSS score can address voiding and storage issues. Associated symptoms like pyuria, urethral discharge, lithuria/graveluria, haematuria and fever with chills can help to rule out many infective differentials. One should probe further if haematuria is present and ascertain whether it is present throughout the stream (suggesting a pathology within the bladder), terminal (suggesting a cause in the posterior urethra or neck) or occurs at the initiation only (suggesting urethral pathology). It is also important to ascertain whether it is associated with pain (usually seen in infective and benign conditions) or painless (usually seen in carcinoma of the bladder).

Past medical history of prior instrumentation, trauma to the genitalia and back and catheterization can be helpful especially in ruling out urethral stricture and neurogenic bladder. Associated comorbidities in the form of diabetes, cardio-vascular morbidity, obesity, erectile dysfunction and other components of metabolic syndrome must be enquired about as they have strong correlation with lower urinary tract symptoms and prostatomegaly.

Examination

Per-abdominal examination should be focused at assessing both the aetiology as well as the consequences of bladder outlet obstruction. It is best suggested to start assessment in the usual manner while keeping the differentials of outlet obstruction as highlighted earlier in mind. The renal angle and back should be examined for renal fullness and palpated for ruling out hydronephrosis. On per abdominal examination suprapubic fullness must be appreciated. It may signify chronic retention if the patient has no pain or urge to void at time of examination or acute retention if the patient also complaints of pain and urgent need to void. A complete pelvic examination should be done in females to rule out compression by pelvic organs and record the state of the urethral meatus. The scheme of per-rectal examination is described below in detail.

Per-rectal Examination

The per-rectal examination offers clinically valuable cases and the abdominal examination is incomplete without it. The examination is commonly done in the left lateral or *Sims position*. In this position the patient is made to lie across the table such that the head lies on the flexed left arm across the edge of the table and the buttocks protrude from the other edge of the table on the examiners side. The upper or right leg and hip is flexed and the left leg is semi extended.

The best position to perform per-rectal examination is the lithotomy position which gives the best and higher access to the finger. The position not only allows the clinician to feel the structures located higher up compared to other positions but also make lower abdominal and pelvic viscera more accessible to examination especially the bimanual palpation. The cons for this position are the need of specialized table with stirrups or lithotomy poles.

The knee elbow position, or prone jack-knife position also referred to as the proctologic position is also a very useful position to perform per-rectal examination. Its exaggeration which is called the pickers position is useful for palpation of the seminal vesicles.

The fourth commonly employed position is the dorsal or supine position with knees flexed. This position is suitable for patients who are frail to assume any other preferred position and useful in most clinical situations. The hand is passed from below the right thigh into the anal canal or alternatively with the knees flexed to the maximum, from between the legs.

In these positions up to 10 cm of the anal and rectal canal can be accessed by the index finger, however, this examination covers only up to 10% of the colorectal mucosal surface area.

It is preferable that the bladder is empty before the per-rectal examination is attempted. A full bladder pushes the prostate down and may give a false positive impression of an enlarged prostate. It also interferes with a bimannual palpation during the anorectal examination.

Per-rectal examination actually begins with inspection of the perianal region. With each hand on the buttocks of the patient, they are gently separated to give a view of the perineal and perianal region. Acutely painful conditions like an anal fissure or prolapsed and thrombosed haemorrhoids preclude further examination per rectum. In the female patient the finger may be directed to the wrong orifice and may be a source of embarrassment for both the doctor and the patient. Common spot diagnosis that are revealed on inspection of the perianal region alone include external haemorrhoids, anal fissure or its sentinel tag, warts, rectal prolapse, papilloma, condylomata, haematomas, fistula, anal melanoma, excoriation, abscesses of the perianal region and blood. At this instance asking the patient to strain gently may reveal hidden internal piles. While the sphincter should relax a bit on straining, failure of relaxation may point to acutely painful conditions like anal fissure which put the sphincter into a state of spasm. The descent of the perineum is also checked during inspection. The perineum is normally an inch higher than the ischial tuberosities and on straining causes the perineum to descend by about half an inch. This maneuver is helpful in diagnosis of abscesses and fistulae. The L1 and L2 integrity can be checked by demonstrating the anal wink reflex on scratching the buttocks on each side with a gloved finger.

A gentle reminder of the anatomy of the rectum and anal canal can be useful to perform a systematic anorectal examination with minimal discomfort to the patient. The anal canal is a 4 cm long and terminal end of the intestines. Anatomically the anal canal and rectum are demarcated by the dentate line or pectinate line which embryonically is the line of fusion of the proctodeum with the postallantoic gut. However, surgically the anal canal and rectum are demarcated by the anorectal ring and thus there is a part of the anal canal which lies above the dentate line. The supra-dentate part of the anal canal bears the anal columns of Morgagni and the anal crypts. On each side of the anal canal are the ischiorectal fossae which meet in the midline posterior to the anal canal. The finger is thus able to trespass all these structures and feel the rectum which is a 10–12 cm long part of the gut. The rectum makes an angle with the anal canal above the anorectal ring and a part of the rectum lying posterior and just above the anorectal ring often is missed during the digital anorectal examination.

The lubricated finger pulp is placed in the midline on the posterior aspect of the anal verge. A gentle pressure is applied posteriorly till the sphincter gives way. The finger is then advanced into the anal canal. The external sphincter feels like a muscle roll and the internal sphincter is felt as a narrowing, an inch above the external sphincter. To truly appreciate the two structures, the finger is rotated and hooked posteriorly and brought out. It tucks at the level of the sphincters. The anorectal ring is felt on the posterior wall and marks the beginning of the rectum. The tone of the sphincter should be assessed at this stage and a laxed tone may be a pointer to neurological deficit.

The finger is followed along the curve of the sacral hollow and the anal and rectal wall is felt for the presence of any induration or growth and any enlarged nodes. The coccyx held between the finger and thumb may be assessed on palpation for coccygodynia. The finger is then gently rotated counterclockwise to feel the anterior surface. In the male patient starting from below upwards, the structures which can be felt anteriorly include the bulbo-urethral glands of Cowper (which are often felt between the finger in the anal canal and thumb placed over the perineum), the prostate gland starting from the apex to the base, the seminal vesicles which are poorly felt when normal, the trigonal portion of the bladder and the recto-vesical pouch. The prostate is felt as a firm bulge encroaching about 1 cm into the rectum. It is easy to appreciate the median sulcus or groove and the two lateral lobes. The prostate may, however, become enlarged with age and is appreciated as an increase in the size of either both or one of the lateral lobes. Obliteration of the median sulcus may be a pointer towards median lobe hypertrophy (Table 22.1).

A vesical calculus can be palpated in the trigonal portion of the bladder. Occasionally there may be induration or hard mass felt in the rectovesical pouch indicating inflammation or abscess and malignancy (rectal shelf of Blumer) respectively. In a male child where prostate is vestigial a bladder stone may be palpated more easily. One may also feel the pelvic colon and other structures of the lower abdomen.

Laterally the ischio-rectal fossae can be felt along with the bony wall of true pelvis, the ischial spines and ligaments and occasionally enlarged internal iliac or hypogastric nodes. Rectal patho-logies like growths, induration of the wall and the normal lowermost valve of Houston may be found on palpation. Faeces may initially be confused with rectal growth but can be indented with the finger. Soft lesions of the rectum may be felt during the downward movement. Movement of the mucosa over the swelling is the best clue to whether the lesion is arising from the rectal wall or outside it.

In the female subject the bladder and urethra are not palpable. A similar firm bulge may be found in the region corresponding to prostate in

Table 22.1: Grading of prostate enlargement					
Gland size		Examination method			Amount of tissue resected during surgery
	DRE (encroachment into rectal lumen)		Cystoscopy findings		
		Intraurethral lateral lobes	Length of urethra between verumontanum and prostatic border	Intravesical prostate covering trigone	
Normal	0–1 cm	Concave lateral walls	1–2 cm	Not reaching up to trigone	Up to 10 grams
Grade I	1–2 cm	Bulging	2–3 cm	Covers up to half of trigone	Up to 20 grams
Grade II	2–3 cm	Touching in midline	3–4 cm	Covers more than half of trigone	20–50 grams
Grade III	3–4 cm	Touching 2–3 cm	4–5 cm	Covers more than trigone	50–125 grams
Grade IV	> 4 cm	Touching more than 3 cm	More than 5 cm	Extends up to fundus	More than 125 grams

males which is the cervix and above it the retroverted uterus. Prolapsed ovaries may be felt in the rectouterine pouch. As one goes down below with one's finger the rectovaginal septum and the perineal body are also palpated. A combined per-rectal and per-vaginal examination may be helpful in a female to rule out pathologies of the recto-vaginal septum and the pouch of Douglas.

Black stools result from degraded blood (melena), iron, licorice, bismuth, rhubarb, or overindulgence in chocolate cookies. Red-colored stools may be due to brisk bleeding known as haematochezia (usually distal to the ligament of Treitz), whereas patients under treatment for tuberculosis may complain of red- or orange-coloured stools due to rifampin. One of the first symptoms of hepatobiliary disease is the develop-ment of tan stools and dark urine. Very rarely, a patient with carcinoma of the ampulla of Vater presents with a complaint of silver stools.

Summary: Scheme of digital ano-rectal examination

- Inspection of the perianal region
  - At rest
  - On straining
- Palpation with index finger (in males)
- Start with gentle pressure posteriorly on sphincter
  - Assess tone of sphincter
  - Rotate finger anteriorly in a gentle fashion
  - Anterior wall
- Prostate
- Seminal vesicles and trigonal region
- Recto-vesical pouch
  - Left lateral wall
  - Posteriorly hollow of sacrum and coccyx
  - Right lateral wall
- Palpation with index finger (in females)
  - Start with gentle pressure posteriorly on sphincter
  - Assess tone of sphincter
  - Rotate finger anteriorly in a gentle fashion
  - Anterior wall
- Cervix (landmark to relate to other structures)
- Pouch of Douglas
- Recto-vaginal septum
- Perineal body
  - Left lateral wall
  - Posteriorly hollow of sacrum and coccyx
  - Right lateral wall
- Inspection of the stool stained finger
- Wipe lubricant and discard gloves.

What is the pathophysiology behind various lower urinary tract symptoms?

Storage Symptoms

Frequency: Frequency is defined as increase in the number of times a patient has to void. Normally a healthy adult voids about 4–5 times during the day with an average voided volume of 300–400 cc. Due to bladder outlet obstruction the patient voids incompletely and a large volume of urine still remains stored within the bladder. Bladder outlet obstruction causes dynamic changes such as detrusor hyperactivity. Due to detrusor overactivity there is increased sensation to void leading to frequency.

Urgency: When about 150 ml of urine collects within the bladder healthy adults have the first desire to void, however, if inhibited due to lack of a suitable time and place the desire can be supp-ressed uptil the bladder is filled to about 400 ml. At this point there is a strong desire which can still be controlled for some time but with difficulty. Dynamic changes caused by outlet obstruction lead to increase in sensitivity of the bladder and detrusor overactivity as described above leading to a strong desire to pass urine even at a low volume. Patients are unable to hold urine and have to rush to the toilet. This is described as urgency. Sometimes it is so severe that detrusor contracts against will leading to loss of urine before the act of micturition starts. This is defined as urge incontinence.

Nocturia: Nocturia can simply be explained as frequency during the night time. While the pheno-menon causative of frequency operate at night as well, additional physiological processes come into play when the position changes from sitting or standing to supine. The dependent edema is relieved and interstitial fluid moves into the circulation causing increase in circulating volume leading to increased urine production.

Urge incontinence: Inability to hold the urine when the patient has desire to micturate.

Voiding Symptoms

Symptoms related stream: These symptoms include narrowing of stream, loss of force in the stream , intermittent stream, straining during micturition, or loss of stream.

Hesitancy: Hesitancy can be defined as a delay to start micturition or difficulty in beginning the flow. Patient has a strong desire to pass urine but he has to wait for a while before he can start the act of micturition. Hesitancy arises due to a mismatch between the pressures generated by detrusor to overcome the resistance offered by the outlet. It is seen in conditions that increase the resistance offered by the bladder outlet. However, it can also be seen in neurogenic bladder if detrusor fails to produce sufficient pressure.

Intermittency: Intermittency is defined as abrupt stoppage of urinary stream in between the act of micturition. Intermittency is also a result of transient mismatch between the pressures generated by detrusor to overcome the resistance offered by the outlet.

Incomplete evacuation of bladder: Patient get sense of incomplete evacuation of bladder after act of micturition attributed to the residual urine.

Terminal dribbling: Terminal dribbling can be defined as leak or involuntary loss of urine after micturition has ceased. It is a sign of a weak sphincter tone or high post-void residual urine which the detrusor tries to expel when the sphincters have contracted. Terminal dribbling is distinguished from post-micturition dribbling in that it occurs at the end of completion of micturition and is a part of the micturition cycle but not when the patient has left the toilet or as a separate event.

Poor urinary stream and duplication of the urinary stream are other important and bothersome voiding symptoms.

What is benign prostatic hyperplasia?

Prostate starts developing in male patients after puberty and grows to the level of obstruction specially after the age of 50 years under the influence of dihydrotestosterone which is a derivate of testosterone resulting from the action of 5α reductase type II enzyme. There is increase in the number of stromal and epithelial components resulting in expansion of the gland and compression of the prostatic urethra which is enclosed by the gland. This leads to dynamic changes leading to detrusor hypertrophy and disordered bladder contraction. Thus both static and dynamic components lead to obstruction.

Benign prostatic hyperplasia commonly originates from the transitional zone in the form of an adenoma. Symptoms may depend upon the region from which the adenoma arises. Median lobe hypertrophy in particular may lead to severe obstructive symptoms even when the overall gland size is small. Histologically adenomas first arise in the region of the periprostatic sphincter and gradually foci spread within the transition or periurethral zone. The presence of the prostatic capsule prevents outward growth leading to production of urinary compression. Other factors like urethral resistance and anatomical variations also play an important role in prostatic symptomatology. Size has been rarely seen to coordinate well with the degree of obstruction and symptoms.

What are the various hormones that play a role in BPH?

Hyperplasia in BPH is not due to an increase in active division of cells but more importantly due to impaired cell aging, which reduces the rate of apoptosis. Androgens which play a major role in development and aging of prostate also inhibit the death of cells. The derived form of androgen, called Dihydrotestosterone (DHT) is the principal androgen acting on the prostate via high affinity androgen receptor protein. It forms 90% of the total prostatic androgen. The real function of DHT consists of promoting the expression of specific genes through a fine molecular mechanism, leading to synthesis of growth-stimulating or growth-inhibiting factors that modulate cell proliferation and function. The complete pattern of molecular factors involved in this mechanism is not yet completely defined but it has been found that after androgen withdrawal and antiandrogen treatment, the androgen responsive prostate cancer cells cease to proliferate and undergo apoptosis, causing tumour regression, and these include essentially the epithelial rather than the stromal cells.

Enzyme 5 alpha reductase is essential for the conversion of testosterone to DHT and is present in two isoforms. Type 1 predominates in liver, skin and other extraprostatic sites and is not affected in 5 alpha reductase deficiency syndrome. Type 2 isoform is present in prostate and unlike type 1 is critical for growth of the gland and BPH. It is essentially located in the stroma. There is evidence that androgens also maintain gland vascularity.

Estrogens also have a unique role to play in BPH. They increase androgen receptor (AR) expression in the aging prostate and contribute to growth despite of normal or decreased levels of androgens in the circulation. Estrogen alpha receptor is present in the stroma while the beta receptor is expressed by the epithelial cells. With age the level of estrogen is seen to increase within the prostate especially in patients with BPH. Currently, the actual role of estrogens in prostatic growth remains largely unclear.

Apart from these two major hormones various growth factors like FGF, VEGF and IGF also play a role in growth of the prostate.

What is international prostatic symptom score?

The IPSS score is an internationally validated scoring system to objectively assess the degree of bother in lower urinary tract symptoms. The scoring system is given in Table 22.2.

Table 22.2: International prostatic symptom scoring system						
	Not at all	Less than 1 time in 5	Less than half the time	About half the time	More than half the time	Almost Always
1. Incomplete emptying: Over the past month, how often have you had a sensation of not emptying your bladder completely after you finished urinating?	0	1	2	3	4	5
2. Frequency: Over the past month, how often have you had to urinate again less than 2 hours after you finished urinating?	0	1	2	3	4	5
3. Intermittency: Over the past month, how often have you found you stopped and started again several times when you urinated?	0	1	2	3	4	5
4. Urge to urinate: Over the past month, how often have you found it difficult to postpone urination?	0	1	2	3	4	5
5. Weak stream: Over the past month, how often have you had a weak urinary stream?	0	1	2	3	4	5
6. Straining: Over the past month, how often have you had to push or strain to begin urination?	0	1	2	3	4	5
	None	1 time	2 times	3 times	4 times	5+times
7. Urinating at night: Over the past month, how many times did you most typically get up to urinate from the time you went to bed at night until the time you got up in the morning?	0	1	2	3	4	5

Symptom Score

1–7 mild, 8–19 moderate, 20–35 severe   Total: _____

Bothersome score due to urinary symptoms						
	Delighted	Pleased	Mostly satisfied	Mixed	Mostly dissatisfied	Unhappy	Terrible
Quality of life due to urinary symptoms: How would you feel if you had to live with your urinary condition the way it is now – no better, no worse – for the rest of your life?	0	1	2	3	4	5	6

What is prostatic specific antigen and what are the important considerations during its interpretation?

However, total Serum PSA is also increased in inflammatory conditions of the prostate like prostatic abscess and acute and chronic prostatitis. It rises transiently after digital rectal examination, prostatic biopsy and transurethral resection. Interpretation of the results should be done with caution. PSA values more than 4 ng/ml should raise concern over prostatic carcinoma and values more than 10 ng/ml are associated with high chances of harboring prostate cancer. In between 4–10 ng/ml chances are equivocal and additional tests like PSA density, PSA velocity, and prostate health index may be useful in further clarifying the need of prostate biopsy in such scenarios. Patients who have findings and PSA levels suspicious of carcinoma of the prostate have to be subjected to a 12 core sextant transrectal ultrasound guided biopsy.

How is the treatment for BPH planned?

The management for BPH includes medical management along with lifestyle changes or surgical management in presence of accepted indications. Medical management is preferred initially in all cases and only if it fails does one switch over to surgery. The accepted indications for switching over to surgery include:

- Poor symptom control with no improvement in IPSS scores with medical management in patients having scores between 8 and 19.

- IPPS scores more than 20 or patient having mainly obstructive symptoms with objective evidence of obstruction like peak flow rate less than 15 ml per second or post-void residual residual urine more than 100–150 ml.

- Recurrent urinary tract infections
- Hematuria, stone formation
- Deterioration of kidney function due to obstruction (obstructive uropathy)
- Acute urinary retention (recurrent)
- Chronic retention of urine

The options for medical management include non-selective and selective alpha blockers. Selective alpha blockers are treatment of choice. The common alpha blockers and their advantages and disadvantages are summarized in Table 22.3.

Patients with PSA > 2.5 ng/ml or volume more than 30 grams have been found to have greater increase in prostate volume and addition of 5α reductase inhibitors like finasteride (inhibits enzyme α reductase type II) or dutasteride (inhibits enzyme 5α reductase type I and II) can be useful in reducing or halting growth of the gland.

Practically the effect of alpha blockers can be seen as early as 3–7 days while 5α-reductase inhibitors take 4–6 weeks to exert effects. These inhibitors also reduce the level of PSA by 50% over a period of 6 months to 1 year and even further over 2–5 years. Hence PSA levels should be cautiously interpreted when patients are on this drug.

Table 22.3: α-blockers and their advantages and disadvantages				
Name	Action	Dose	Advantage	Disadvantage
Tamsulosin	α_1 A blocker	0.4 mg HS	Effective symptom control	Retrograde ejaculation, rhinitis, postural hypotension, nasal congestion, floppy iris syndrome
Alfuzosin	α_1 A blocker	10 mg HS	Effective control preferred in sexually active males	Postural hypotension, asthenia, headache, drowsiness
Naftopidil	α_1 D blocker	50 mg HS	Effective nocturnal control	Postural hypotension, dizziness, flushing, palpitations
Silodosin	α_1 A blocker	8 mg HS	Effective control	Rhinitis, postural hypotension, nasal congestion, retrograde ejaculation
Terazosin	α_1 blocker	2 mg HS	Useful in hypertensives	Rhinitis, dizziness, drowsiness, dyspnea postural hypotension, nasal congestion, chest pain
Doxazosin	α_1 blocker	10–20 mg	Useful in hypertensives	Headache, fatigue, pain, hypotension, edema, dry mouth, dyspnea, muscle weakness, tinnitus, rhinitis, vision anomalies, sexual dysfunction and impotence

The available surgical therapies for management of benign prostatic hyperplasia include:

- Minimally invasive therapies
  - Transurethral microwave heat treatment
  - Transurethral needle ablation of the prostate
  - Prostatic urethral stenting
  - UroLift
- Surgical therapies
  - Transurethral resection of the prostate
  - Transurethral electrovaporization
  - Transurethral incision of the prostate
  - Transurethral holmium laser resection/enucleation
  - Transurethral laser vaporization
  - Transurethral laser coagulation
  - Open prostatectomy

How is transurethral resection of the prostate performed?

TURP is the gold standard in surgical management of the prostate and involves the removal of the prostate through the urethra. The resectoscope is a special instrument using which chips of the prostate are removed piecemeal using electric current from within the urethra. Chips are resected uptil the prostate capsule is seen on all sides and no resection is performed beyond or distal to the verumontanum as just below it lie the fibers of the external sphincter. Resection below the verumontanum risks injury to the external sphincter. After the surgery an empty fossa is created within the capsule of the prostate that slowly gets covered by urothelium and contracts. Continuous irrigation with 1.5% glycine is used for performing the procedure to keep a good vision.

What are the common complications of TURP?

The common complications associated with TURP include:

Early complications:
- Haemorrhage
- Rectal injury
- Capsular perforation
- Bladder injury
- Dysuria
- Clot retention (3.5%):
  - Cystoscopy and clot evacuation should be done
- Capsular perforation (2%):

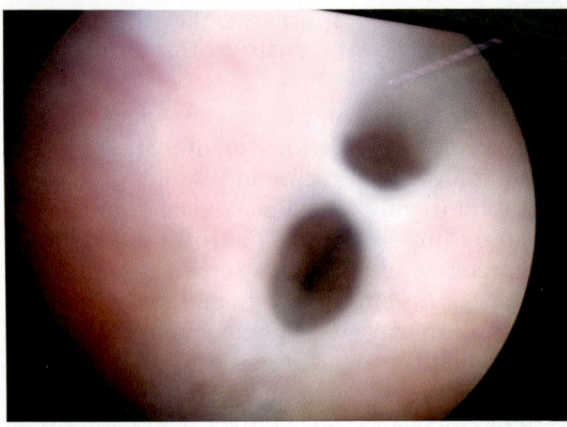

Fig. 22.5: Endoscopic view of a case of stricture urethra

- It is characterized by extravasation of fluid
- Manifested by restlessness, nausea, vomiting and abdominal pain despite anaesthesia
- Once detected haemostasis must be secured and procedure terminated
- An SPC may be done if significant extravasation is suspected.
- Transurethral resection (TUR) syndrome (2%):
  - It becomes symptomatic usually when serum sodium falls below 125 mEq/l
  - Usually occurs if resection time exceeds more than 90 min usually in gland volume of more than 75 mg.
  - TUR syndrome is manifested by confusion vomiting, hypertension with bradycardia.
  - 20 ml per minute fluid is absorbed by patient amounting up to a total of 1000 ml during the complete procedure

Late complications:
- Bladder neck contracture
- Urethral stricture (Fig. 22.5)
- Incontinence
- Secondary or delayed haemorrhage
- Urinary tract infection
- Retrograde ejaculation.

What are the indications of doing an open prostatectomy?

Open prostatectomy has the advantage of a more complete removal of the gland under vision with no incidence of TUR syndrome and lower rates of recurrence and reoperation. It employs a lower midline incision with disadvantage of more blood loss and longer postoperative stay. The procedure has fallen out of vogue as it is associated with more morbidity with regards to the presence of an incision line and prolonged hospitalization, but it results in better IPSS, PFR improvement, less re-operation rate, and less dysuria.

Open prostatectomy is a useful alternative when transurethral resection cannot be done. These indications include:

- Huge prostate size more than 100 grams (higher chances of TUR syndrome in prolonged surgery)
- Associated cardiac conditions like CHF in a setting of fluid overload
- Pathology of hip joint precluding lithotomy position
- Large size diverticulum that cannot be managed endoscopically (both can be managed by open surgery)
- Large bladder stones that cannot be managed endoscopically
- Associated urethral conditions like complicated stricture or previous hypospadias repair (trans-urethral route is not possible)
- Patients requiring simultaneous ureteric reimplantation
- Associated inguinal hernia along with BPH
- Patients with known coagulopathy (bleeding is easier to control during open surgery)

The following methods are used for open pro-statectomy:

- Suprapubic (Frayer's procedure)
- Retropubic (Millin's procedure)
- Trans-perineal (Young's procedure)

How can benign prostatic hyperplasia be differentiated from prostatic carcinoma?

Benign prostatic hyperplasia originates from the transitional zone while carcinoma arises from the peripheral zone of the prostate. Prostatic cancer can be suspected on the basis of positive family history, suspected digital rectal examination findings and serum PSA levels. Due to peripheral origin digital examination carries utmost value. Nodules may be palpable which are distinct, non-tender and hard. Rarely rectal mucosa may be fixed to these nodules signifying possibility of malignancy. Total serum PSA is increased in patients with carcinoma prostate and the amount of free PSA is reduced. Even though prostatic cancer cells do not produce more PSA compared to the normal cell there is increased access to the blood stream leading to increased level of PSA. Free PSA levels are decreased as total PSA escapes

proteolytic cleavage in cancer cells. The ratio of free to total PSA or percentage of free PSA is decreased (cutoff <18% provides high sensitivity and specificity).

How is prostate cancer diagnosed?

The diagnosis of prostate cancer is mainly based on PSA screening in the modern times. Occasionally it may also be diagnosed incidentally on histopathological examination of the TURP chips. If the PSA is raised, patients are subjected to transrectal biopsy of the prostate guided by ultrasound. A minimum of 12 cores should be taken. The sensitivity and specificity of 6–8 cores is low and the standard sextant biopsy provides just the right balance between invasion and results. If the PSA is high and the biopsy turns out to be negative, the PSA is followed up to observe a decline. Otherwise, the biopsy is repeated with special precautions like, use of transperineal biopsy rather than transrectal biopsy, MRI and TRUS fusion biopsy, additional sampling from the transitional zone and anterior regions and satura-tion biopsy (20–24 cores). Use of multiparametric MRI may be used to direct the biopsy needle to the suspected sites and to support the possibility of prostate cancer.

What is the natural course of prostate cancer?

The incidence of prostate cancer rises as age progresses and at the age of 90 years and above the risk of harboring prostate cancer as found at the time of autopsy is 90% and higher. In most patients, however, the cancer is low grade and indolent and patients usually die with the disease than of it. There are two forms of the cancer, namely sporadic and hereditary. Hereditary prostate cancer presents earlier in life and detected at an age younger than 50 years. Hereditary cancer is more aggressive and may be associated with higher chances of recurrence. A recurrent prostate cancer shows excellent response to locally ablative therapy in the form of radiotherapy or radical prostatectomy for a period of 7–10 years, after which the disease burden may rise again. At this conjuncture androgen deprivation therapy may be needed and the growth is suppressed for a period of another 5 years. However, due to the develop-ment of hormone resistance rescue therapy needs to be started to take care of the increasing disease burden. The cancer eventually metastasizes and chemotherapy and second line hormonal agents may prolong the survival in androgen independence recurrence.

What are the risk factors for prostate cancer?

Older age and African American race are important risk factors for prostate cancer. Hereditary factor has an important role and up to 15% of prostate cancer is hereditary with disease starting below the age of 50 years. Obesity or higher BMI is also associated with a higher risk of prostate cancer. Other risk factors have not been proven in the causation of prostate cancer but have been implicated as associations which include high calcium, high fat intake, prostatitis, and even vasectomy.

How is prostate cancer staged?

TX: Primary tumour cannot be assessed

T0: No evidence of primary tumour

T1: Clinically inapparent tumour neither palpable nor visible by imaging

- T1a: Tumour incidental histologic finding in 5% or less of tissue resected
- T1b: Tumour incidental histologic finding in more than 5% of tissue resected
- T1c: Tumour identified by needle biopsy (for example, because of elevated PSA)

T2: Tumour confined within prostate

- T2a: Tumour involves one-half of one lobe or less
- T2b: Tumour involves more than one-half of one lobe but not both lobes
- T2c: Tumour involves both lobes

T3: Tumour extends through the prostate capsule

- T3a: Extracapsular extension (unilateral or bilateral)
- T3b: Tumour invades seminal vesicle(s)

T4: Tumour is fixed or invades adjacent structures other than seminal vesicles, such as external sphincter, rectum, bladder, levator muscles, and/or pelvic wall

NX: Regional lymph nodes were not assessed

N0: No regional lymph node metastasis

N1: Metastasis in regional lymph node(s)

M0: No distant metastasis

M1: Distant metastasis

- M1a: Non-regional lymph node(s)

- M1b: Bone(s)
- M1c: Other site(s) with or without bone disease

Staging of prostate cancer

Group	T N M PSA Gleason
Stage I	T1a–c: N0 M0 PSA <10 Gleason ≤6
	T2a: N0 M0 PSA <10 Gleason ≤6
	T1–2a: N0 M0 PSA X Gleason X
Stage IIA	T1a–c: N0 M0 PSA <20 Gleason 7
	T1a–c: N0 M0 PSA ≥10<20 Gleason ≤6
	T2a: N0 M0 PSA ≥10<20 Gleason ≤6
	T2a: N0 M0 PSA <20 Gleason 7
	T2b: N0 M0 PSA <20 Gleason ≤7
	T2b: N0 M0 PSA X Gleason X
Stage IIB	T2c: N0 M0 Any PSA Any Gleason
	T1–2: N0 M0 PSA ≥20 Any Gleason
	T1–2: N0 M0 Any PSA Gleason ≥8
Stage III	T3a–b: N0 M0 Any PSA Any Gleason
Stage IV	T4: N0 M0 Any PSA Any Gleason
	Any T N1 M0 Any PSA Any Gleason
	Any T Any N M1 Any PSA Any Gleason

What is Gleason's score and what is its importance?

The Gleason scale was developed by physician Donald Gleason in the 1960s to help predict the aggressiveness of prostate cancer. Based on glandular differentiation at low power Grade/pattern is differentiated into grades varying from 1 to 5. Based on Gleason grade of the first and second most predominant patterns on examination a score is provided. The range of scores is from 2 to 10. Well-differentiated tumours with a score of 2–4 are indolent and rarely aggressive while patients with a Gleason's score of 8–10 have high likelihood of dying from the disease. If only one pattern can be recognized on the tissue the primary and secondary patterns are given the same grade, e.g. 4+4 or 3+3. Secondary patterns are also not reported if they are present in <5% of the tumour in presence of a higher grade. However, Gleason score is unable to predict the aggressiveness and prognosis if there is only minimal tumour on biopsy (1 mm or less). When Gleason's scoring is done for specimens of radical prostatectomy, any tertiary pattern if present must be mentioned by the pathologists but they are not considered in the final scoring. There is a marked difference in the prognosis of 4+3 cancer compared to 3+4 cancer even though the total score for both is 7.

What are the various treatment options for patients with prostatic cancer?

Treatment options for prostate cancer depend upon the stage of the disease at presentation but grossly there are two forms of management strategies: curative and palliative.

- If the disease is localized to the prostate and the patient has a reasonable life expectancy of more than 10 years based on his current performance status and associated comorbidities, the patient can be offered treatments to ablate or remove the tumour. The procedure of choice is radical prostatectomy. Lymph nodes are removed only if the chances of involvement are high (>5% as per Partin's Normograms). Radical prostatectomy is offered to patients with PSA < 20 ng/ml, Gleason score 7 and disease confined to the capsule. A higher PSA is an indicator of widespread disease and a Gleason score more than 7 is an aggressive disease with no better results with radical prostatectomy. But in carefully selected patients with cT3a cancer, Gleason score 8–10 or PSA >20 ng/ml radical prostatectomy is a reasonable treatment modality. Extended lymph node dissection involves removal of the nodes over external iliac artery and vein, within the obturator fossa, and nodes around the internal iliac artery. Adjuvant therapy is needed when more than two nodes are involved with the tumour.

- Active surveillance can also be offered as a treatment modality to patients with very low risk prostate cancer that is patients with over 10 years of life expectancy, cT1-2, PSA <10 ng/mL, Gleason score <6 with <2 positive biopsies positive for tumour and minimal biopsy core involvement (<50% cancer). These patients are followed up with 6 monthly digital examination, PSA measurement and repeat biopsy. If there is any progression, patients can be offered radical surgery.

- Patient who have a short life expectancy can be offered watchful waiting. It can also be offered to those patients who are unwilling for any intervention for their condition.

- Intensity-modulated radiotherapy (IMRT), with or without image-guided radiotherapy (IGRT), is the gold standard for external beam radiotherapy of the prostate and it can be offered to patients with localized cancer who decline surgery. For locally advanced disease ERBT can be offered in combination with androgen deprivation therapy. In patient with very high risk disease T3–T4 with N1, pelvic external irradiation and immediate long-term adjuvant hormonal treatment is the recommended modality of management.

- In patients with localized prostate cancer unwilling for surgery or radiotherapy, high-intensity focused ultrasound can be offered with counselling regarding lack of prospective data on survival beyond a decade.

The other form of therapy available is palliative therapy which can be offered to patients with metastatic tumour or high risk tumours with short life expectancy and adverse prognostic factors. Such patients can be offered bilateral orchiectomy, or medical castration in the form of estrogens, LHRH agonists and anti-androgens apart from special focus on bone health, anaemia and other oncological emergencies like spinal cord compression.

What are the agents available for androgen deprivation therapy?

Both surgical and medical alternatives are available for androgen deprivation therapy and a comprehensive list of these agents has been presented below. Some medical alternatives may produce a transient upsurge or flare in the levels of testosterone and this has been prevented by the addition of anti-androgens to medical and surgical therapy. Such a combination is referred to as combined androgen blockade (CAB). Whether this combination has a definite advantage over castration is a matter of debate. Only a marginal decrease in the death rate has been demonstrated by adding anti-androgens. Combined androgen blockade has an important role in patient with symptomatic bony metastasis and impending cord compression where flare may produce severe symptoms and life threatening complications. These symptoms can also be prevented by a week prior administration of non-steroidal anti-androgens before initiation of LHRH agonist therapy.

What are the side effects of androgen deprivation therapy?

The side effects of androgen deprivation therapy include, diminished libido, erectile dysfunction,

Table 22.4: Side effects of androgen deprivation therapy

Class	Drug name	Mechanism of action	Notable side effects
Drugs acting on the pituitary			
GnRH agonists	Leuprolide Goserelin Triptorelin Histrelin	Desensitization of LHRH receptors	Flare reaction
GnRH antagonists	Abarelix Degarelix	Inhibition of LHRH receptors	Anaphylaxis
Drugs acting on the adrenal gland Adrenal ablating agents	Aminoglutethimide Ketoconazole Abiraterone	Decreases androgen synthesis from steroid precursors	Adrenal insufficiency
Drugs acting on the prostate			
Androgen receptor antagonists	Steroidal: Cyproterone acetate	Competitively inhibit androgen receptor ligand binding domain	Liver dysfunction, gynaecomastia, breast tenderness
	First generation non-steroidal: flutamide, bicalutamide, nilutamide Second generation non-steroidal: Engalutamide RD 162		
5α–reductase inhibitors	Finasteride Dutasteride	Inhibits conversion of testosterone to dihydro-testosterone	Sexual side effects, erectile dysfunction
Oestrogen	Diethylstilbestrol	Direct apoptotic effect on prostate cells, exploits the anti-androgen effects of oestrogen	Cardiovascular complications, DVT, transient ischaemic effect, oedema, gynaecomastia

hot flashes, weight gain of 10 to 15 pounds, mood swings, depression, fatigue, anaemia (normocytic normochromic), osteoporosis, memory loss, elevated cholesterol and breast and nipple tenderness. To reduce these effects the concept of intermittent androgen deprivation (IAD) came into existence. IAD was also proposed to delay the emergence of hormone resistance. With the current amount of data in hand the benefits seem limited with no beneficial advantages in sexual function and quality of life. The reduction in adverse myocardial events and osteoporosis also appear to be comparable with IAD vs. conventional ADT. Intermittent androgen deprivation is being increasingly used as an alternative to continuous ADT in advanced and recurrent prostate cancer. There is level I evidence supporting the oncologic equivalence of intermittent and continuous blockade in patients with biochemical failure. Compared with CAD, IAD is associated with better quality of life and less side effects; however,

patient selection is important to maintain good results. IAD must be administered with caution in men with bone metastases. In patients who have a complete biochemical response, a trial of IAD can be given. If there is a rapid rise in PSA, these patients can be restarted on continuous therapy.

Hot flushes are the most common side effect of ADT affecting the majority of patients. Loss of libido is also a common side effect, with only about 20% patients being able to maintain sexual activity. Loss of muscle mass and increase in body fat can lead to change in body habitus and also predispose to metabolic syndrome, diabetes and cardiovascular morbidity. Painful gynaecomastia can be cured by prophylactic radiation. Cosmetic concerns are managed by subcutaneous mastectomy or liposuction. Management of all complications is essentially symptomatic and discontinuation of therapy is rarely indicated. Interestingly patients who develop resistance to therapy still remain on ADT (Table 22.4).

How is androgen deprivation therapy monitored?

Serum PSA and serum testosterone are two important indicators for monitoring ADT. Agents must be able to inhibit testosterone synthesis from the major sources and this is reflected by a reduction in serum testosterone levels to less than 50 ng/dL. If the levels are more than this, the androgen ablation may be insufficient and prostatic growth may be taking place. The degree of fall in PSA is also an important predictor of the response to androgen deprivation therapy. Monitoring PSA levels can predict progression and emergence of hormone resistant disease. The absolute PSA levels 6 months after therapy has also been found to be a useful predictor of response.

What is radical prostatectomy and what are its complications?

Radical prostatectomy consists of removal of the prostate along with surrounding fascia, seminal vesicles, ejaculatory duct and 2–4 cm of the vas on each side. Transperineal and trans-abdominal routes (open, laparoscopic and robotic) are available options and trans-abdominal route is preferred when lymphadenectomy is indicated. Radical prostatectomy involves mobilization of the prostate and freeing it from the pelvic floor and its blood supply. It is separated from the rest of the urethra after ligation of the dorsal venous complex and from the bladder by incision over the bladder neck. The membranous urethra and the bladder neck are then anastomosed to form the new vesico-urethral junction.

The common complications associated with radical prostatectomy and lymphadenectomy include haemorrhage involving injury to major vessels, injury to the cavernous nerves leading to impotence, rectal injury, bladder injury, urinary incontinence and anastomotic strictures.

How are patients with prostate cancer followed up?

Patients with prostate cancer require regular follow up on conservative and palliative therapy as well as after definitive therapy. Patient who are asymptomatic should undergo history and examination including rectal exam and PSA measurement at 3, 6 and 12 months after treatment followed by 6 monthly for 3 years and then annually. After surgery the PSA levels should fall to undetectable levels but a rise to more than 0.2 ng/ml after surgery denotes recurrence or residual tumour. After management with radiation therapy rise in PSA values by 2 ng/ml or three consecutive rises in PSA is significant and warrants further therapy.

If PSA levels rise after androgen ablation and testosterone levels are within castrate limits, consideration needs to be given to hormone refractory prostate cancer which may require initiation of chemotherapy with docetaxel or initiation of abiraterone to prolong survival.

23

Soft Tissue Sarcoma

What is sarcoma?

The word sarcoma is derived from the greek word "srax" meaning flesh. The sarcomas are malignancies of connective tissue arising from fatty tissue, muscle, blood vessels or bones. Most of these are mesodermal in origin except Ewing sarcoma, neuro-sarcoma and the primitive neuroetodermal tumour (PTEN).

What is the common clinical presentation?

Clinical presentation depend upon the site and most common presentations are:

1. Painless lump in extremity which is rapidly growing firm to hard in consistency. In case of lump on extremity the overlying skin temperature may be raised to increased vascularity with lot of engorged veins over the tumour. Pain is seen at presentation in one-third of cases only. On physical examination size of swelling, relation to deeper structures like fascia or muscle, mobility of mass and proximity to neurovascular structures or bone should be noted. As a rule any soft tissue which is rapidly enlarging or symptomatic, any deep seated lump irrespective of size or superficial mass more than 5 cm should be biopsied.

2. Debilitating pain due to involvement of nerves.

3. Site specific symptoms due to compression or involvement of neurovascular structures.

4. Intestinal obstruction in cases of leiomyosarcoma of intestine.

5. Symptoms due to haematogenous spread, e.g. haemoptysis.

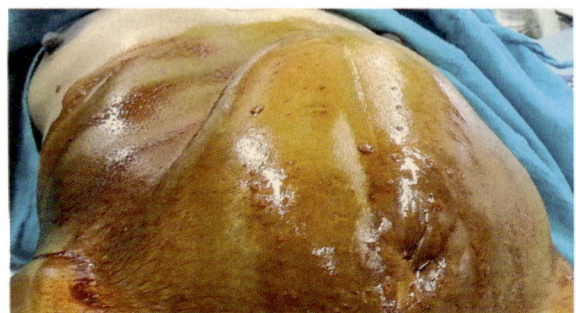

Fig. 23.1: Retroperitoneal tumour presenting as an abdominal mass

6. Patient may have nonspecific symptoms like weight loss or anorexia.

7. Abdominal lump displacing the gut (Fig. 23.1).

What is incidence of STS?

It accounts for <1 % of all adult malignancies and 15% of paediatric malignancies.

What are the risk factors for STS?

Risk factors for STS are:

1. *Radiation:* Radiation induced sarcoma generally occurs at least 3–4 years to decades later near the site of external beam radiation. Radiation induced sarcomas are generally malignant fibrous histiocytoma (MFH), angiosarcoma or osteosarcoma. Sarcoma arises in heavily irradiated extremities (50 Gy or more).

2. *Chemical:* Exposures to phenoxyacetic herbicides, chlorophenols and dioxins predisposes to development of STS.

3. *Genetic factors*:
   a. *Neurofibromatosis*: 2% of patients with neurofibromatosis develop malignant nerve sheath tumour.
   b. *Familial adenomatous polyposis (FAP)*: Desmoid can occur in patients with FAP.
   c. *Li-Fraumeni syndrome*: 36% of patients with this syndrome develop soft tissue sarcoma or bone sarcoma.

What is the mode of spread to these tumours?

The tumours most commonly metastasize by haematogenous route to lungs. But the soft tissue sarcomas which also metastasize to lymph nodes are epitheloid sarcoma, clear cell sarcoma, angiosarcoma, lymphosarcoma, rhabdomyosarcoma and malignant fibrous histiocytoma (MFH).

Enumerate various common STS in various sites.

The most common extremity tumour in adult is MFH followed by liposarcoma and leiomyosarcoma.

The most common retroperitoneal sarcoma is liposarcoma.

In children, the most common extremity sarcoma is the rhabdomyosarcoma.

How will you prove the diagnosis?

- The investigation of choice for establishing the diagnosis is core cut tissue biopsy. If core cut tissue biopsy yields negative result repeatedly, then incisional biopsy is preferred.
- In incisional biopsy of an extremity tumour, the incision should be longitudinal centred over the mass so that during definitive surgery the previous incision can be included in the resection. During incisonal biopsy adequate haemostasis should be achieved and flaps should be minimally raised to prevent cellular dissemination of the tumour cells by haematoma. Drain placement should be avoided.
- Excision biopsy is indicated only for small cutaneous or subcutaneous lesions if the tumour size is <5 cm.
- Fine needle aspiration biopsy has no role in diagnosing extremity STS but may have a role in evaluation of recurrence.
- In cases of retroperitoneal sarcomas classical CT or MRI findings are sufficient to take up the patient for definitive surgery. Image guided biopsy has limited role in the initial diagnostic evaluation of these tumours. CT guided biopsy is indicated if initial diagnosis of lymphoma, germ cell tumour or carcinoma is strongly suspected. Preoperative CT-image guided biopsy is also an indicator if patient has distant metastasis or locally advanced disease and patient is planned for preoperative chemotherapy.

How will you evaluate the extent of disease?

- In radiological imaging, MRI is preferred for the extremity and trunk tumour as it provides exact anatomical delineation. On T1 weighted images, the tumour appears as low signal intensity and on T2 weighted imaging; it appears as heterogenous high signal intensity lesion. It accurately defines tumour size, multiplicity, location and three-dimensional definitions of fascial planes (Fig. 23.2).
- CECT abdomen is preferred in cases of retroperitoneal and visceral sarcomas as it defines involvement of the contiguous structures and vascular involvement. MRI is less accurate in this perspective.
- Ultrasonography is useful only for guiding core cut biopsy and for the assessment of recurrence.

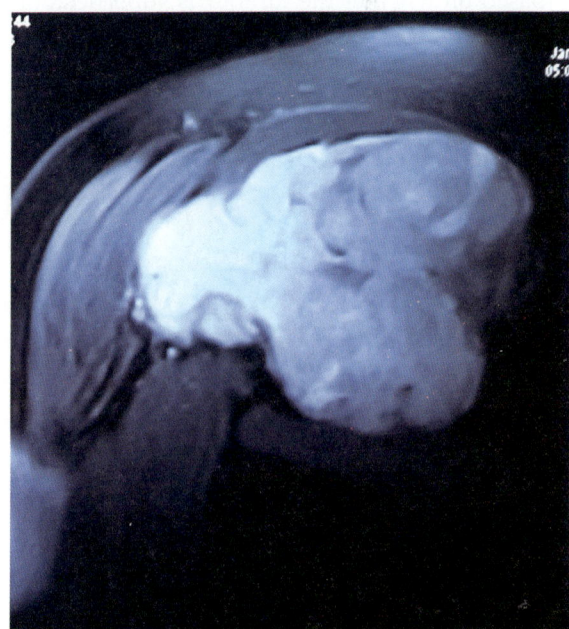

Fig. 23.2: Magnetic resonance imaging showing soft tissue sarcoma arising from the infraspinatus muscle

- Only in myxoid liposarcoma of the extremity, CECT abdomen and pelvis is indicated to assess for metastases.
- HRCT chest is indicated if there is suspicion on chest X-ray, tumour size >5 cm and if it is a high grade tumour.

What is the histopathological classification of STS?

The histopathological classification of STS are as follows:

1. Sarcomas with no malignant potential
   a. Well differentiated liposarcoma
   b. Dermatofibrosarcoma protuberans
2. Sarcomas with intermediate malignant potential
   a. Myxoid liposarcoma
   b. Extraskeletal chondrosarcoma
3. All other sarcomas are associated with high recurrence.

What is AJCC staging system?

The staging system as per the 7th AJCC is as follows:

A. *Grade*: G1—low; G2 —intermediate and G3—high
B. T1—tumour size ≤5 cm
   T2—tumour size >5 cm
   The tumour is further divided into 'A' and 'B' based on whether the tumour is superficial or deep to deep fascia respectively. The retroperitoneal and visceral sarcomas are considered 'B' lesions.
C. Lymph node involvement
   N0—no involvement and N1—lymph node involvement present
D. Metastasis
   M0—absent and M1—present

Staging

1. Stage Ia: T1a/b G1 N0 M0
   Stage Ib: T2a G1 N0 M0
2. Stage IIa: T1a/b G2/3 N0 M0
   Stage IIb: T2a G2/3 N0 M0
3. Stage IIIa: T2b G2/3 N0/1 M0
4. Stage IV: Any T Any G Any N M1.

Outline the basic principles of treatment for STS.

The basic management of soft tissue sarcoma consists of surgery followed by radiotherapy. Surgery for STS of limb should aim for maximum function preservation with limb sparing surgeries.

- Surgery typically consists of wide excision with a normal tissue margin of 1–2 cm. The deliberate removal of major neurovascular structures or bone should be avoided. In case sarcoma is in close association with bone, removal of periosteum is sufficient.
- In cases of myxoid fibro-sarcoma (previously known as myxoid MFH) more liberal excision is required as tumour is often multifocal and may spread for considerable distance along fascial planes. These tumours require excision of extensive lateral margins (2–3 cm) and 1–2 cm of deep soft tissue margins. The aim should be to include all suspicious areas of enhancement on MRI.
- Amputation is rarely needed in extremity STS (in less than 5% of cases). It should be resorted in patients in whom tumour cannot be excised by any other means but have good prospects of long-term survival like without evidence of metastatic disease with large low grade tumour causing significant functional or cosmetic deformity.
- For retroperitoneal sarcomas surgery is the mainstay of treatment. Preoperative or postoperative RT can be added. However, full dose radiation (60–66 Gy) is difficult to deliver due to the large targeted area and adjacent structures like kidney, spinal cord, bowel and liver which are sensitive to radiation.
- The radiotherapy can be delivered in the form of external beam RT, brachytherapy or intensity modulated RT.
- RT is indicated for deep, high grade sarcomas, tumour more than 5 cm, if tumour margin is close, if there is extra-muscular involvement or if there is suspected chance of local failure especially near major neurovascular structures.
- The role of chemotherapy in STS is only in cases of recurrent high grade disease and in case of systemic disease.
- The drug of choice for chemotherapy is doxorubicin.
- The treatment plan as per staging is as follows:
  - *Stage I*: Surgery and follow-up
  - *Stage II*: Surgery with or without radiotherapy
  - *Stage III*: Surgery with radiotherapy with or without chemotherapy
  - *Stage IV*: Chemotherapy followed by surgery and radiotherapy based on response.

24

Scrotal Swelling

What are the differential diagnoses of a scrotal swelling?

- Painful scrotum, tender testis
  - Epididymitis
  - Orchitis
  - Testicular torsion
  - Trauma, e.g. hematocoele
- Painful scrotum, non-tender testis
  - Incarcerated hernia
  - Insect bite
  - Inflammatory skin lesions (Fig. 24.1)
  - Torsion of testicular appendix
- Painless scrotum, testis enlarged
  - Genetic syndrome, e.g. fragile X syndrome

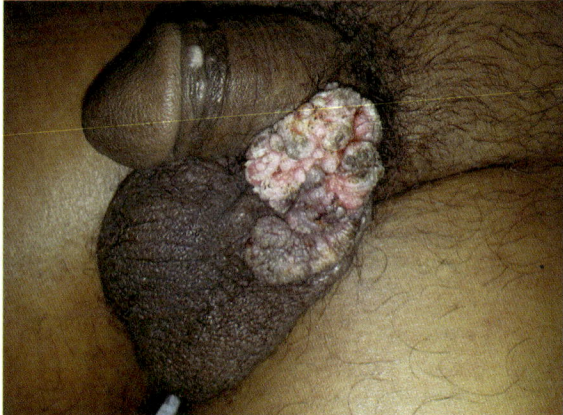

Fig. 24.2: Clinical picture of an epididymal mass infiltrating into the skin

  - Testicular torsion in newborn
  - Tumours of the testis, e.g. primary and secondary
- Painless scrotum, testis normal sized
  - Henoch-Schönlein purpura
  - Hydrocoele
  - Varicocoele
  - Scrotal edema—idiopathic or generalised
  - Paratesticular tumour (Fig. 24.2)

TESTICULAR TUMOURS

What are the predisposing factors for testicular tumours?

The recognised risk factors for testicular tumours are:

- Cryptorchidism (4–6 times more risk)

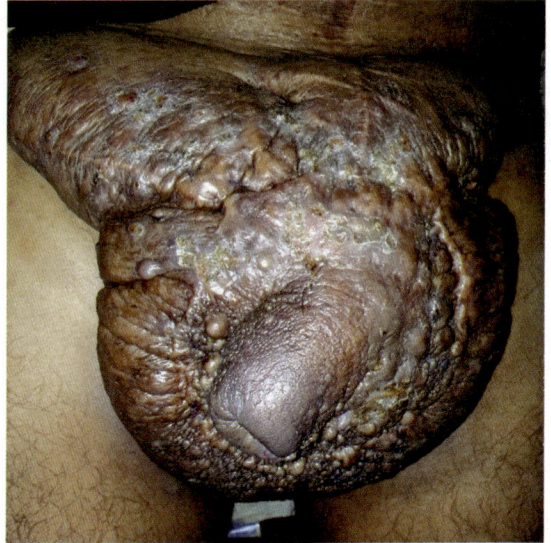

Fig. 24.1: Clinical picture of scrotal filariasis presenting as a scrotal mass

- Intra-testicular germ cell neoplasia
- Personal history of testicular tumour
- Family history of testicular tumour

How are testicular tumours classified?

WHO classification of testicular tumours is the standard classification of testicular tumours based on histological characteristics:

- Intra-tubular germ cell neoplasia

Tumors of one histologic type (pure forms):

- Seminoma
    - Seminoma with syncytiotrophoblastic cells
    - Spermatocytic seminoma
- Embryonal carcinoma
- Yolk sac tumour
- Trophoblastic tumours
    - Choriocarcinoma
    - Trophoblastic neoplasms other than chorio-carcinoma
    - Monophasic choriocarcinoma
    - Placental site trophoblastic tumour
- Teratoma (Fig. 24.3)
    - Dermoid cyst (Fig. 24.4)
    - Monodermal teratoma
    - Teratoma with somatic type malignancy (malignant transformation)

Tumours of more than one histologic subtype (mixed forms).

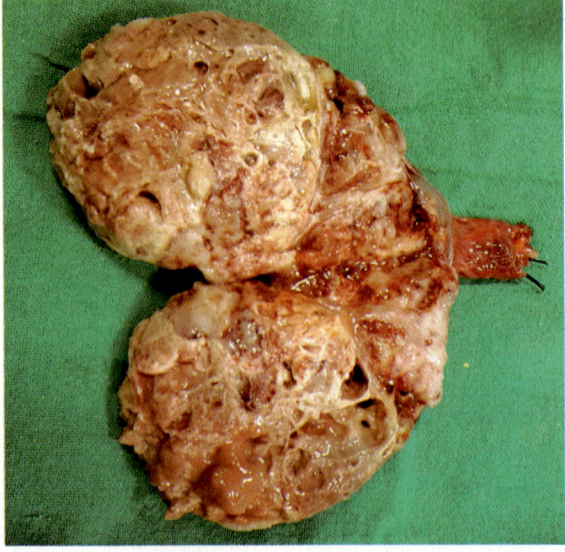

Fig. 24.3: Bisected testicular tumour (teratoma) showing variegated appearance

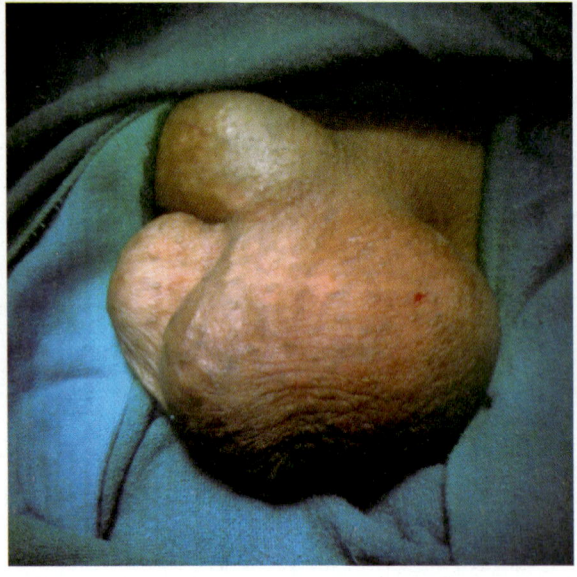

Fig. 24.4: Clinical picture of a dermoid cyst presenting as a scrotal mass

What are the various types of seminomatous germ cell tumours?

Seminomas have been classified as:

- Pure seminoma
- Spermatocytic seminoma
- Anaplastic seminoma

Seminomas occur a decade later than non-seminomatous germ cell tumours and in 15% syncytiotrophoblasts are present in pure semino-matous tumours which are responsible for elevation of β-hCG. On histopathology the cells are arranged as a sheet with clear cytoplasm and intervening fibrovascular septae. Seminomas are positive for CD30 and placental alkaline phos-phatase (PLAP).

What are the various types of non-seminomatous germ cell tumours (NSGCT)?

Non-seminomatous germ cell tumours consist of embryonal carcinoma, yolk sac tumour, chorio-carcinoma, teratomas or the mixture of these neoplasms.

Embryonal carcinoma is an aggressive tumour with high rates of metastasis. It is the most undifferentiated of all NSGCTs and can mature into other forms of NSGCT. This tumour secretes both AFP and HCG.

Yolk sac tumour often occurs as a part of mixed NSGCTs and pure yolk sac is rarely encountered.

These tumours produce AFP. These tumours exhibit hyaline globules and Schiller-Duval bodies and presence of these is associated with a lower risk of relapse.

Teratomas range from well differentiated to poorly differentiated tumours. They may show mild elevations of AFP. Embryonal tumours may transform to teratomas and proliferate at meta-static sites. Since teratomas are chemotherapy resistant, it is essential to resect them surgically. Teratomas are histologically benign but they may occasionally turn malignant and become highly aggressive and chemoresistant.

Choriocarcinoma is relatively rare and aggressive NSGCT. Usually the disease presents as a metastatic disease spreading through the hematogenous route. It is usually strongly positive for HCG.

How do testicular tumours present?

A hard painless mass in the scrotum is often the presenting symptom. It is usually pain-free unless the growth is too rapid or there is associated haemorrhage or infarction. Non-seminomatous tumours are more vascular and grow rapidly, making it more probable for them to be painful. In approximately 20% of cases the first symptom is scrotal pain and up to 27% of patients with testicular cancer may have local pain. Important differentials are other scrotal masses like hydro-coele, hematocoele and chronic epididymo-orchitis.

On examination, it is important to look for an abdominal mass as retroperitoneal lymphadeno-pathy and metastasis may be present in up to 60% of these tumours. Supraclavicular lymph nodes may be involved in some cases. Altered hormonal milieu may result in gynaecomastia (7% of NSGCTs) and decreased fertility. Secondary hydrocoele and inguinal lymphadenopathy may also be found. Loss of testicular sensation is an important sign.

What are the laboratory investigations required for diagnosis of testicular tumours?

Ultrasonography is helpful in ruling out the other differentials, ascertain presence of hydrocoele, look at the contralateral testis for presence of tumour (2% GCTs are bilateral) and occasionally to rule out a burnt primary tumour. It is advocated for all cases of testicular tumours as sensitivity in detecting a testicular tumour is almost 100%, and it has an important role in determining whether a mass is intra- or extra-testicular. Ultrasound is also indicated in follow-up of the contra-lateral testis. MRI of the scrotum may be useful in differen-tiating seminomatous from non-seminomatous lesions.

LDH, AFP and hCG are recommended in every case of suspected testicular cancer (Table 24.1). Pre-orchiectomy levels are essential. Up to 50% of tumours have been found to be associated with raised markers like LDH. PLAP is an optional marker for testicular tumours.

The initial aims of diagnosis and workup are to establish a baseline level of markers, and meta-static status into lungs, brain, bones and nodes. Abdominopelvic CT is the investigation of choice to evaluate suspicious retroperitoneal nodes (Fig. 24.5). In cases of doubt an MRI of the abdomen may be useful. A chest CT is mandatory in all patients with NSGCT as up to 10% may harbour metastasis. There is no role of CT of the head in initial workup except for cases with highly elevated hCG (>10,000 IU/L).

Table 24.1: Testicular tumour markers			
Marker	Half life	Testicular tumour	Other differentials
LDH	24 hours	All GCTs (20% of low grade and up to 60% of high grade)	Diseases of smooth, cardiac and skeletal muscles, haemolytic syndromes
AFP	5–7 days	50–70% low grade NSGCT 60–80% advanced NSGCTs (embryonal and yolk sac)	Stomach, liver, pancreatic, biliary and lung cancer, benign liver conditions and infections
hCG	24–36 hours	20–40% low stage NSGCTs 20–60% advanced NSGCTs (embryonal and choriocarcinoma) 15% of seminomas	Liver, biliary, stomach, pancreatic, lung, breast, kidney cancer

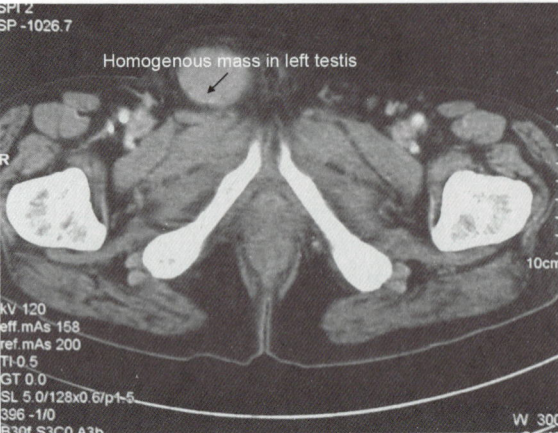

Fig. 24.5: Abdominal CT scan showing homogenous testicular mass

What is the initial management of testicular tumours?

High inguinal orchiectomy is the recommended initial therapy (Fig. 24.6). Every patient is initially subjected to inguinal exploration and orchiectomy with division of the cord at the level of the internal

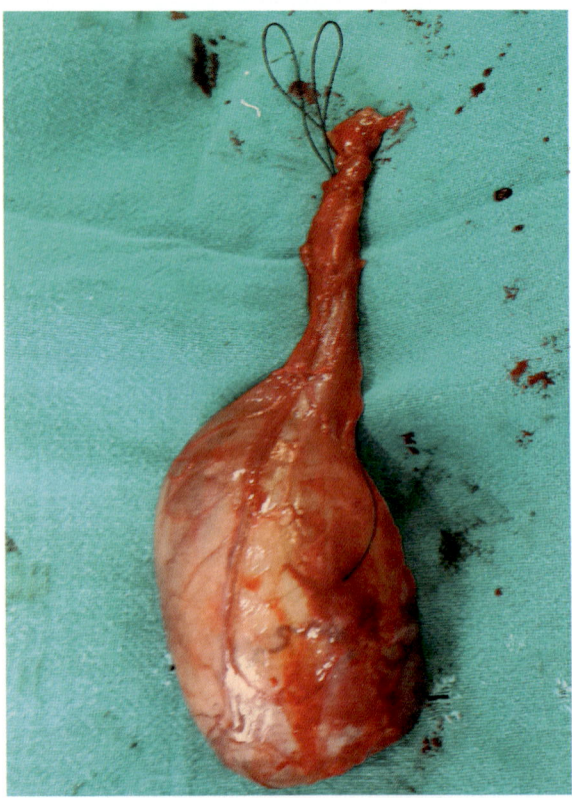

Fig. 24.6: Excised testicular tumour

inguinal ring. Only in life-threatening conditions may up-front chemotherapy be started and orchiectomy delayed for later. In synchronous bilateral testicular tumours, metachronous contra-lateral tumours or in a tumour in a solitary testis with normal preoperative testosterone levels, organ preserving surgery can be performed if tumour volume is less than 30% of testicular volume.

It is recommended that sperm preservation be offered to all patients prior to orchiectomy with potential for future families as virtually all patients develop azoospermia after chemotherapy. The recovery of fertility may take 2–5 years after chemotherapy or radiation. Similarly, surgery in the form of retroperitoneal lymph node dissection may lead to ejaculatory dysfunction in up to 80% of the patients.

What is the TNM Staging for Testicular Tumours?

pT Primary Tumour

pT   Primary tumour cannot be assessed

pT0   No evidence of primary tumour (e.g. histological scar in testis)

pTis   Intra-tubular germ cell neoplasia (carcinoma *in situ*)

pT1   Tumour limited to testis and epididymis without vascular/lymphatic invasion: Tumour may invade tunica albuginea but not tunica vaginalis

pT2   Tumour limited to testis and epididymis with vascular/lymphatic invasion, or tumour extending through tunica albuginea with involvement of tunica vaginalis

pT3   Tumour invades spermatic cord with or without vascular/lymphatic invasion

pT4   Tumour invades scrotum with or without vascular/lymphatic invasion

N Regional Lymph Nodes Clinical

Nx   Regional lymph nodes cannot be assessed

N0   No regional lymph node metastasis

N1   Metastasis with a lymph node mass 2 cm or less in greatest dimension or multiple lymph nodes, none more than 2 cm in greatest dimension

N2   Metastasis with a lymph node mass more than 2 cm but not more than 5 cm in greatest dimension, or multiple lymph nodes, any one mass more than 2 cm but not more than 5 cm in greatest dimension

N3   Metastasis with a lymph node mass more than 5 cm in greatest dimension

pN Pathological

pNx   Regional lymph nodes cannot be assessed

pN0   No regional lymph node metastasis

pN1   Metastasis with a lymph node mass 2 cm or less in greatest dimension and 5 or less positive nodes, none more than 2 cm in greatest dimension

pN2   Metastasis with a lymph node mass more than 2 cm but not more than 5 cm in greatest dimension; or more than 5 nodes positive, none more than 5 cm; or evidence or extranodal extension of tumour

pN3   Metastasis with a lymph node mass more than 5 cm in greatest dimension

M Distant Metastasis

Mx   Distant metastasis cannot be assessed

M0   No distant metastasis

M1   Distant metastasis

M1a   Non-regional lymph node(s) or lung

M1b   Other sites

S Serum Tumour Markers

Sx   Serum marker studies not available or not performed

S0   Serum marker study levels within normal limits

	LDH (U/l)	hCG (mIU/ml)	AFP (ng/ml)
S1	<1.5 × N	<5,000	<1,000
S2	1.5–10 × N	5,000–50,000	1,000–10,000
S3	>10 × N	>50,000	>10,000

How is risk stratification of testicular tumours done?

The testicular tumours are classified into various risk groups based on International Germ Cell Consensus Classification.

IGCCC Risk Classification for advanced NSGCT is as follows:

Good risk group

- Testis/retroperitoneal primary
- No non-pulmonary visceral metastases
- AFP <1,000 ng/ml
- hCG <5,000 IU/L (1,000 ng/ml)
- LDH <1.5 × ULN

(contd.)

Intermediate risk group

- Testis/retroperitoneal primary
- No non-pulmonary visceral metastases
- AFP >1,000 and <10,000 ng/ml or
- hCG >5,000 and <50,000 IU/L or
- LDH >1.5 and <10 × ULN

Poor risk group

- Mediastinal primary
- Non-pulmonary visceral metastases
- Poor serum markers
  - AFP > 10,000 mg/ml
  - hCG > 50,000 IU/L
  - LDH > 10x ULN (upper limit of normal)

IGCCC Risk Classification for advanced seminoma is as follows:

Good risk group

- Any primary site
- No non-pulmonary visceral metastases
- Normal AFP
- Any hCG
- Any LDH

Intermediate risk group

- Any primary site
- Non-pulmonary visceral metastases
- Normal AFP
- Any hCG
- Any LDH

Note that there is no poor risk category for seminomatous germ cell tumours.

What are the management guidelines for NSGCT?

Stage I NSGCT

Surveillance, Retroperitoneal Lymph Node Dissection (RPLND) and chemotherapy are all viable options in the management of early stage NSGCT. If put on surveillance, up to 30% of patients experience relapse. Up to 80% of these relapses occurs within the first year and despite surveillance up to 10% of patients present with large volume recurrent disease. Lymphovascular invasion has been found to be the important risk factor for occult metastasis from amongst advanced pathological T stage, predominant embryonal carcinoma, absence of yolk sac tumour, MIB-1 staining, patient age and tumour size. The rate of occult metastasis with lymphovascular invasion is 45–90% and that with predominant embryonal component is 30–80%. If these risk factors are absent the risk of occult metastasis is less than 20%.

Chemotherapy with Bleomycin, Etoposide and Cisplatin (PEB) as primary treatment for high-risk patients is an attractive and reliable option. Relapse rates of less than 3% have been reported with minimal toxicity in a large series, but these relapses are more difficult to treat with subsequent surgery. There is minimal impact on the quality of life and fertility. The cost effectiveness is not essentially clear and there is a risk of late chemoresistant relapse with slow growing teratomas which needs to be kept in mind. Overall chemotherapy is the single best modality that can be administered in any setting, however, it requires surveillance and has the risk of long-term toxicity.

RPLND is the other treatment possibility for clinical stage I NSGCT. Since most relapses and metastasis are retroperitoneal and the procedure offers an almost complete cure, it should be offered to the patient, at high volume centers. In more than 75% patients chemotherapy can be avoided and even if relapse occurs, the salvage rates with chemotherapy are high. Since up to 25% of the patients have teratoma in the metastasis RPLND offers the best chance of cure. If RPLND is offered to these patients, up to 30% may be found to have lymph node metastasis that corresponds to pathological stage II disease. If the nodes turn out to be negative, 10% of these patients are still found to relapse at distant sites. Risk of retroperitoneal relapse after a properly performed nerve-sparing RPLND is very low (less than 2%) and the follow up is much less costlier. If a relapse occurs, it is generally in the chest, neck or at the margins of the surgical field. Pulmonary relapses occur in 10–12% of patients and more than 90% of those relapses occur within 2 years of RPLND.

Patients without vascular invasion constitute about 50–70% of the CS1 population, and these patients have only a 15–20% risk of relapse on surveillance, compared with a 50% relapse rate in patients with vascular invasion.

As a part of risk adapted treatment patients with vascular invasion are recommended to undergo adjuvant chemotherapy with two cycles of BEP and those without vascular invasion may be put on surveillance. These patients may still

Why not RPLND	Why RPLND
Additional therapy needed in up to 50% patients	15–35% patients have no disease and avoid chemotherapy
Up to 15% have persistent disease and require full induction chemotherapy	Ejaculatory function is preserved in 70–90%
Not possible at all institutions	30% have chemoresistant teratoma
Why avoid induction chemotherapy	*Why give induction chemotherapy*
Long-term toxicity	Up to 80% have a complete response
Risk of relapse with chemorefractory GCT	95–100% cancer specific survival
	Available at all institutes

have to follow with abdominal CT as the risk of relapse in retroperitoneum is unclear. One course of adjuvant PEB is superior to RPLND with regard to recurrence rates in patients unstratified for risk factors.

Management of Clinical Stage 1S Tumours

Post-orchiectomy markers are followed up closely. Markers that rise or do not fall after orchiectomy are suggestive of residual disease. In these patients nearly 90% are pathologically positive nodes on RPLND. These patients are managed with induction chemotherapy on similar lines as those with clinical stage IIC or III disease.

Stage II NSGCT

The management of Stage II and beyond non-seminomatous tumours depends upon the histological characteristics and the prognostic grades as defined by the IGCCCG. The acceptable treatments include RPLND with or without adjuvant chemotherapy or induction chemotherapy with post-chemotherapy RPLND (PCS RPLND). Stage IIA/IIB tumour without elevated markers can be treated with initial chemotherapy, primary RPLND or surveillance. Based on the extent of the disease combination of cisplatin-based chemotherapy and surgery (aggressive multimodality) achieves cure rates between 65% and 85%. Tumours that are associated with elevated markers should be managed with chemotherapy (three or four cycles of BEP). Alternatively RPLND with adjuvant chemotherapy may be offered to these patients where risk of teratoma is high and chance of systemic involvement is low. However, high tumour markers post-orchiectomy or retroperitoneal lymphadenopathy greater than 3 cm have been correlated with increased risk of systemic relapse after RPLND.

The BEP regimen consists of cisplatin 20 mg/m², days 1–5, etoposide 100 mg/m², days 1–5, and bleomycin 30 mg administered on days 1, 8, 15. If bleomycin is contraindicated due to some reason, four cycles of EP may be administered. Alternatively VIP may be substituted for BEP in poor risk patients with pulmonary compromise or thoracic surgery. 3 cycles are given in good prognosis patients, while patients with intermediate prognosis are given 4 cycles of BEP. 5-year survival in this group is about 80%. Patients with poor risk are also served best with 4 cycles of BEP chemotherapy, but 5 year progression free survival is in the order of 45–50%. These patients may be enrolled in ongoing prospective trials for high dose chemotherapy. Management should be done preferably at a referral center.

Stage IIC and III NSGCT

The initial therapy recommended in these patients is induction chemotherapy. 4 cycles of BEP is the standard regimen. Once complete remission is achieved with chemotherapy, surgery is not indicated. Such a scenario arises in 25–60% of patients. If any residual mass is left (30% of cases), it should be removed preferably using nerve sparing RPLND within 4–6 weeks of chemotherapy

(PCS). In these specimens only 10% have viable cancer, while 50% contain mature teratoma and 40% contain fibrosis and necrotic tissue. Absence of teratoma in the primary tumour and good response to chemotherapy are useful predictors of necrosis in the PCS specimen. A complete resection of all visible masses is critical. If the resected specimen shows presence of mature teratoma or necrosis, no further therapy is instituted. In case of incomplete resection of teratoma or vital tumour, two cycles of adjuvant cisplatin based chemotherapy is beneficial. Unresected teratoma may grow rapidly (growing teratoma syndrome) and undergo malignant change.

How are patients with seminomas managed?

Based on clinical staging in patients with non-seminomatous tumours, clinical stage I tumours can be offered surveillance, chemotherapy and dog leg radiotherapy (20–30 Gy in para-aortic region and ipsilateral pelvis). Patients with clinical stage IIa and IIb disease are best served by 3 cycles of BEP specially if the disease is bulky and multifocal disease or alternatively by dog leg radiotherapy. Good prognosis clinical stage IIc and III disease are managed with 3 cycles of BEP while those with intermediate prognosis are administered 4 cycles of BEP.

What are the boundaries of the Nerve Sparing RPLND ?

The boundaries of modified template nerve sparing RPLND are depicted in Fig. 24.7.

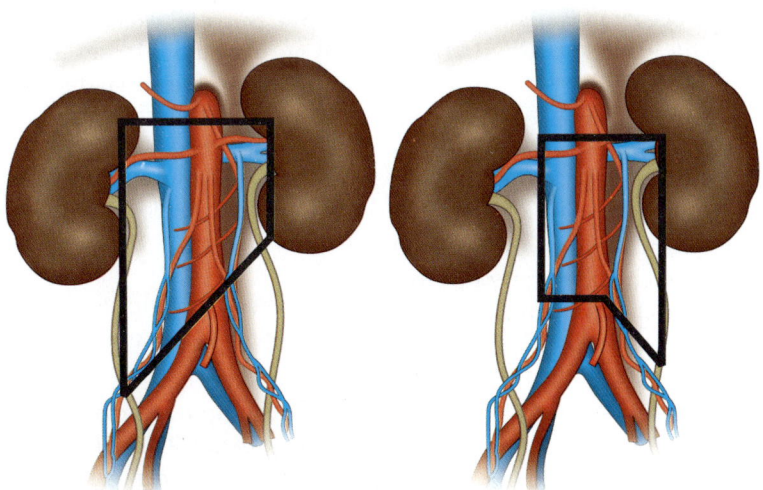

Fig. 24.7: Boundaries of modified template nerve sparing RPLND

How are patients with NSGCT followed after definitive treatment?

Follow up protocol for surveillance of stage I NSGCT:

Procedure	First year	2 year	3–5 year	6–10 year
Physical examination	3-monthly	3-monthly	Twice/year	Once/year
Tumour markers	3-monthly	3-monthly	Twice/year	Once/year
Chest X-ray	Twice/year	Twice/year		
Abdominopelvic CT scan	Once/year	Once/year		

Follow up protocol for RPNLD of stage I NSGCT:

Procedure	First year	2 year	3–5 year	6–10 year
Physical examination	3-monthly	3-monthly	Twice/year	Once/year
Tumour markers	3-monthly	3-monthly	Twice/year	Once/year
Chest X-ray	3-monthly	3-monthly	Twice/year	Once/year
Abdominopelvic CT scan	Twice/year	Twice/year	Once/year	Once/year
Chest CT and Brain CT	As indicated			

How are patients with seminomatous GCT followed after definitive treatment?

Procedure	First year	2 year	3–5 year	6–10 year
Examination	4-monthly	4-monthly	Once yearly	Once yearly
Markers	4-monthly	4-monthly	Once yearly	Once yearly
Chest X-ray	6-monthly	6-monthly		
CT Abdomen/pelvis	6-monthly	6-monthly		

What are the guidelines for management of recurrence/relapse in NSGCT?

For recurrent disease or relapse, induction chemotherapy is the treatment of choice using agents like VIP, VeIP or TIP. Long-term remission may be achieved in up to 40% of patients. These patients have bulky retroperitoneal lymphadenopathy, elevated markers and occasional distant metastasis. In the absence of these features, RPNLD may be offered as the first line treatment.

Prognostic indicators of response to salvage therapy include location and histology of the primary tumour, response to first-line treatment, duration of remissions, level of AFP and hCG at relapse. 10% improvement in survival is noted with the use of high dose chemotherapy but this benefit is doubtful. After chemotherapy surgery should be performed in 4–6 weeks after markers have declined. If the markers do not decline resection of residual tumours ('desperation surgery') should be considered if complete resection of all tumours seems feasible.

Late relapse is defined as any patient relapsing more than 2 years following chemotherapy for metastatic disease. These patients should be subjected to radical surgery as early as possible. Late relapse may be due to viable malignancy (most commonly yolk sac tumour), teratoma (20–30%) or malignant transformation to adenocarcinoma (10–20%). History of prior relapse and teratoma in PCS specimen are predictors of late relapse. Surgical excision of all tumour gives the best cure as late relapses are usually chemoresistant. If there is residual disease following surgery, salvage chemotherapy should be started based on histological results. These cases should be managed at high volume centres and surgery should be done once response to chemotherapy has been achieved.

What are the guidelines for management of recurrence/relapse in seminomatous GCT?

Patients who have residual disease >3 cm after chemotherapy are offered post-chemotherapy surgery if the PET CT shows positive activity, otherwise they can be observed. Patients who relapse after radiotherapy can be given first line chemotherapy.

What are the various non-germ cell tumours that affect the testis? (*see* Table 24.2)

Table 24.2: Non-germ cell tumours affecting the testis			
Leydig cell tumour	20–60 years 90% are benign	Feminising characteristics, gynaecomastia precocious puberty	Exhibit Rienke's crystals
Sertoli cell tumours	Any age 90% are benign	Gynaecomastia	Epithelial elements organised into tubules
Granulosa cell tumours	Any age Mostly benign	Gynaecomastia with raise oestrogen	Adult type granulosa cells
Gonadoblastoma	Intersex patients at young age 30% bilateral	Female phenotype with primary amenorrhoea or males with cryptorchidism	Large germ cells intermixed with small immature Sertoli cells
All these tumours are best managed with radical inguinal orchiectomy. Gonadoblastomas may require bilateral prophylactic orchiectomy			

What are paratesticular tumours?

Paratesticular tumours are the tumours arising from testicular adenexa. The most common paratesticular tumour is adenomatoid tumour which is a benign tumour commonly arising from the epididymis. It presents a small painless mass in the scrotum and is managed by inguinal exploration and excision. Cystadenoma is another paratesticular tumour found commonly in patients with von Hippel-Lindau syndrome. Mesotheliomas and sarcomas are malignant paratesticular tumours that require radical inguinal orchiectomy and RPLND with chemotherapy. Embryonal rhabdomyosarcoma is the most common sarcoma in patients less than 30 years while liposarcoma is the commonest adult paratesticular sarcoma.

25

Penile Lesions

How should one approach a case of penile lesions?

History in patients presenting with penile lesions should focus on points like duration of the lesion, rate of growth, age of onset, associated symptoms like pain, urethral discharge, inability to retract prepuce, urinary complaints, pain, foul odour, presence of inguinal swellings and detailed sexual history including exposure to multiple partners, lesions in partner, pain and extent of sexual activity possible with the lesion. History must also include questions regarding status of circumcision (religion of patient may provide important clue), presence of similar lesions off and on (indicating recurrent balanoposthitis), ballooning of preputial sac at micturition, bleeding, and presence of antecedent trauma.

Visual inspection of the lesion if often enough to clinch a diagnosis in penile lesions but it requires that the prepuce be completely retracted when possible and the penis stretched (Fig. 25.1). The external genitalia is examined as a whole and the following points are to be noted on inspection:

- Secondary sexual characters
- Status of the prepuce (retractable or not)
- Preputial glands
- Glans and corona
- Meatus location and calibre (adequate or inadequate)
- Lesions over the penile shaft
- Secondary sexual characters (pubic hair as per tanners staging)
- Scrotum (well developed with preserved rugosity/underdeveloped)
- Testicular volume in bilateral testis

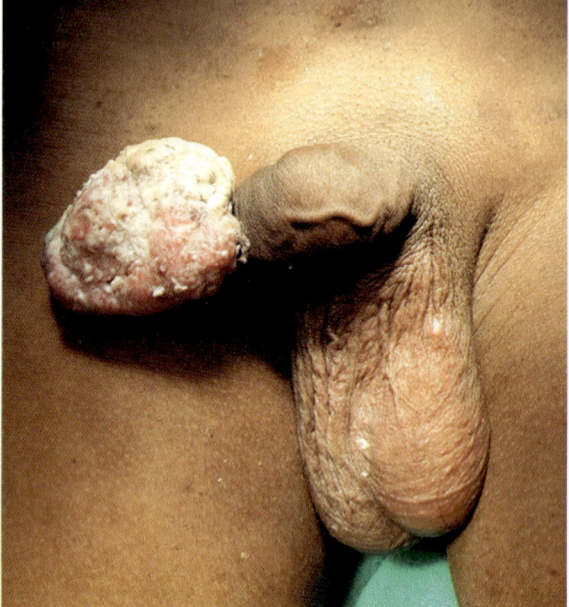

Fig. 25.1: Clinical picture of carcinoma of the penis

- Any obvious scrotal swelling
- Inguinal swelling
- Hernial orifices

All the above findings are then confirmed by palpation. Prepuce should be manually retracted to ensure absence of adhesions. The shaft should be palpated in its entirety for any induration, plaque or mass. Many penile lesions may be contagious and examination should not be done with bare hands. The glans should be held between the thumb and index finger and penis stretched before palpation to expose the structures near the base of penis. If an obvious growth is present over the penile shaft or glans, surrounding induration signifies probability of involvement of the corpora. On the ventral aspect of the penis the urethra must be palpated in its entirety to rule out its involvement by a penile lesion or distinct lesions or malignancies involving the urethra as primary. Rectal examination must also be done in cases of penile carcinoma to rule out the involvement of the perineal body and presence of any pelvic mass. Also check for any induration of the scrotum which suggests direct involvement by tumour. The inguinal regions must be palpated for presence of lymph nodes and any nodes larger than 1.5 cm should be considered significantly enlarged. A thorough inguinal examination is the most important part of examination as the prognosis and survival depends upon the presence of inguinal metastasis. Associated tenderness in these nodes may point to the inflammatory nature of these nodes but hard painless and fixed nodes are pointers to malignant involvement. The nodal examination should be reported in the following format: Node consistency; location; diameter; unilateral or bilateral; number of nodes identified on each side; mobile or fixed; relationship (e.g. infiltration or perforation) to other surrounding structures like skin and inguinal ligament; associated oedema of leg and/or scrotum.

What is the differential diagnosis of penile lesions?

Penile lesions are a cause of worry as they affect a private organ which defines sexuality and associated with fear of impotence. Penile lesions may range from benign infective to malignant diseases and to the point history and detailed examination can delineate almost all penile conditions. Cutaneous lesions often occur on the penis and may require dermatological opinion. These conditions have been discussed briefly while surgical conditions are described at length.

Differential diagnosis of penile lesions:
- Benign tumours of the skin of the shaft
  - Congenital cysts
  - Acquired cysts
  - Retention cysts
  - Neurilemomas
  - Syringomas
- Benign tumours of adventitial tissue
  - Angioma
  - Fibroma
  - Lipoma
  - Myoma
  - Neuroma
- Inflammatory lesions
  - Pseudotumours (caused by self intracorporeal injection of drugs)
  - Pyogenic granuloma
  - Peyronie's disease
  - Lymphangitis
  - Phlebitis
- Cutaneous lesions
  - Coronal papillae
  - Pearly penile papules
  - Zoon's balanitis
  - Sexually transmitted infections
- Premalignant lesions
  - Cutaneous horn
  - Keratotic balanitis
  - Pseudoepitheliomatous micaceous balanitis
  - Balanitis xerotica obliterans
  - Leukoplakia
- Infective lesions
  - Condyloma acuminata
  - Bowenoid papulosis
  - Kaposi sarcoma
  - Tuberculosis
- Malignant lesions
  - Buschke-Löwenstein tumour (Verrucous carcinoma)
  - Carcinoma *in situ*
  - Squamous cell carcinoma
  - Basal cell carcinoma
  - Melanoma
  - Adenosquamous carcinoma
  - Paget's disease
  - Sarcoma
  - Secondaries

What are the common benign lesions of the penis?

Many benign tumours arise from the skin overlying penile shaft like inclusion cysts, nerve tumours that arise from dermal nerves, syringomas, and retention cysts. These lesions affect the sebaceous and sweat glands and other appendages of the skin. Angiomas, fibromas, neuromas, lipomas, and myomas arise from the supporting structures of the penis as small firm lesions. Pseudotumours may result from self-administered drugs within the penis. Rarely inflammatory vascular lesions like phlebitis, lymphangitis, and angiitis may also produce subcutaneous nodules in the penis. Often painless, small and smooth surfaced; these lesions are managed by excision. When a diagnosis is in doubt, these lesions are best treated with local excision and histologic evaluation to uncover malignant transformation.

What are the various premalignant lesions of the penis?

Up to 40% of penile lesions may arise from a precursor premalignant lesion of the penis. These have been enlisted in the differential diagnosis of penile lesions. Leukoplakia presents as a whitish plaque often near the meatus. It has been shown to be associated with both *in situ* squamous cell cancer and verrucous cancer of the penis. Early detection of the lesion and management in the form of removal of chronic irritants and circumcision may be protective. The lesion may increase the odds of developing a penile cancer by up to 10 times and regular follow-up is advocated even after complete excision.

Balanitis xerotica obliterans is genital form of Lichen Sclerosus et atrophicus which presents as a diffuse whitish patch on the prepuce, glans or meatus that often extends up to the fossa navicularis. The lesion is associated with pain, pruritis and urethral strictures and is a premalignant condition. Even after the condition has been treated squamous cell carcinoma of the penis has been reported. Management of this lesion is in the form of topical and injectable steroids and occasionally excision of the indurated white lesion.

Pseudoepitheliomatous Micaceous and Keratotic Balanitis are also premalignant lesions that present as micaceous growths on the glandular penis associated with hyperkeratosis. These lesions are recurrent and may lead to the formation of fibrosarcoma.

Cutaneous horns over the penis represent extreme hyperkeratosis and usually develop over pre-existing warts, abrasions or other lesions. They are related to HPV 16 infection and managed with excision from the base and close follow-up.

What is verrucous carcinoma of the penis?

Verrucous carcinoma is a malignant low grade squamous carcinoma that is locally aggressive but rarely metastatic. It was initially described by Buschke and Löwenstein in 1925 and later by Löwenstein in 1939 in the United States. Verrucous carcinoma is thus also known as Buschke-Löwenstein tumour or giant condyloma acuminatum. This tumour does not metastasize even to the lymph nodes but grows by destruction of surrounding tissue leading to necrosis and secondary infection. Excisional biopsy or multiple deep biopsies can help to differentiate the lesion from penile carcinoma and treatment consists of excision while sparing as much of the penis as possible. Large lesions may require total penectomy. As with other premalignant lesions recurrence is common, and close follow-up should be done. Topical therapy in the form of Podophyllin and 5-fluorouracil is ineffective. Radiation therapy induces malignant change within the lesion and should also be avoided. Among minimally invasive options for management of verrucous carcinoma, cryotherapy and laser therapy are viable options.

What is erythroplasia of Queyrat or Bowen's disease?

Erythroplasia of Queyrat is the other name for carcinoma *in situ* (CIS) of the penis involving the glans penis and prepuce. When it involves the shaft of the penis or other parts of the genitalia, it is known as Bowen's disease. Carcinoma *in situ* represents an intraepithelial malignant process that has not breached the basement membrane. Histologically the lesion is characterised by mitotic figures, hyperchromatic nuclei, atypical hyperplastic cells and vacuolations. There is a surrounding inflammatory infiltrate that consists mainly of plasma cells. Carcinoma *in situ* may progress to invasive carcinoma in 10% of the patients although rates as high as 33% have been reported and metastasis has not been reported as yet with CIS.

Management of CIS is by organ preserving wide local excision with a safety margin of 5 mm around the lesion. For lesions located on the foreskin circumcision can be performed. Local application of 5 fluorouracil cream or topical Imiquimod cream can also be done. Lasers like Nd:YAG, carbon dioxide and KTP have also been used to ablate the lesions. Radiation therapy can be offered to patients unwilling for surgery.

What are the predisposing and protective factors in carcinoma penis ?

The various recognised predisposing factors are:
1. HPV infection
2. Penile trauma
3. Genital UV radiation exposure

Other suspected factors that have not been found to have a definitive link include venereal diseases, alcohol abuse, marijuana and occupational hazards.

Protective factors are hygienic practices, circumcision and avoidance of tobacco.

How does penile carcinoma present?

Penile carcinoma presents as a penile lesion which is usually in the form of an induration, papule, wart or exophytic lesion. There is also an ulcerative variant which presents as a non-healing but painless ulcer with elevated edges. Most commonly the tumour is found on the glans and prepuce. Shaft of the penis is less commonly involved.

Rarely the patient may present with inguinal nodes that have ulcerated or become infected. Occasionally there may be malaise, weight loss and fatigue resulting from chronic infection. Sometimes the lesion develops in a phimosed penis and is thus not subject to the patient's observation. Up to half of the patients neglect the problem at first and majority of patients die within a period of 2 years if untreated. Death is usually from metastatic enlargement of the inguinal nodes leading to skin breakdown and chronic suppuration, sepsis or haemorrhage.

Distant metastasis without involvement of regional lymph nodes in the inguinal region is rare. Systemic sites of metastasis include the lung, liver, bone and brain.

What is the lymphatic drainage and pathway of spread of penile cancer?

Penile cancer metastasizes using the lymphatic channels. The earliest nodes to get involved are the superficial inguinal lymph nodes followed by the deep inguinal lymph nodes and subsequently the pelvic lymph nodes. There is crossover to the lymph nodes on the contralateral side also, hence positive nodes on any one side require subsequent exploration of the other side during surgery. The superficial deep and pelvic nodes are in close continuity; hence if the superficial nodes turn out to be positive on FNAC, excisional biopsy or lymph node dissection, then the deep inguinal and pelvic nodes also need to be removed on that side. In such an event the contralateral superficial inguinal dissection is also done as there is high chance of involvement of the opposite side. If the opposite side comes out to be positive on frozen section, then deep inguinal and pelvic nodes are also removed on this opposite side.

What are the various investigations that should be done in such cases?

Apart from the routine laboratory investigations the diagnosis is confirmed by biopsy. Laboratory investigations may reveal hypercalcemia which is a result of parathyroid hormone and related hormones produced by the tumour. Rarely urethral involvement and obstruction may lead to renal failure in these patients and kidney function tests are required during initial work up. Patients may have associated anemia and poor nutritional status can be uncovered by basic laboratory work up.

A biopsy that proves the diagnosis is the mainstay for instituting therapy. Since many lesions have associated phimosis a dorsal slit has to be given in many cases. A wedge biopsy must be done with adequate depth to assess the histological depth of invasion, grade and the presence of vascular invasion.

For adequate TNM staging examination suffices almost 90% of the times but occasionally additional imaging modalities may have to be employed. When in doubt regarding corporeal invasion, an ultrasound can be helpful. Alternatively magnetic resonance imaging may also be used to see the extent of corporeal invasion, however, most of the times clinical examination suffices. MRI may be useful when organ preserving surgery is planned in a scenario of large growth where corporeal involvement cannot be clinically assessed.

Computerised tomography scan has been used to assess the inguinal and pelvic nodes in patients with palpable nodes to see the level of involvement. However, its value in patients with no palpable nodes is insignificant. CT scan may be used in obese patients or those who have undergone prior inguinal surgery as clinical examination in these cases may be difficult.

What precautions should be taken while taking a biopsy from the lesion?

The biopsy taken should be in the form of a wedge biopsy which includes the periphery of the lesion along with a part of the healthy penile tissue. If it is taken from the centre of the lesion it may show only necrosis. The biopsy should be of adequate depth to comment upon the depth of invasion of the tumour and vascular invasion.

What are the histological features of penile cancer and how are they histologically graded?

Most penile cancers are squamous cell cancers demonstrating keratinization, keratin pearl formation, and various degrees of mitotic activity. Basiloid variants and anaplastic variants are associated with poorer survival. Broders classification is used to grade squamous cell carcinomas of the penis based on degree of keratinization nuclear pleomorphism number of mitosis, hyperchromatic nuclei and other features. Most commonly found cancer of the penis is low grade 1–2. They demonstrate presence of keratin pearls and intercellular bridges.

More than half of the high grade tumours are associated with nodal involvement. Vascular involvement and perineural invasion are significant prognostic factors in penile carcinoma.

What is TNM Staging of penile cancer?

T   Primary tumour

Tx   Primary tumour cannot be assessed

T0   No evidence of primary tumour

Tis   Carcinoma *in situ*

Ta   Non-invasive verrucous carcinoma, not associated with destructive invasion

T1   Tumour invades subepithelial connective tissue

T1a   Tumour invades subepithelial connective tissue without lymphovascular invasion and is not poorly differentiated or undifferentiated (T1G1-2)

T1b   Tumour invades subepithelial connective tissue with lymphovascular invasion or is poorly differentiated or undifferentiated (T1G3-4)

T2   Tumour invades corpus spongiosum/corpora cavernosa

T3   Tumour invades urethra

T4   Tumour invades other adjacent structures

N   Regional lymph nodes

Nx   Regional lymph nodes cannot be assessed

N0   No palpable or visibly enlarged inguinal lymph node

N1   Palpable mobile unilateral inguinal lymph node

N2   Palpable mobile multiple or bilateral inguinal lymph nodes

N3   Fixed inguinal nodal mass or pelvic lymphadenopathy, unilateral or bilateral

M   Distant metastasis

M0   No distant metastasis

M1   Distant metastasis present

Staging of Penile Carcinoma

Stage 0: The cancer has not grown below the superficial (surface) layer of skin, and does not involve the lymph nodes or distant structures (Tis or Ta; N0, M0).

Stage I: Low-grade cancer that has invaded the superficial layer of skin but has not spread to lymph nodes or distant structures (T1a, N0, M0).

Stage II: Invasive high grade and/or invaded into blood or lymph vessels and/or into the corpora/ or the urethra but has not spread to lymph nodes or distant structures (T1b, T2, or T3; N0, M0).

Stage IIIa: Invaded up to the urethra, and spread to one inguinal lymph node, but has not involved distant structures (T1, T2, or T3; N1, M0).

Stage IIIb: Invaded up to the urethra and has spread to more than one inguinal lymph node, but not pelvic lymph nodes or distant structures (T1, T2, or T3; N2, M0).

Stage IV: Any of the following:

Involving distant structures (T4, any N, any M).

Fixed inguinal nodal mass or pelvic lymphadenopathy (any T, N3, any M).

Involvement of at least one pelvic node (any T, N3, any M) and/or distant lymph nodes outside the pelvis or distant structures (any T, any N, M1).

What is Jackson Staging of penile carcinoma?

Jackson classification is the older classification system used for carcinoma of the penis.

Stage I: Confined to glans or prepuce

Stage II: Invasion into the shaft or corpora

Stage III: Operable inguinal lymph node metastasis

Stage IV: Inoperable inguinal lymph node metastasis/ invasion of tumour into adjacent structures.

What are the surgical options for management of penile cancer?

Organ preserving surgeries are performed in patients with low grade and low T stage tumours. A 2 centimetre margin has been suggested as safe for patients undergoing partial penectomy. Since skip lesions have not been encountered in penile carcinoma, partial penectomy is the surgical procedure of choice for squamous cell carcinoma.

Partial amputation of the penis: Partial amputation of the penis is performed using the penile disassembly technique. In this technique a degloving circumcision incision is given around the corona and dissection is done up to the tunica albuginea. The corpora are separated and amputation or division is done at a safe margin of 2 centimetres from the edge of the tumour. The urethra is split ventrally and fixed to the ligated corpora. The urethral margins are sutured to the margins of the skin to form a cosmetically acceptable penis.

In total penectomy the penis is divided at the level of the suspensory ligament. A long segment of the urethra is spared and brought down into the perineum using a modified lambda incision. In these patients scrotum and testis are also sometimes removed to minimise libido and avoid the hanging scrotum from obstructing the urinary stream through the perineal opening. However, most surgeons do not advocate orchiectomy due to the useful role of testosterone in elderly patients. The patient is asked to squat and void after the surgery.

In patients where corporal bodies are involved up till the root of the penis, a radical penectomy may be required. In this surgery the corporal bodies are dissected up to the tips of the crura. 2–3 centimetres of the urethra is spared to perform a perineal urethrostomy.

What is Mohs' micrographic surgery (MMS)?

Mohs' micrographic surgery is a technique that allows excision of the tumour in thin layers. Each layer is analysed under the microscope for presence of carcinoma. Frozen sections are cut horizontally to examine the depth of involvement by the tumour. The process is continued till the entire malignant tumour has been completely excised. This procedure is organ sparing and provides excellent local control. For small lesions less than 1 cm the cure rates approach 100%. Mohs'

micrographic surgery should be offered to patients with carcinoma *in situ* or small superficial tumours of the penis. This technique should be performed by experts and is relatively time consuming. Possibility of meatal stenosis and disfigurement of the glans must also be explained to the patients. Multiple sessions of the procedure may be needed at times. The surgery should not be advised in patients with locally advanced tumour >3 cm or history of prior treatment failure.

How are the lymph nodes managed?

In up to half of the patients inguinal lymph node enlargement is due to inflammatory response. In such patients of 4 to 6 weeks course of antibiotics was earlier recommended.

Fine needle aspiration cytology may be useful in patients with enlarged inguinal lymph nodes and low-grade tumours, however, the false negative rate of cytology has been reported to be 20 to 30% in some series.

Patients with lesions up to T1 grade 1–2 without lymph node involvement can be safely observed. Those with positive lymph node are given 4–6 weeks of antibiotics followed by FNAC if adenopathy persists. If the FNAC is negative but the lymph nodes do not subside with therapy excisional biopsy of the lymph nodes is done. If the FNAC or biopsy is positive, the patients are subjected to ipsilateral superficial and deep inguinal lymphadenectomy along with pelvic lymphadenectomy. Contralateral superficial inguinal node dissection is also done and subjected to frozen section analysis. If it turns out to be positive, similar dissection is done on the contralateral side as well.

In patients with high-grade or T2–4 lesions with no positive nodes, bilateral superficial inguinal dissection and frozen section analysis is still performed due to high possibility of involvement. If it comes out to be positive for malignancy, a complete inguinal dissection along with pelvic node dissection is performed on that side, else the patient is observed. If nodes are positive on one side and <4 cm and mobile, a complete dissection is performed on that side along with superficial inguinal dissection on the contralateral side. If positive on frozen section, the contralateral nodes are also dissected completely. If patient presents with bilaterally positive inguinal nodes an FNAC is first performed. If it is negative, then superficial inguinal dissection is performed on both side but if positive, then a complete dissection is performed on the positive side with superficial dissection on opposite side. Alternatively neo adjuvant chemotherapy as described below may also be offered for bilaterally node positive tumours.

If the nodes are >4 cm and fixed or the CT scan shows positive pelvic nodes induction chemotherapy is started and surgery of nodes is deferred for later.

What is the role of sentinel node biopsy in patients with penile cancer?

Sentinel node biopsy was introduced by Cabanas as a means of limiting inguinal dissection and avoiding related morbidity. The success described by Cabanas could not be reproduced in other series and the procedure has become less popular compared to the modified and standard ilioinguinal dissection. In the technique described by Cabanas, a 2 inch incision is made parallel to the inguinal crease and a finger is inserted under the upper flap towards the pubic tubercle. The node is encountered there and excised and sent for histopathology. The technique has been supplanted by ultrasonographic and lymphoscintigraphic detection but still resulted in a significant false negative rate of up to 5–25%.

What are the boundaries of inguinal and pelvic lymph node dissection?

Ilioinguinal radical lymphadenectomy is performed in patients with positive nodes 4–6 weeks after penectomy. The inguinal dissection area is often referred to as the Dressler's quadrilateral. The classical ilioinguinal dissection is done in the area bound superiorly by a line from superior margin of the external inguinal ring to the anterior superior iliac spine (ASIS), laterally by a similar line from ASIS extending 20 cm inferiorly, medially by a parallel line from pubic tubercle to 15 cm below along the medial side of thigh and inferiorly a line joining the inferior ends of the two vertical lines. An oblique incision is made 3 cm below and parallel to inguinal ligament to expose the nodes. The saphenous vein is sacrificed and sartorius is mobilised from the ASIS and used to cover the femoral vessels.

Modified inguinal lymphadenectomy is used for initial staging and has several advantages over the radical ilioinguinal lymphadenectomy like smaller skin incision and preservation of the saphenous vein and sartorius. The area of dissection is minimised by avoiding the area lateral to the femoral artery and below the fossa ovalis.

What is the role of radiotherapy in carcinoma penis?

Radiation therapy to the penile region is a useful alternate to surgery in patients who require organ preservation. In such patients a dose of 60–74 gray is administered over 25 to 40 fractions. Brachytherapy in the form of Radium–Iridium and Caesium may also be given with successful penile conservation in up to 80% of the patients.

Radiotherapy may lead to formation of fistula, strictures and occasionally penile necrosis, edema and pain. Brachytherapy may be used in tumours less than 4 centimetres in size. Radiotherapy may also be given to the inguinal nodes with an acceptable rate of survival, however, surgery is the most commonly employed treatment modality in patients with carcinoma penis as radiation therapy to the inguinal area has not been found to be as effective as surgical therapy. It may be useful in inoperable cases and those requiring palliation. There is no role of prophylactic radiation therapy in patients with lymph node negative disease.

What is the role of chemotherapy in carcinoma penis?

Patients with advanced penile cancer who have unresectable regional disease or widespread metastasis are subjected to chemotherapy. The optimal chemotherapy regimen is still under investigation but cisplatin containing regimes have been shown to improve surgical outcomes. In patients with fixed nodal metastasis, pelvic nodal metastasis and nodes more than 4 centimetres in size induction chemotherapy may be given. If the lesion responds to chemotherapy, extensive radical–surgical resection should be done. In patients who do not respond to induction chemotherapy, palliative chemotherapy in the form of BMP regime may be given along with radiation. TIP regime has been shown to be better tolerated than bleomycin based regimes.

Commonly employed regimes include:

- BMP: Bleomycin, methotrexate and cisplatin
- TIP: Paclitaxel, ifosfamide and cisplatin
- Paclitaxel and carboplatin.

What is the most important prognostic factor in penile carcinoma?

The presence and extent of lymph node metastasis is the most important prognostic factor for survival. Even in presence of inguinal nodal metastasis with timely surgery, 5-year survival of up to 80% can be achieved. Similarly presence of vascular invasion on the histopathological examination also carries poor prognosis. Prognosis also worsens with increasing age and grade of the lesion.

Good prognostic factors include no nodal involvement and unilateral involvement with no extranodal extension and absence of pelvic nodes.

How is a patient with penile carcinoma followed up?

Patients who have undergone penile preserving treatment should be followed up 3 monthly for the first two years and then six monthly for up to 5 years. At every visit, the patient should undergo regular examination and also taught self-examination. Patients who have undergone total penectomy should be examined six monthly for the first two years and then yearly up to 5 years.

Patients who were having positive inguinal lymph nodes should also be examined 3 monthly for the first two years and six monthly for up to 5 years. These patients should be subjected to ultrasound and fine needle aspiration cytology (if positive on ultrasonography) at the time of visit. Patients who had no positive nodes are followed on the lines of patients who have undergone total penectomy.

How is basal cell carcinoma of the penis managed?

Basal cell carcinoma is a rare carcinoma of the penis. Very few cases have been reported and they have been managed by local excision. The prognosis of basal cell carcinoma is extremely good with almost 100% success rates. It differs from the squamous cell carcinoma in its site being the penile shaft as opposed to the prepuce and glans in squamous cell carcinoma. Basal cell carcinoma also grows more slowly and rarely undergoes metastasis.

What are the common malignancies metastasising to the penis?

The most common organs from which metastasis may arise are the bladder, prostate and rectum. Other sources include the gut, testes and kidneys. Penile metastasis usually represents advanced form of disease which is rarely amenable to surgical therapy and most patients die within the first year of diagnosis.

Metastasis to the penis is unusual and often manifests as priapism. It may also lead to penile swelling, ulceration or formation of nodules and indurated patches. Occasionally there may be haematuria and features of urinary obstruction. Malignant cells usually deposit into blood rich corpora leading to priapism.

26

Hypospadias

What is hypospadias and how does it develop?

Hypospadias is a clinical condition resulting from arrested penile development that leads to a ventrally placed or proximal urethral meatus. It consists of three parts: Ventral opening of the meatus, ventral curvature, and dorsal hood of prepuce.

In the male the genital tubercle starts to lengthen at about 9 weeks of gestation. Penis develops from this enlargement and elongation of the genital tubercle and fusion of the folds of urethra occurs under the influence of testosterone. The cloacal endoderm grows along the midline of the genital tubercle ventrally to form the primitive urethral plate. The medial endodermal folds fuse in the midline to form the male urethra ventrally. The lateral extension of this plate, the lateral ectodermal leads to formation of the skin of the penile shaft and prepuce. The layers fuse from posterior to anteriorly forming the median raphe in the midline. Arrest in fusion leads to hypospadias. Causative factors for hypospadias may be polygenic in nature resulting from abnormal production of androgen or abnormal androgen sensitivity. Abnormal development of the growth plate, disproportionate corpora and fibrosis may lead to penile curvature.

How is hypospadias classified?

Commonly used classification system divides hypospadias into:
- *Anterior*:
  - Glanular
  - Coronal (Fig. 26.1)
  - Subcoronal

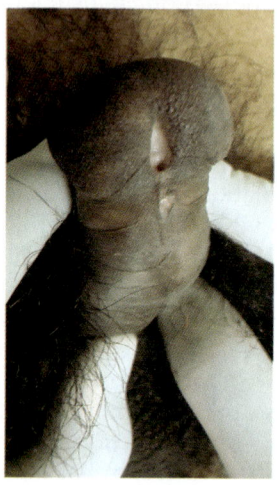

Fig. 26.1: Clinical picture of distal coronal hypospadias

- *Middle*:
  - Distal penile
  - Midshaft
  - Proximal penile
- *Posterior*:
  - Penoscrotal (Fig. 26.2)
  - Scrotal
  - Perineal

Anterior hypospadias is the most common presentation accounting for up to 50–70% of the cases. Posterior hypospadias accounts for only 10–15% of the cases.

How is a patient presenting with hypospadias evaluated?

The presenting scenario is a child brought by the patient or referred by a paediatrician with

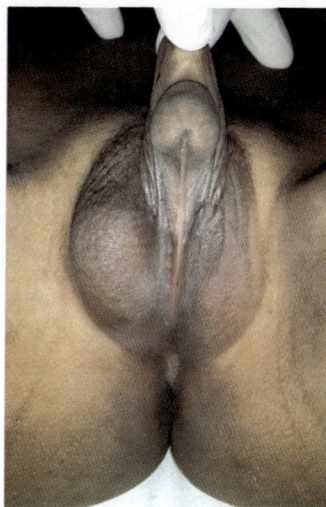

Fig. 26.2: Clinical picture of penoscrotal hypospadias showing chordee and dorsal hooded prepuce

complaints of abnormal opening of the meatus. The urinary stream is normal but there may be associated defects that have to be ruled out by history and examination. Hypospadias is a part of over 50 different syndromes and associated commonly with undescended testis, inguinal hernia, hydrocele and micropenis. Hypospadias may be a presentation of disorders of sexual differentiation and proximal hypospadias associated with unilateral or bilateral undescended testis must undergo thorough investigations for possible intersex states.

Ask for the character of the stream, position of the meatus, deviation of the penis, associated inguinal swellings and location of the testis. Also ask for anorectal defects and problems with defecation. History of similar problems in siblings and maternal health during course of pregnancy should be ascertained. Hypospadias may be more commonly found in babies conceived with artificial reproductive technique. Prior history of surgery in the form of circumcision may be a problem at the time of eventual reconstruction. In many cases the hypospadiac meatus is revealed after this surgery.

On examination there is a need to rule out associated conditions and ascertain how the eventual repair will be done. Apart from the location and size of the meatus, the size of the phallus, state of the prepuce and its dimensions, presence of penile deviation or chordee must be assessed at the time of examination. In a variant

of hypospadias megalomeatus with intact prepuce (MIP) the meatus is large and often no surgical therapy is needed. It is important to retract the prepuce as much as feasible if it is not hooded to assess the glans and meatal location. Examination on the same lines as undescended testis should be done to rule out the same.

What are the investigations required in a patient presenting with hypospadias?

Routine preoperative investigations including the hemogram, kidney function and electrolytes along with urine examination and coagulation profile is mandatory and part of the pre-anaesthetic workup. For patients with distal hypospadias and no testicular anomalies, this workup is sufficient to proceed for surgery. In patients with posterior hypospadias, ultrasonography, genitography and chromosomal and biochemical testing should be done. Micturating cystourethrogram and cystoscope should be done to look for the presence of prostatic utricle.

What are the treatment options in a patient with hypospadias?

Hypospadias repair is a surgical procedure that is comprised of three components;
- Orthoplasty (chordee correction)
- Urethroplasty
- Meatoplasty and glanduloplasty

Prior to the surgical repair of proximal hypospadias androgen stimulation may be given when the penis appears small in the form of hCG 6 to 8 weeks pre-operatively in a dose of 250–500 IU as intramuscular injections. This may lead to the increase in penis size and vascularity of skin flaps. Locally applied creams containing testosterone can also be used. Alternatively two to three intramuscular injections of testosterone 2 mg/kg over a 6 to 12 weeks can be administered.

The penis is first degloved using a circumcision incision which is extended on the ventral aspect proximally to spare the urethral plate. Preservation of the urethral plate is an important step as earlier surgeons used to excise it thinking that it was maldeveloped and degenerated. After degloving the penis the inherent chordee is reflected as the fibrous adhesions and adhesions caused by other tissues are relieved. The residual deviation is then assessed and orthoplasty is performed. Orthoplasty is followed by urethroplasty and second layer incorporation and eventually meatoplasty and glanuloplasty. Skin incision is then closed and antiseptic dressing is applied. For the procedure fine absorbable sutures like PDS are used and bipolar cautery is preferred for coagulation along with optical magnification especially in pediatric patients.

What are the aims of surgery in a patient with Hypospadias and when should it be performed?

The aims of surgery are to achieve micturition in standing position, sexual intercourse and ability to inseminate effectively. Achievement of a near normal looking phallus is also important.

The optimal timing of surgery was suggested to be between the fourth to fifth year in older times based on psychological development, but presently the best time for surgery is considered to be between 6 and 12 months.

What is chordee and how is it corrected?

Chordee is the deviation of penis or formation of penile curvature that can be truly appreciated in an erect penis. It may lead to painful erections and dyspareunia often precluding intercourse. Chordee is an important component of hypospadias and the first defect that requires correction in hypospadias repair.

Orthoplasty: The aim of orthoplasty is to correct the penile deviation. The first step of this surgery is to assess the penile curvature using the Gittes and Mc Laughin technique where a vascular tape or sling is applied tightly at the root of the penis and normal saline is injected through a butterfly cannula on the lateral aspect of the corpora causing artificial erection to take place. Erections can also be induced pharmacologically by intracorporeal injection of prostaglandin E1 or alprostadil.

- Nesbit technique may be employed wherein a vertical incision is made and part of tunica albugenia is excised from the convex side.
- Heineke Mikulicz procedure involves a number of transverse incisions followed by longitudinal closure on the concave side to lengthen the penis.
- Tunica albugenia plication (Duckett's and Baskin) involves making transverse incisions over the tunica albugenia followed by closure of albugenia on the convex side.
- Koff's Corporal Rotation can be used in severe curvature where the corpora are rotated medially and fixed using a suture to each other.

- Devine and Horton Dermal graft can be placed after incising the tunica albugenia on the convex side. Grafts are used when the penis is short and plication will lead to further shortening of the phallus. Dermal graft is harvested from non-hair bearing skin. Other grafts that can also be placed include tunica vaginalis graft, small intestinal submucosal graft, etc.
- *Penile disassembly*: Perovic technique of penile disassembly and corporoplasty involves separation of the three corpora after degloving the penis which corrects the chordee without the use of substitution.

What are the various methods used for urethroplasty?

Urethroplasty requires taking of a graft or flap to reconstruct the urethra. Grafts are free tissues without a defined vascularity that survive due to imbibition followed by neovascularization. Flaps have their vascularity preserved and thus have a better chance at survival.

The second layer of coverage can be provided by use of a subcutaneous or dartos flap, Tunica Vaginalis flap or paraurethral spongiosal approximation. Grossly the correction of distal hypospadias repair is based on tubularized incised plate. The other commonly used procedures for distal hypospadias include MAGPI (meatoplasty and glanduloplasty integrated), urethral advancement and Mathieu perimeatal flip flop technique.

For proximal hypospadias the reconstructive procedures include tubularized and onlay preputial flaps and koyanagi flap. Alternatively two stage repair can also be performed using preputial graft and Byars flaps.

Denis-Browne repair: Orthoplasty (chordee correction) at the age of 2 years is followed by neo-urethral construction at 3–5 years.

What is Snodgrass or Tubularized Incised plate repair (Fig. 26.3)?

Distal tubularized incised plate repair or Snodgrass repair is one of the most commonly performed repairs for distal hypospadias. The steps of the surgery are as follows:

1. A degloving incision is made approximately 2–5 mm below meatus.
2. Vertical incision is made on the urethral plate.

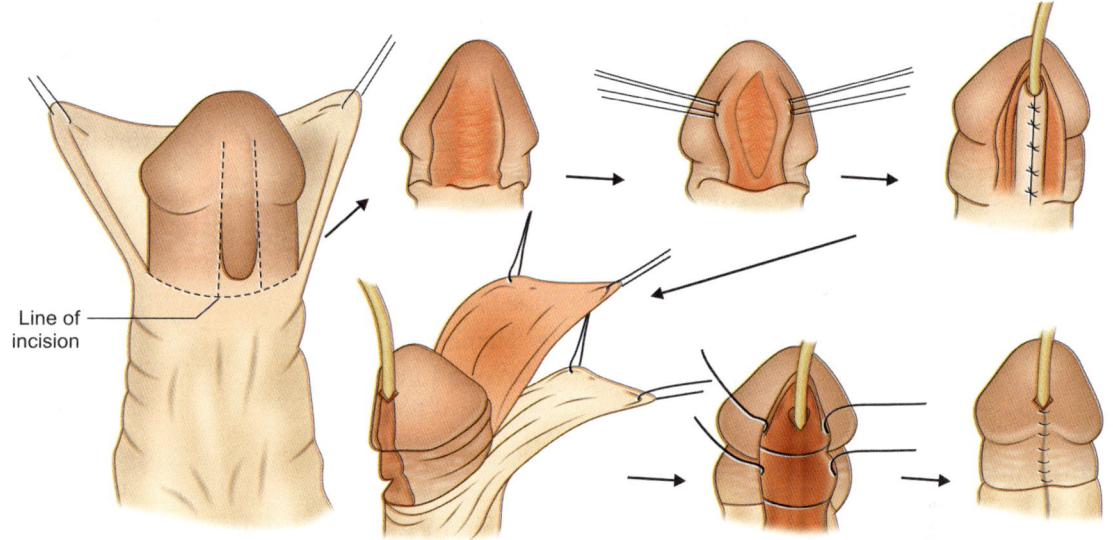

Fig. 26.3: Operative steps of Snodgrass repair for distal hypospadias

3. Over a foleys catheter the urethral plate is tubularized up to the tip of the glans.
4. Dartos flap is harvested from the preputial skin and shaft skin and brought ventrally to cover the neo-urethra.
5. A flap can usually be developed from the ventro-lateral dartos in patients with no foreskin.
6. Incised part of the glans is approximated and glansplasty is performed.
7. Shaft skin closure and approximation using absorbable sutures is done.

What is Mathieu perimeatal flip flop technique (Fig. 26.4)?

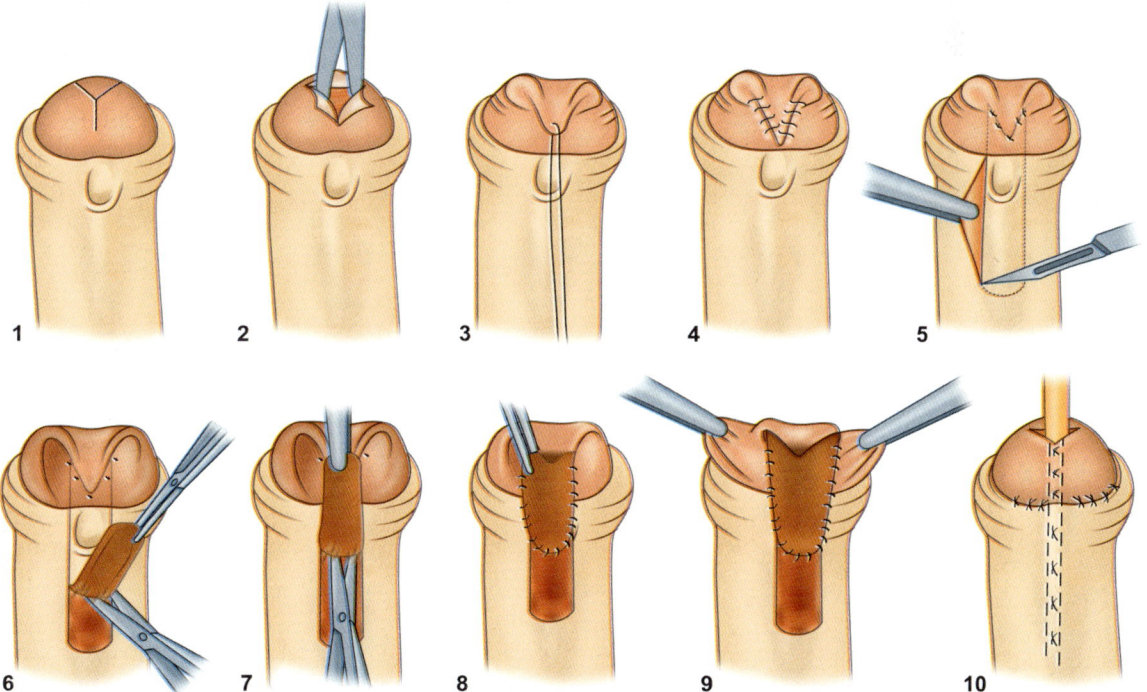

Fig. 26.4: Operative steps (1 to 10) demonstrating Mathieu repair for distal hypospadias

In the Mathieu technique a penile shaft skin flap is mobilized to create the neo-urethra. Two lateral incision are made between the neomeatus and the hypospadiac meatus and the intervening tissue of 7 to 8 mm is measured for the proximal flap gradually tapered to 5–6 mm at the meatal tip. Skin of the shaft is degloved and the subcutaneous tissue of the flap is dissected carefully. The flap is flipped and brought to the tip of the glans. Flap is approximated to the lateral lines of the urethral plate and the meatus is matured. A dartos flap tissue is used as a second layer to cover the flap and the glans wings are approximated. Incision is closed using absorbable sutures

What are the common procedures used for proximal hypospadias?

Ducketts preputial island flap and the Asopa's Procedure are commonly used one-stage procedures for mid and proximal hypospadias.

In the Ducketts' procedure penis is degloved and orthoplasty is performed. Inner layer of the prepuce is dissected off and raised as a pedicle flap. The flap is placed ventrally over the urethral plate. In the Asopa modification, the inner prepuce is used as a flap, but the neo-urethra is left attached to the underneath surface of the foreskin from which it was dissected.

What are the complications of surgery for Hypospadias?

Early complications include:
- Hemorrhage
- Wound infection
- Painful erections

Late complications:
- Stricture urethra
- Urethrocutaneous fistula
- Meatal stenosis
- Residual chordee/recurrent curvature
- Urethral diverticulum
- Hair ball formation.

27

Undescended Testis

How will you evaluate a patient presenting with undescended Testis (Fig. 27.1)?

Undescended testis is the absence of one or both testes in normal scrotal position. Practically it includes palpable cryptorchid testes and non-palpable testes, which are either cryptorchid or absent. Examination should be aimed at determining the testicular presence, its location and association with other syndromes.

The presenting complaint is straightforward but many times the parents may notice the absence of testis only later after birth. It is imperative to ask for maternal co-morbidities such as pre-eclampsia and eclampsia in patients with undescended testis and the use of any drugs like steroids during the gestational period. It must be ensured on history that the testis was undescended since birth and did not go missing sometime later during life as that may portray torsion. History of

surgery especially of the groin hernia may be useful as there can be injury to testicular artery leading to testis atrophy. Also ask about history of cryptorchidism in family members. If the patient presents in an adult phase of life, questions should be asked regarding fertility as paternity can significantly compromised in men with bilateral undescended testis.

Examination must be done in the supine position, upright cross legged and standing position. Examination should be done with warm hands, with adequate distraction. With the legs adducted the cremasteric muscle is relaxed and examination is facilitated. One should look for size position and mobility of the testis along with associated hernia and hydrocele. Cremasteric reflex should be elicited and genitalia should be examined for ambiguity. The hand is slid from the ipsilateral anterior superior iliac spine towards the external inguinal ring along the inguinal canal and gentle attempt made to push the testis through the canal. With the help of the other hand, the distal most extent to which the testis can be brought down is ascertained. In up to one-fourth of the patients cryptorchidism is bilateral. Ectopic sites should be thoroughly checked for the presence of ectopic testis. Examination especially under anaesthesia can definitively locate the testis in up to 70–80% cases and is as sensitive as ultrasound examination in deciphering the location.

Association with Down syndrome, Eagle-Barrett/prune belly syndrome, cerebral palsy, spigelian hernia, meningomyelocele, umbilical hernia, posterior urethral valve, imperforate anus, and gastroschisis, renal and spinal anomalies has

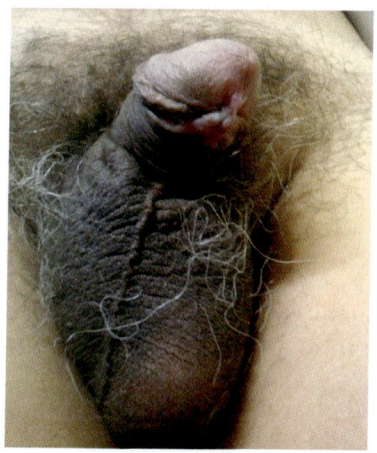

Fig. 27.1: Clinical picture right undescended testis

been found. Abnormalities of the spine, abdominal wall, central nervous system and urogenital system have a common origin. Genital anomalies resulting from androgen insensitivity may also be present during examination. All these associations must be ruled out.

What are retractile testes?

Retractile testes are testes that retract out of the scrotal sac but can be easily replaced manually in a stable scrotal position and remain there for some period of times even after letting them free.

How can one differentiate between ectopic testis and undescended testis?

Ectopic testis is defined as the testis that deviates from its normal path of descent. It is most commonly located in the superficial inguinal pouch. The other common locations are suprapubic (near the pubic symphysis at the root of penis), perineal, femoral and in the opposite scrotum. The following points are useful in differentiating ectopic from undescended testis:

- Testis has descended but in an abnormal location.
- The scrotum on the side of ectopic testis is well developed.
- The cord length is adequate.
- Spermatogenesis and seminal parameters are normal.
- Testis becomes more prominent on asking patient to raise legs (Carnett's test).

What are tails of Lockwood?

The gubernacular ligament was proposed to have multiple tails by Lockwood which terminated in the superficial inguinal, pubic, perineal and femoral regions. The persistence of any of the tails was considered as responsible for driving the testis to its respective abnormal location.

What is the difference between vanishing testis and testicular agenesis?

Agenetic testis can be defined as a testis that was never formed and is marked by the presence of mullerian structures on that side. A vanishing testis is formed initially and is subsequently lost due to torsion or vascular accident.

Presence of blind-ending spermatic vessels in the abdomen, inguinal canal, or scrotal sac is mandatory for the diagnosis of vanishing testis.

What is a normal descended testis?

Normal scrotal position has been defined as positioning of the midpoint of the testis at or below the midscrotum.

What is the pathogenesis of undescended testis?

Testicular descent is a complicated process and many theories have been proposed that include the role of gravity, muscular and endocrine factors and intra-abdominal pressure. Various phases of testicular descent have been proposed (1) intra-abdominal nephric phase which involves the degeneration mesonephros at 6th to 7th week, (2) trans-abdominal phase where the testis descends and reaches the inguinal ring, (3) inguinal phase where the testis moves down to its final position in the scrotum at about 28 weeks and (4) the scrotal phase. Occasionally the intra-abdominal and trans-abdominal phases are considered as one and a total of three phases of descent are described. The role of cranial suspensory ligament and gubernaculum that acts as a rudder during the descent of testis has been described but is controversial. Testosterone plays an important role in trans-inguinal descent and errors in its synthesis that are seen in enzyme deficiencies like 17α-hydroxylase/17, 20-lyase , 3β-hydroxysteroid dehydrogenase type 2, and 17β-hydroxysteroid dehydrogenase type 3. Levels of mullerian inhibiting substance are low in these patients. Abnormalities of the genito-femoral nerve and calcitonin gene-related peptide have also been postulated in causation of undescended testis. Epididymal anomalies have been found in up to 90% cases of undescended testis.

What are the complications associated with undescended testis?

If left untreated the most dreaded complication associated with undescended testis is development of testicular tumours like seminoma, embryonal carcinoma and gonadoblastoma. Due to the lack of any symptom in an intra-abdominal testis, these lesions are detected during the late stage of disease when they have metastasized. Up to 2% patient with undescended testis have been found to have carcinoma *in situ*.

Infertility is another irreversible complication that affects undescended testis. Many unilateral cryporchid patients have near normal semen parameters but most patients with bilateral undescended testis are infertile. Undescended testis is intrinsically defective with higher risk of spermatodysgenesis, it is thus often debated whether infertility is due to subsequent dysregulation of spermatogenesis or this intrinsic defect. Leydig cell hypoplasia is seen as early as 1 month after birth in the undescended testis and peritubular fibrosis starts by as early as one year. Early orchidopexy is instrumental in preservation of fertility. Decrease in the number of Leydig cells, Sertoli cells, germ cells and primary spermatocytes, delayed appearance of spermatogonia and persistence of gonocytes are some histological features observed in undescended testis as early as 1 to 2 years.

Torsion is common in undescended testis compared to the normal testis due to free lying narrow mesentery and lack of a fixed axis within the abdomen. Torsion often leads to testicular atrophy 'vanishing testis' and associated with episode of acute abdomen or acute scrotum. Orchidopexy is the best way of preventing this complication.

Hernia is an associated comorbidity in up to 90% patients and during surgery it is necessary to diligently look for the sac and dissect and ligate it followed by orchidopexy. Failure to identify the sac may lead to hernia formation and need for re-operation which is more difficult than the primary repair.

Inguinal testis is more susceptible to trauma because of its fixed and non-mobile location.

How will you work up a patient of undescended testis?

Patients with bilateral cryptorchidism and genital anomalies like hypospadias must have a karyotype analysis and hormonal analysis done. The risk of chromosomal and metabolic anomalies increases as the hypospadias becomes more proximal. The level of testosterone, luteinising hormone and follicle stimulating hormone should be done to assess the functional status of the gonads.

Imaging in the form of ultrasound and magnetic resonance imaging (MRI) has a little to contribute to the diagnosis. Ultrasound may help in identification of an inguinal testis if it is non-palpable on initial examination. MRI may not be able to visualise the testis in a large number of cases. It may be indicated when laparoscopy is unable to visualize an ectopic testis within the abdomen. Diagnostic laparoscopy is the investigation of choice for localising intra-abdominal testis.

What is the role of hCG stimulation test?

The presence of testis can be identified in some cases using the hCG stimulation test. 5000 IU of hCG is administered as 6 divided doses over 3 weeks. Levels of testosterone, dihydrotestosterone, FSH, and LH levels are attained before the start of the test and 24–48 hours after completing the dose. If there is an increase in level of testosterone and DHT and FSH and LH levels fall, the presence of at least one testis may be implied. False-negative response without a rise in testosterone and dihydrotestosterone can occur if the Leydig cells are unresponsive to hCG. The test is not needed if the baseline testosterone, LH and FSH levels indicate primary testicular failure indicating absence of testicular tissue (raised LH and FSH in presence of reduced testosterone).

What is the role of hormonal therapy in patients with undescended testis?

Exogenous hCG and exogenous GnRH or LHRH have been administered in patients with undescended testis. These agents increase the levels of serum testosterone by acting at different stages of hypothalamo-pituitary-gonadal axis. hCG is the most commonly available agent that bears homology to luteinizing hormone. Some studies have found favourable results with hormonal therapy while others relate the presence of various favourable factors as the cause of success of hormonal therapy. Hormonal therapy has a role in young patients with palpable testis (the lower the position, better the results). In these patients a twice weekly intramuscular injection of 1500 IU/m^2 is given for 4 weeks. Alternatively intranasal spray of GnRH analogues may be given in a dose of 1–1.2 mg daily for a period of 4 weeks. The overall success of treatment varies from 10 to 20% and is dependent upon the pre-treatment position of testis. Hormonal therapy is not recommended for non-palpable testis and surgery remains the gold standard.

The therapy is contraindicated in immunocompromised patients, those who have undergone prior scrotal surgery, patients with ectopic testis or associated hernia. Hormonal manipulation may lead to increase in penile size and appearance of secondary sexual characters along with increase in scrotal pigmentation and rugosity.

How is a case of nonpalpable testis managed?

Patients who present with a non-palpable testis should be managed by laparoscopy to rule out the presence of an abdominal viable testis. Laparoscopy can be avoided if a nubbin is palpable within the inguinal canal on examination. On laparoscopy the testis is located and is usually found near the internal ring in many cases. If the testis cannot be found during laparoscopy, the vessels are followed up to the internal inguinal ring. The following possible findings may be present:

1. *Normal testis near the internal ring*: Brought down into the scrotum using single stage/staged orchidopexy.
2. *Normal testis high up in the abdomen*: Staged orchidopexy.
3. *Only blind ending vessels*: No further treatment needed.
4. *Vessels seen passing into internal ring but no testis seen*: Inguinal exploration and orchiopexy/ excision of nubbin.
5. *Small testis or short atretic vas*: Consider orchidectomy.

What are the various surgeries that can be done for orchidopexy?

Inguinal orchidopexy with repair of concomitant inguinal hernia is the treatment of choice for undescended testis. The surgery is performed after 6 months of age as spontaneous descend can occur up till this time. Beyond 6 months there are a little chances of further descent.

If the testis is palpable a trans-scrotal approach may also be used to fix the testis to the scrotum. The incision is placed along the superior border of scrotum and the hernia is dealt through the same incision.

Open transabdominal orchidopexy can be performed using an extended inguinal incision. In this procedure a muscle splitting incision is used and peritoneum is incised to expose the testis. The testis is fixed to the scrotum using a tunnel made through the scrotum.

Laparoscopic orchidopexy is the procedure of choice for non-palpable intra-abdominal testis. During this procedure the testis is localized and mobilized. The gubernaculum is dissected and used as a support to hold the testis and prevent direct handling. If the vessels and vas are long enough, the testis is brought down into the internal ring. Hernias then pulled back in and the ring closed.

What manoeuvres can be done to bring the testis into the scrotum during open orchidopexy?

Many a times the cord attached to the testis may fall short and it may be difficult to bring down or retain the testis into the scrotal or subdartos pouch. In such situations the following manoeuvres can be performed in the given order:

- Dissection of attached sac formed by tunica vaginalis
- Most commonly the mobility of the testis is limited by the cremasteric fibres and fascia that form a part of the cord. These may be gently separated from the cord or dissected to gain additional length.
- Medialization of the spermatic vessels.

If the testis lie at a distance greater than 4 cm from the internal ring or the testis cannot be mobilized up to the opposite internal ring, it may be difficult to bring the testis down to the scrotum. These additional manoeuvres can be helpful in these situations:

- *Prentiss manoeuvre*: The spermatic cord is brought medially by incising floor of inguinal canal and ligating internal epigastric vessels. Testis may be passed under the inguinal floor and brought from just above the pubic tubercle bypassing the whole inguinal canal.
- External nylon fixation button.
- *Albert and Presky operation*: This is a two-staged approach, where testis is mobilized up to the external ring or pubic tubercle and mobilized again as a second stage procedure after 6–12 months after placing the cord structures in a sialastic sheet.
- Fowler-Stephens test followed by Fowler Stephens procedure. This procedure is based on the principle that testis derives its blood supply from three sources, namely testicular artery, cremasteric artery and artery to the vas. Occasional certain scrotal vessels may also provide some blood supply to the testis. Testicular artery can thus be ligated in the presence of collaterals 1–3 cm proximal to the testis. Initial clamping of the testicular artery is done for 5 minutes and colour change is noted. Absence of change of colour is a useful predictor of presence of collaterals. This is referred to as

the Fowler-Stephens test. A two-staged Fowler Stephens procedure provides time for collateral formation and provides mobility to bring the testis down to the scrotum.

- *Silber and Kelly's procedure*: This procedure is more popularly known as testicular auto-transplant wherein the testis is removed and vascular continuity is restored by anastomosis with the inferior epigastric artery. Up to 80% salvage rates have been reported when the procedure was performed in patients more than 2 years old where the two arteries were large enough for a more successful microscopic anastomosis.

How is the testis fixed within the scrotal sac?

Space is created through a small subcentimetric mid-scrotal incision and a superficial sub-dartos pouch is created with the help of an artery forceps where the testis placed. Occasionally if the tension on the cord prevents safe placement into the scrotal sac and there is fear of retraction sutures have to be placed between the testis and scrotal fascia. Non-absorbable monofilament sutures are taken through the tunica albugenia and transparen-chymal sutures should be avoided. However, when there is clinical torsion of the spermatic cord or a nylon button is required to keep the testis in its location due to tension on the cord transparen-chymal sutures may have to be taken. Disruption of the blood testis barrier and formation of antisperm antibodies are the main concerns behind avoiding sutures through the testicular paren-chyma.

The various other methods for fixing testis to the scrotal sac include:

1. *Keetley-Torek technique*: A space is created superficial to the fascia lata and the testis is brought out through the scrotal incision into the pounch on the thigh fixing the gubernacular tail to the fascia lata and scrotum fixed with the thigh. After a period of 4–6 months the gubernacular stitch is released such that the testis lies within the scrotum.

2. *Ladd and Gross technique*: The testis is fixed to the scrotal skin and the suture brought out and fixed to a nylon button or rubber sheath at the base of the scrotum. The suture is removed after 2–4 weeks.

3. *Ombredanne's technique*: The undescended testis is mobilized and placed into the opposite scrotal sac along with the normal testis after making a window in the transverse scrotal septum.

What is the role of orchidopexy in adolescent patients?

Orchidopexy has not been found to prevent the development of a testicular tumour but there is some evidence that prepubescent orchidopexy may lessen the risk. The main aim of orchidopexy is to make the testis more amenable to examination so that any cancer can be detected earlier and treated with better chances of cure. Orchidopexy also pro-vides psychological support to the patient of presence of both testis within the scrotum. The most common tumour that develops in the undescended testis is seminoma which must be screened for by regular self-examination of the testis. Orchidopexy also minimizes the chances of testicular torsion to which undescended testis are more prone and repairs the concomitant inguinal hernia which is present in as many as 80–90% of the patients.

Should the contralateral testis also be fixed at the time of surgery for ipsilateral testis?

During surgery for torsion of the testis, both testes are fixed due to the belief that Bell Clapper deformity is bilateral in a large number of cases; however, in cases of undescended testis the issue is controversial. Many surgeons prefer to fix the contralateral testis for the fear of Bell Clapper deformity that may lead to torsion of the opposite testis, however, it is not mandatory based on available evidence.

28

Male Infertility

How is infertility of a couple defined?

Infertility can be defined as the failure of conception in a couple engaging in regular and unprotected coitus for 1 year. A simpler definition can be inability to bear a child within 1 year of marriage. There are many old definitions that extend this period to two years. Normally the rates of conception are 20 to 25% per month and cumulate to 75% by 6 months and 90% by 1 year. Infertility has been classified broadly into primary and secondary infertility. Couples without a prior pregnancy are classified into primary, whereas couples with prior fertility are classified into secondary infertility.

One may also choose to evaluate these couples earlier than 1 year if any of the following conditions are present:

Male factors	Female factors
History of surgery on testis	Elderly female >35 years
History of undescended testis	Present or previous ectopic pregnancy
Varicocele	STD or pelvic inflammatory disease
Sexually transmitted diseases	Irregular periods
Prior chemo or radiotherapy	Uterine fibroids

How many percentage of cases male factors are responsible for infertility?

Male factors are responsible for infertility in more than fifty percent of cases.

What are the relevant points on history in a case of an infertile couple?

In the case of an infertile couple the husband is often referred to the surgeon for assessment of fertility. Often there is a problem in conception and history relevant to all aspects of sexual health must be sought. History should focus on points like:

- What is the occupation of the patient?
- Does it involve long term standing, exposure to herbicide pesticides, radiation or heavy metals, or chronic heat (as subtle as laptop use)?
- Does the patient co-inhabit with his wife?
- Has there been sufficient number of attempts to conceive?
- Was the wife on any form of birth control?
- What is the sexual technique and the timing of intercourse?
- Is the female partner being evaluated concomitantly and what have been the significant findings in her case?
- Is the patient suffering from any form of sexual dysfunction like premature ejaculation, erectile dysfunction or sexually transmitted diseases?
- Are there any associated urinary complaints suggesting recurrent UTIs?
- Has the patient had any trauma to the back or genitalia?
- Is there history of any congenital diseases like cryptorchidism, hypospadias or spinal dysraphism?
- How has been the growth in the puberty period?
- Has there been any history of systemic illnesses like fevers, mumps, epididymitis or orchitis?
- Any history of anosmia, recurrent respiratory tract infections or sinus infections? (Kallmann syndrome)
- Is there history of hospitalization for any chronic disease or long term?

- Is there history of any drug intake for diseases like tuberculosis?

- Is there history of drug abuse in the form of antibiotics for long duration steroids like testosterone and recreational drugs or excessive intake of alcohol as these commonly interfere with spermatogenesis, erection, or ejaculation?

- History of chemotherapy or radiotherapy for a previous malignancy?

- Surgical history especially of hernia repair, testicular torsion, orchidopexy, hypospadias repair, sympathectomy, vasectomy or any other procedure on the scrotum may risk injury to the male reproductive tract and entrapment of the vas or history of transurethral resection surgery that may lead to retrograde ejaculation?

On examination the habitus may be suggestive of chromosomal anomalies like Klinefelter's syndrome. Secondary sexual characters and gynaecomazia may be useful clues to primary testicular dysfunction. Examination of the external genitalia and abdomen should be undertaken next. Look for the presence of scars on the lower abdomen and scrotum. Hernial sites should be inspected. Note the stage of penile growth and pattern of secondary sexual characters. Note the location of the meatus to rule out hypospadias. Inspect the penis for chordee or any deformity that may preclude intercourse. Patients with a proximal hypospadias may be capable of coitus but unable to deposit semen in the vagina. Examine the scrotum to first ascertain the presence of both the testis. Undescended testis has been explained in a separate chapter in this book. The size or volume of the testis should be ascertained clinically. The consistency, presence of testicular sensations, and absence of any mass must be looked for. Occasionally in cases of obstructive azoospermia the epididymis is bulky. It may also be involved in tuberculosis. The epididymis continues into the vas which should be palpated on each side to rule out congenital absence of the vas deferens. Any obvious anomalies like dilated veins (varicocele), hydrocele, sinuses and previous scars should be noted. Per-rectal examination is also essential to look for dilated seminal vesicles, or midline prostatic cysts that may cause obstruction to the ejaculatory ducts.

How can sexual maturity be assessed using Tanner staging?

5 stages of sexual maturity have been described by Tanner. At the time of examination it is useful to mention the staging. In hypogonadism secondary sexual characters may be regressed.

Stage I: Fine hair in pubic region as in rest of the body
Testicular volume less than 5 cc.

Stage II: Sparse straight hair along root of penis
Change in texture of the skin with reddening, and increase in size of the testis to >5 cc.

Stage III: Hair become coarser darker and thicker growth in length of penis but testis remain smaller and scrotum is hypopigmented.

Stage IV: Adult like pubic hair confined to an area smaller than normal.
Subnormal testicular volume with pigmented scrotal skin.

Stage V: Adult pubic hair, curly thick and coarse spread over the genital region and medial aspect of thigh, with normal adult genitalia.

What are the basic biochemical investigations required during the workup of a patient of Infertility?

Initial workup of the infertile male includes routine investigations like haemogram, random blood sugar, renal function tests, urine analysis and semen analysis. Based on the reports of semen analysis and examination further battery of tests can be decided.

In moderate to severe oligospermia with counts less than 10 million/ml, hormonal profile should be evaluated. These include FSH and testosterone but if abnormal assay of LH, prolactin and thyroid hormones are also done. Assay of antisperm antibodies in serum is required in patients with abnormal mobility of the sperms and presence of clumping. Imaging in the form of transrectal ultrasound is needed in patients with low semen volume to look for causes of ejaculatory duct obstruction. Scrotal ulrasonography may reveal presence of varicocele and epididymal pathology. If a central cause of infertility is suspected, imaging of the hypothalamus and pituitary is also indicated in the form of an MRI or CT scan. If the semen parameters are adequate, the compatibility with the female and sperm function assay are indicated.

These advanced semen parameters include post-coital test, sperm cervical mucus penetration test, acrosome reaction test and zona-free hamster oocyte sperm penetration assay. In patients with leukocytospermia and necrospermia, evaluation of oxidative stress and DNA integrity assay may also be needed.

What precautions must be undertaken when interpreting semen analysis?

The specimen may be collected at lab or at home but delay should be minimal preferably not more than 1 to 2 hours. If semen has been collected at home it should be brought to lab while keeping it in the shirt pocket next to the body to keep it at near body temperature. The specimen is usually collected by masturbation and collection using coitus interruptus should be avoided. Semen collected by masturbation closely but not accurately represents the semen release during normal coitus as semen released at coitus results from adequate excitation and foreplay. Semen is collected in a wide mouthed container and patient needs to be instructed to squeeze out the semen completely in order to collect the complete ejaculate without missing the post-seminal portion of semen. Most important aspect when ordering semen analysis is to ascertain adequate abstinence. The patient should practise abstinence for 2–7 days prior to giving the semen sample. Both shorter and longer duration of abstinence can cause erroneous results in a patient with normal semen.

What are the features of normal semen?

Based on the criteria by WHO the lower reference range limits for semen parameters are shown in Table 28.1.

What are the various terms used to describe the semen parameters?

- Normozoospermia—normal semen parameters
- Oligozoospermia—reduced sperm number <15 million/ml
- Asthenozoospermia—reduced sperm motility
- Teratozoospermia—increased abnormal forms of sperm
- Oligoasthenoteratozoospermia—all sperm variables are abnormal
- Azoospermia—no sperms seen in semen
- Leucocytospermia—increase white blood cells in semen

Table 28.1: Features of normal semen

Semen parameter	Lower reference limit
Semen volume (ml)	1.5 (1.4–1.7)
Total sperm number (10^6 per ejaculate)	39 (33–46)
Sperm concentration (10^6 per ml)	15 (12–16)
Total motility (progressive + non-progressive, %)	40 (38–42)
Progressive motility (PR, %)	32 (31–34)
Vitality (live spermatozoa, %)	58 (55–63)
Sperm morphology (normal forms, %)	4 (3.0–4.0)
pH	7.2
Peroxidase-positive leukocytes (10^6 per ml)	1.0
MAR test (motile spermatozoa with bound particles, %)	50
Immunobead test (motile spermatozoa with bound beads, %)	50
Seminal zinc (mol/ejaculate)	2.4
Seminal fructose (mol/ejaculate)	13
Seminal neutral glucosidase (mU/ejaculate)	20

- Necrozoospermia—non-viable sperms present in semen
- Aspermia—no ejaculation or ejaculate formation

What is Azoospermia and how is it classified and managed?

Azoospermia can be defined as the absence of sperms in the semen. It is broadly classified into obstructive and nonobstructive azoospermia. When there is a lack of sperm production in the testis due to primary testicular failure or lack of stimulation from the hypogonado-pituitary axis, the causes are classified under nonobstructive azoospermia (NOZA), whereas diseases that lead to physical obstruction to the outflow of sperms lead to obstructive azoospermia.

Low semen volume is an important clue to obstruction. The causes of low semen volume are discussed below along with appropriate management. If the semen volume is normal, the usual approach is to obtain serum hormone levels like FSH and testosterone. Their levels can be helpful to differentiate obstructive azoospermia from reduced testicular function. Low FSH associated with low testosterone is suggestive of hypogonadotrophic hypogonadism. Serum LH, prolactin, cranial CT and MRI are indicated in such patients as the part of work up. In patients with normal testicular size, elevated FSH (>2 times of normal) and normal testosterone, primary testicular failure should be ruled out. Testicular biopsy or fine needle aspiration can be useful in these cases. If the testicular histopathology shows normal spermatogenesis, obstruction should be considered as a cause of azoospermia. If there is arrest in the development of sperms, *in vitro* fertilization has to be considered after sperm extraction if feasible.

What are the important causes of obstructive azoospermia?

Absence of sperms in the semen in the presence of normal testicular function (as evidenced by normal physical characters, hormonal profile and fine needle aspiration cytology) is an indicator towards obstructive azoospermia. To label a patient as having azoospermia at least 2 centrifuged speci-mens should be observed. The common causes of obstructive azoospermia are:

Obstruction within the epididymis:
- Acute or chronic epididymitis
- Iatrogenic trauma resulting from previous scrotal surgery
- Previous fertility intervention (PESA, MESA)
- Young syndrome (sinobronchial disease with azoospermia)
- Congenital complete or partial absence of epididymis
- Secondary to vassal obstruction from increased pressure

Obstruction of the vas deferens:
- Vasectomy or any other diagnostic intervention on the vas
- Congenital bilateral/unilateral absence of vas deferens
- Prior inguinal or scrotal surgery

Obstruction to the ejaculatory duct:
- Partial ejaculatory duct obstruction
- Prostatic, utricular or seminal vesicular cysts
- Endourological intervention
- Prostatic infections

What are the causes of low volume on semen analysis and how does one manage such patients?

Low volume on semen analysis is often a result of improper collection of semen. A repeat semen analysis is warranted in such cases. The other causes include:

- Drugs
- Retroperitoneal or bladder neck surgery
- Ejaculatory duct obstruction, CBAVD
- Diabetes mellitus
- Spinal cord injury
- Androgen deficiency
- Psychologic disturbances
- Idiopathic

It must be ascertained that the abstinence period is adequate for production of good volume ejaculate. Occasionally retrograde ejaculation may result in low volume antegrade ejaculation as a large part of the semen is reposited in the bladder and post-ejaculatory urinalysis is the next logical step in evaluation. Sympathomimetics or sperm harvest and artificial reproduction are simple and useful options for treatment. If no sperms are obtained on post-ejaculatory urinalysis, etiologies like partial or total ejaculatory duct obstruction must be considered. Transurethral ultrasound is the initial minimally invasive treatment in such cases. If the seminal vesicles are found to be dilated on transrectal ultrasound semen with viable sperms can be aspirated from the vesicle or trans-urethral, resection of ejaculatory, duct can be done. If no abnormality is found, then the aetiology of failure to ejaculate semen is managed by electro-ejaculation or sympathomimetics.

What is varicocele (Fig. 28.1)?

Varicocele can be defined as an abnormal dilata-tion and tortuosity of the veins draining the testis

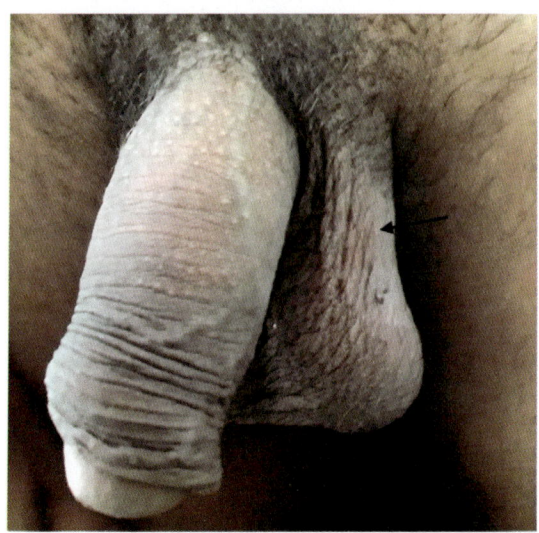

Fig. 28.1: Clinical picture of varicocele

and epididymis that form the pampiniform plexus of the spermatic cord. It often results from renal venous hypertension and defect in the valves of the testicular vein. The aetiology also includes genetic predisposition, inherent defect in the veins and the body habitus of the patient.

What is the clinical presentation of varicocele?

Varicocele presents in the young age or early adulthood with complaints of pain, swelling and often as infertility. Many patients also present for the reason of medical fitness.

What are the common differential diagnoses of varicocele?

The common differential diagnosis of varicocele includes:
- Encysted hydrocele of the cord
- Lipoma of the cord
- Vaginal hydrocele
- Epididymal cyst
- Inguinal hernia
- Lymph varix
- Spermatocele

Why is varicocele more common on the left side?

Up to 90% of the varicoceles occur on the left side. This is due to various anatomical and physiological reasons:
- Left testicular vein drains into the renal vein perpendicular to it while the right drains into the IVC at an acute angle. The opening is more superior to the location on the right and thus a longer column of venous blood stays in the left vein increasing its pressure.
- *Nut cracker phenomenon*: The left renal vein is often placed between the abdominal aorta and the superior mesenteric vein and its compression leads to varicocele.
- Compression of the renal vein by the testicular artery and the pelvic colon may also lead to varicocele.
- As adrenal and renal metabolites drain via the renal vein to which the left testicular vein is directly exposed there is increased reflux.

What is secondary varicocele?

Varicocele arising secondary to obstruction to the testicular veins is called secondary varicocele. It often results from extrinsic compression or venous hypertension due to involvement by tumours like renal tumour invading into the renal vein and testicular vein and retroperitoneal tumours.

Clinically it is differentiated from primary varicocele in that primary varicocele appears insidiously while secondary varicocele appears in a short span of time. Primary varicocele disappears on lying supine while secondary varicocele may still persist. Secondary varicocele may be associated with an abdominal mass.

Primary varicocele can be emptied in lying down on raising the scrotum but secondary varicocele cannot be emptied on raising the scrotum in lying down position.

How is varicocele graded clinically?

Clinically varicocele may be graded as follows:
- *Grade 0*: No evidence of varicocele clinically but detected on ultrasound of the scrotum. It is also called subclinical varicocele and management is indicated only if associated with pain or discomfort.
- *Grade I*: Varicocele is not appreciable on inspection but can be felt on valsalva manoeuvre.
- *Grade II*: Varicocele is not appreciable on inspection but can be felt without performing valsalva.
- *Grade III*: Varicocele can be appreciated on inspection.

What are the indications of surgery in a case of varicocele?

The indications of surgery in a patient with varicocele include:
- Pain
- Scrotal swelling
- Infertility
  - Abnormal semen analysis with high grade varicocele
  - Varicocele with disparity in testicular size on affected side >2 cm
- Medical clearance.

What are the surgical procedures available for management of varicocele?

The surgical procedures for management of varicocele include:

Retroperitoneal varicocele repair (Palomo's operation): One of the most popular procedures in the earlier times retroperitoneal repair has fallen out of favour in the present time. This procedure involves high ligation of the testicular vein above the level where it receives multiple tributaries. This procedure is associated with the highest risk of hydrocele formation as lymphatics that drain into the vein are also obstructed. Recurrence is observed in 2–4% of the cases. The advantages of this approach are that vein is easier to identify and only a single vein needs to be ligated. The procedure can also be performed laparoscopically.

Inguinal approach (Ivanissevich's procedure): The inguinal approach gained popularity owing to the familiarity of the surgeon with inguinal anatomy. Much like the inguinal hernia surgery the inguinal canal is opened and the spermatic cord is isolated and opened. Testicular artery is identified either by its pulsations or using a Doppler probe and veins are ligated. Occasionally a single vein adjacent to the artery may be spared to maintain venous return. This procedure is cumbersome due to the large number of veins to be ligated and is associated with high rates of both recurrence and hydrocele formation.

Subinguinal approach (Lemack): Spermatic cord in the sub-inguinal approach is accessed at the level of the external inguinal ring or below at the root of the scrotum. Using a small transverse incision the spermatic cord is exposed and explored. The rest of the technique is similar to the inguinal approach. The advantage of this procedure is the cosmetic appeal even though the chances of recurrence are the highest with this technique. There are chances of testicular atrophy if the testicular artery is accidentally ligated.

Microscopic sub-inguinal varicocelectomy: This is the gold standard for management of varicocele today. This procedure combines the cosmetic advantage and reduced rates of recurrence and complications. It requires an optical microscope but many studies have shown comparable results with use of surgical loupes as well.

Sclerotherapy: Sclerotherapy is another minimally invasive technique for management of varicocele. Both antegrade and retrograde approach can be used to inject the sclerosant into the spermatic veins. Sclerotherapy is associated with high rates of recurrence.

What are the complications of surgery for varicocele?

The common complications of surgery for varicocele include:

- Hemorrhage
- Testicular atrophy
- Hydrocele
- Recurrence.

Skin
and Subcutaneous
Tissue

Section 5

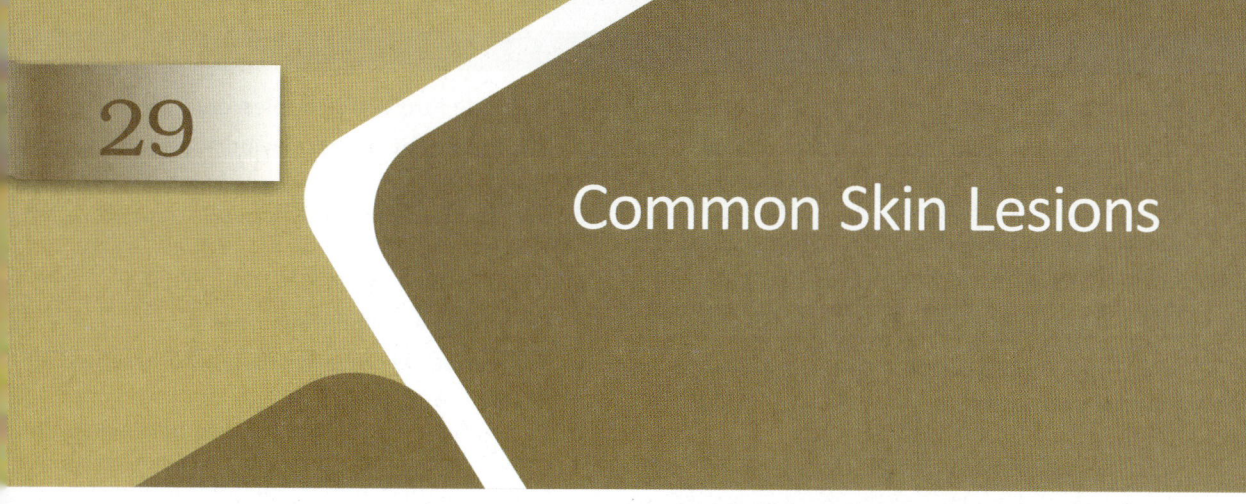

29

Common Skin Lesions

What are the different layers of skin?

The skin is the largest organ in the body and comprises epidermis and dermis. The epidermis is mainly derived from keratinocytes and comprises stratified squamous epithelium. The distinct cell layers of epidermis are (a) stratum basale (single cell layer) with columnar or cubical cells, (b) stratum spinosum (5–15 cell thick), (c) stratum granulare (1 to 3 cells thick), (d) stratum corneum (5–10 cells thick). Dermal fibers are predominantly made of type I and type III collagen in 4:1 ratio.

What is a dermoid cyst and what are its types?

A dermoid cyst is located deep to the skin and primarily consists of structures derived from primitive ectoderm. They are mostly congenital in origin except post-traumatic implantation dermoid. They are mostly cystic on the body surface but sometimes may be solid, e.g. mediastinal dermoid.

Types of dermoid (Fig. 29.1) are:

a. *Sequestration dermoid*: It results from sequestration and inclusion of an island of skin deep to the normal skin along embryonic lines of fusion. It contains toothpaste like sebaceous material frequently with tufts of hair and desquamated material. The lining of the cyst wall is stratified squamous epithelium with hair follicles, hair, sweat and sebaceous gland and papillary of dermis. The papillary layer of dermis is absent in implantation dermoid.

b. *Implantation dermoid*: This occurs when the skin get buried in the dermis due to trauma.

c. *Tubulodermoid*: It is cystic swelling arising from the unobliterated persistent portion a congenital ectodermal duct or tube used in development.

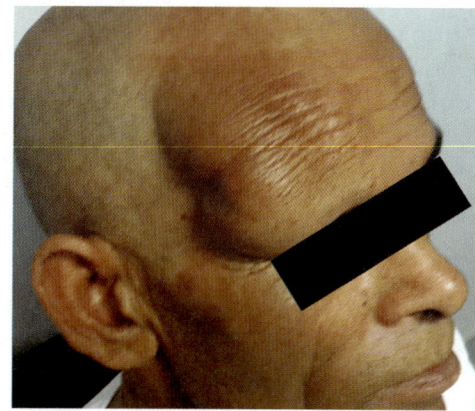

Fig. 29.1: Clinical picture showing angular dermoid

The examples are thyroglossal cyst, urachal cyst and postanal dermoid.

d. *Teratomatous dermoid*: This denotes cystic swelling arising from the totipotent cells with preponderance of ectodermal cells. The common sites are mediastinum, sacrococcygeal, ovary, retroperitoneum and testis. The contents are cartilage, bone, tooth, hairs, muscle and glandular tissue. They are prone undergo carcinomatous or sarcomatous changes.

What are the sites of a dermoid cyst?

They can occur anywhere on the body surface along the lines of fusion. Common sites are forehead, root of nose, brow areas, and post-auricular regions of scalp, median raphe of scrotum and perineum. Dermoid of the nasoglabellar region may have meningeal connection. Dermoid sometimes can occur in lateral situation like shoulder or buttock possibly due to displacement or dislocation of tissue to a site distant from fusion line.

What is sebaceous cyst (Fig. 29.2)?

It is retention cyst due to obstruction of the opening of the duct of the sebaceous gland. The duct of these glands opens most commonly in the hair follicle but sometimes on to the skin surface. Sebaceous glands are known as holocrine glands and produce secretions by fatty degeneration of their central cells. This secretion is known as sebum and can block the mouth of the duct of gland if gets dried up.

What is the function of sebaceous gland?

The sebum secreted by sebaceous glands keeps the skin soft and oily.

What are sites where sebaceous glands can occur?

They can occur on any hairy part except palm and sole where the sebaceous glands are usually absent. The most common sites are scalp, face, scrotum, vulva, back of the trunk and limbs.

Describe the pathology of sebaceous cyst.

Pathologically they are regarded as epidermoid cyst when the obstruction of sebaceous duct is followed by down growth and accumulation of desquamated epidermal cells. The content of sebaceous cyst is yellowish white material composed of fat and epithelial cells and the consistency is putty like.

How does one identify a sebaceous cyst?

Clinical features of sebaceous cysts are following:

a. They are slow growing and can occur in any age group.

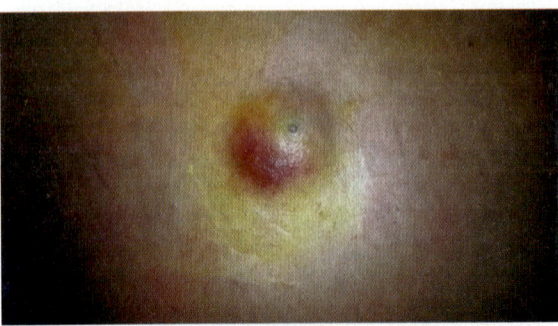

Fig. 29.2: Clinical picture of sebaceous cyst

b. They are rare before adolescence.

c. They present as hemispherical round well defined swelling.

d. The size of the swelling depends upon duration of the cyst.

e. They are firm or elastic in consistency.

f. They have a well-defined margin.

g. The surface is smooth but can be indented by finger.

h. The punctum which is the site of blockage of external opening of the duct is seen as bluish point. The punctum is adherent to the cyst.

i. The swelling is fixed to the overlying skin but is free from underlying structures.

j. In the scalp the swelling is more prominent as it cannot bulge backwards in the solid skull bones.

What is the differential diagnosis?

Sebaceous cyst must be differentiated from dermoid cyst. A sebaceous cyst is a swelling in the skin and a dermoid is a swelling deep to the skin.

What are the complications of sebaceous cyst?

Complications of sebaceous cyst are:

a. *Infection*: Infected cyst is characterised by rapidly enlarging painful cyst with overlying red and hot skin.

b. *Calcification*: Calcified sebaceous cyst is also known as benign calcifying epithelioma. They are commonly seen in scrotum as subcutaneous hard tumour which are calcified radiological examination.

c. *Cock's peculiar tumours*: Infection is followed by suppuration and rupture with escape of purulent and sebaceous material. This leaves a granulating ulcer or a mass of edematous granulation tissue giving an appearance of epithelioma. It is not a real tumour but has appearance of malignant ulcer. Biopsy is required to settle the diagnosis. The local lymph nodes may be enlarged and tender.

d. *Sebaceous horn*: It results from escape and inspissation of the sebaceous material in successive layers on the skin resulting in horny projection. It is commonly seen in scalp or scrotum.

e. *Malignant change*: Malignant change in sebaceous cyst is rare and can result in adenocarcinoma.

What is the treatment of sebaceous cyst?

Excision of sebaceous cyst is advised due to its tendency to grow and become infected. The cyst should be excised completely in order to avoid recurrence. If the cyst is small and the overlying skin is healthy, a linear incision is employed. If the cyst is markedly protuberant or if the skin is thin and unhealthy or if there is an overlying punctum, an elliptical incision is used. The punctum should be in the centre of the ellipse which should be equal in length to the diameter of cyst. If the skin overlying the cyst is stretched, the width of the ellipse can be wider to avoid excess skin folds and dog ears when closing the wound. After the skin ellipse is incised, a plane is developed between the cyst wall and the surrounding skin by sharp or blunt dissection, preferable without opening the cyst. After dissection all around, the cyst is easily shelled out. An alternative method is avulsion of the cyst. This is particularly suited for removal of cysts on the scalp. A comparatively small incision is required and cutaneous scarring is less. A skin flap is raised on only one side. The cyst is then deliberately opened and contents squeezed out. A pair of non-toothed dissecting forceps with one blade outside the cyst and one blade inside, cyst wall is grasped at its deepest part and by traction on the forceps; the entire cyst wall can be avulsed easily. The cyst wall is held at the deepest portion because the deeper part is tougher than the superficial portion and will not tear easily. The wound is sutured and a pressure dressing is applied to prevent hematoma formation in the cavity.

If the sebaceous cyst is infected, removal is deferred until the inflammation subsides. If there is abscess formation, it should be incised and pus drained. Curettage of the abscess cavity or swabbing with pure carbolic acid may prevent the cyst from reforming. Infected sebaceous cysts should not be excised as wound complication rates are high and the resulting scars are unsatisfactory. They often do not recur after incision because infection frequently destroys the lining of the cyst.

What is Pott's Puffy tumour (Fig. 29.3)?

Sir Percivall Pott in 1760 first described it. It is a rare clinical entity characterized by subperiosteal abscess associated with osteomyelitis of frontal bone. This results in a swelling on the forehead. The abscess can extend inwards, leading to an

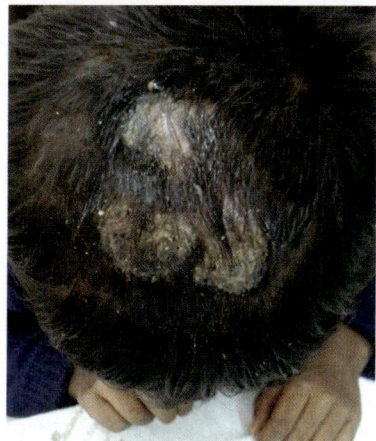

Fig. 29.3: Clinical picture of Pott's puffy tumour

intracranial abscess. It can be associated with cortical vein thrombosis, epidural abscess, subdural empyema, and brain abscess. The vein thrombosis results through extension of infection through diploic veins, which communicate with the dural venous plexus. The septic thrombi can potentially evolve from foci within the frontal sinus and propagate through this venous system. Although it can affect all ages, it is mostly found among teenagers and adolescents. It is usually seen as a complication of frontal sinusitis or trauma.

What is a pyogenic granuloma (Fig. 29.4)?

Pyogenic granuloma is also known as:
a. Eruptive haemangioma
b. Granulation tissue-type haemangioma

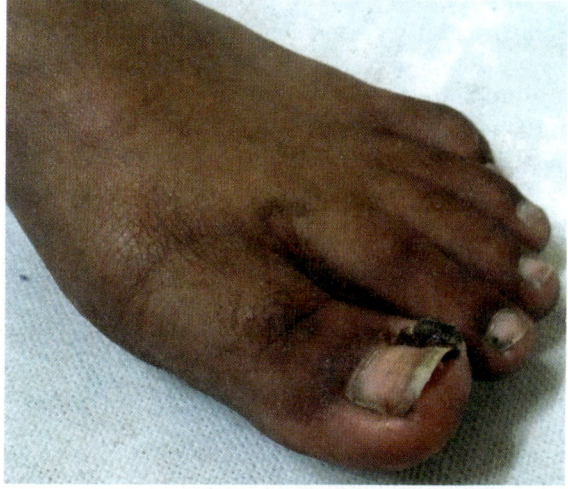

Fig. 29.4: Clinical picture of pyogenic granuloma of left great toe

c. Granuloma gravidarum

d. Lobular capillary haemangioma

It was first described by two French surgeons, Poncet and Dor in 1897.

The name pyogenic granuloma is misnomer as it is not a true granuloma. In reality it is a capillary haemangioma of lobular subtype which is prone to bleeding. It is not truly pyogenic in nature as the cause is traumatic and not infectious. It is a lesion that occurs on both mucosa and skin, and appears as an overgrowth of tissue. It results from irritation, physical trauma or hormonal factors.

Common sites of occurrence are the gums, the skin and nasal septum, in the distal extremity. They occur as a solitary, glistening red papule or nodule which can bleed or ulcerate. Pyogenic granuloma typically grows rapidly over a period of a few weeks, most often on the head, neck, extremities, and upper trunk. Pyogenic granuloma can arise in pregnancy (or rarely with oral contraceptive usage), particularly on the gingival or elsewhere in the oral mucosa, and then is termed the "pregnancy tumour." Systemic retinoids may occasionally trigger pyogenic granuloma-like lesions. Antiretrovirals have been associated with the development of pyogenic granuloma, predominantly of the great toes. Periungal pyogenic granulomas occurring during epidermal growth factor receptor inhibitor therapy are a mounting problem for oncology patients, arising after 2 months of drug exposure.

The typical solitary pyogenic granuloma (lobular capillary haemangioma) is a bright red, friable polypoid papule or nodule ranging from a few millimeters to several centimeters. The average size is 6.5 mm. The classic exophytic raspberry like lesion has a moist surface and an epithelial collarette at the base. Bleeding, erosion, ulceration, purulence, and crusting frequently are noted. Regressing lesions appear as a soft fibroma.

Topical Imiquimod cream and Alitretinoin gel have both been successfully used to treat pyogenic granulomas. Injectable sclerosing agents, chemical cauterization with silver nitrate, topical phenol for periungual lesions, and photodynamic therapy with 5-aminolevulinic acid, intralesional injection have all been used.

What is a pilonidal sinus (Fig. 29.5)?

Pilonidal disease was described way back in 1833, by Mayo is a hair-containing cyst located just below the coccyx. Hodge coined the term "pilonidal". Pilonidal includes a spectrum of clinical presentations, ranging from asymptomatic hair-containing cysts and sinuses to large symptomatic abscesses of the sacrococcygeal region that have some tendency to recur. Pilonidal sinus has also been known occur in hands and in axilla.

The pilonidal disease has been studied on an embryologic basis and is considered to be of congenital origin. Excision of the lesion was thought to be fundamental to removing all embryologic remnants. It came to be known as Jeep disease as nearly 80,000 US soldiers were admitted and treated at US Army Hospitals between the years 1941 and 1945 for this problem.

Patey and Scarf hypothesized the origin of pilonidal disease was acquired by penetration of hair into the subcutaneous tissue with consequent granulomatous reaction, basing this theory on the high incidence of recurrence, as well as occurrence of disease in other areas of the body, such as the hands of a barber or sheep shearer. An acquired aetiology of the disease is now the prevailing theory in the medical world.

It has been postulated that hair penetrates into the subcutaneous tissues through dilated hair follicles, which is thought to occur particularly in late adolescence, though follicles are not found in the walls of cysts. A sinus develops with a short tract, with a not clearly understood suction mechanism involving local anatomy, eventually

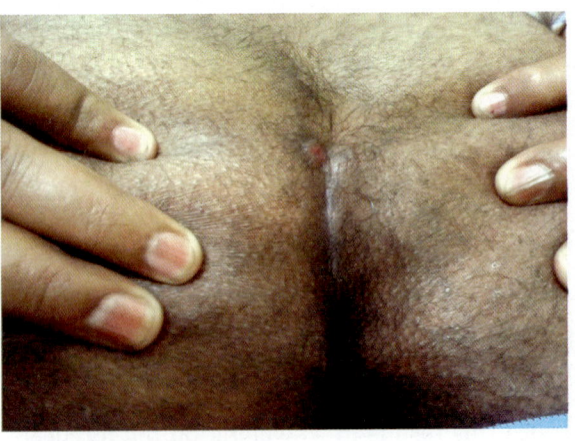

Fig. 29.5: Clinical picture of pilonidal sinus

leading to further penetration of the hair into the subcutaneous tissue. A foreign body-type reaction may then lead to formation of an abscess. If given the opportunity to drain spontaneously, this may act as a portal of further invasion and eventually formation of a foreign body granuloma.

Microscopically, the sinus where the hair enters is lined with stratified squamous epithelium with slight cornification. Additional sinuses are frequent. Cyst cavities are lined with chronic granulation tissue and may contain hair, epithelial debris, and young granulation tissue. Cutaneous appendages are not seen in the wall of cysts. Cellular infiltration consists of PMNs, lymphocytes, and plasma cells in varying proportions. Foreign body giant cells in association with dead hairs are a frequent finding.

The three factors are important in development of pilonidal sinus (1) the invader, hair; (2) the force, causing hair penetration; and (3) the vulnerability of the skin.

What is neurofibromatosis and what are its types?

Neurofibroma is a benign tumour of nerve sheath origin which comprises mixture of fibrous (mesodermal) tissue and neural (ectodermal) tissue. This is not a true tumour or neuroma but is regarded as hamartoma.

Types of neurofibroma are:
a. Solitary neurofibroma
b. Generalised neurofibromatosis (Fig. 29.6)
c. Plexiform neurofibromatosis (Fig. 29.7)
d. Elephantisis neuromatosa
e. Cutaneous neurofibromatosis

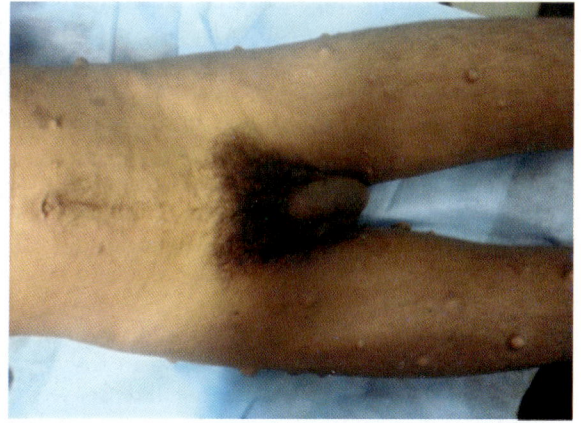

Fig. 29.6: Clinical picture of generalized neurofibromatosis

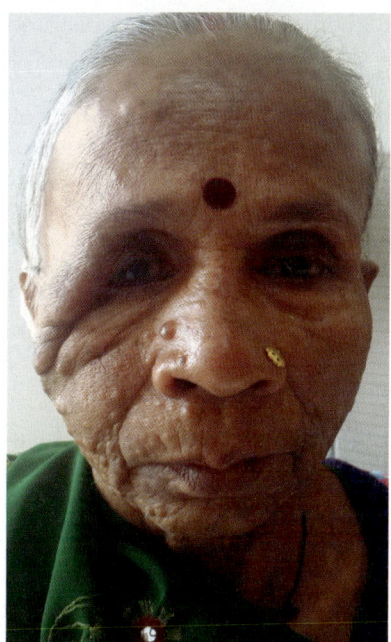

Fig. 29.7: Clinical picture of plexiform neurofibromatosis

What is solitary neurofibroma?

a. It appears along the course of a peripheral nerve as a solitary well defined, smooth painful nodule.
b. It can be moved in lateral direction but not in the direction of nerve.
c. Pain or paraesthesia may occur from the pressure of the tumour on nerve fibers.
d. Cystic degeneration or sarcomatous changes may occur some times.

What are the nerves which are commonly involved in solitary neurofibroma?

Following nerves are commonly involved:
1. Peripheral nerves like median, ulnar, lateral popliteal
2. Cranial nerve like acoustic neuroma
3. Cord of brachial plexus.

What is von Recklinghausen's disease and what are its diagnostic features?

This disease was first described by Friederich Daniel von Recklinghausen, the pathologist, in 1882. It is one of the most frequent human genetic diseases, with a prevalence of one in 3,000 births. This is a condition of generalised neurofibromatosis in which neurofibroma are scattered throughout the body giving Cobble Stone appearance. There is diffuse proliferation or thickening of the nerve sheath. The clinically patient present with widespread nodular or elliptical swelling of nerves. There is overgrowth in relation to endoneurium with epineurium remains unchanged. They comprise spindle cells with whorled appearance. It is an autosomal dominant disease caused by a spectrum of mutations that affect the NF1gene located at the 17q11.2 chromosome. Only 50% of the NF1 patients have a positive family history of the disease. The rest of the patients represent spontaneous mutations.

Diagnosis requires the presence of 2 or more major criteria:

a. 6 or more café au lait spot (>0.5 cm in prepubertal children, >1.5 cm in post-pubertal individuals), axillary or inguinal freckling. Café au lait spots are hyperpigmented flat spots that are oval or rounded with fairly smooth borders. They are present at birth in many individuals and increase in size and number over the first 5 to 7 years of life.

b. Two or more cutaneous neurofibroma. Cutaneous or dermal neurofibroma are tumours of the nerve sheath comprised of Schwann cells, fibroblasts, perineural cells, mast cells, axons, and blood vessels. They may appear in childhood but more commonly develop in teenagers or adults. They may be purplish depressions in the skin or pedunculated lesions.

c. At least 1 plexiform neurofibroma which are histologically similar to cutaneous neurofibroma but have more extra-cellular matrix. They often arise from the dorsal spinal roots, nerve plexi, large nerve trunks, or sympathetic chains. Plexiform tumours may be discrete, homogeneous, and well circumscribed or diffuse, heterogeneous, and infiltrative. They may involve superficial skin or be entirely internal.

d. The characteristic bony lesions (pseudarthrosis, sphenoid wing hypoplasia).

e. An optic glioma.

f. 2 or more iris Lisch nodules, or a first-degree relative with NF1.

In some, the diagnosis can be made at birth, whereas others must be observed for a few years for the presence of additional criteria.

What is lipoma?

Lipomas are slow-growing benign, adipose tumours derived from adipocytes that are most often found in the subcutaneous tissues but may be seen anywhere in the body where fat cells are present.

What are common sites of lipoma?

Lipomas are known as universal tumour and can occur anywhere in the body. They most commonly occur on the nape of the neck, paravertebral region, shoulder, buttock, and check. They are seldom seen in eyelid, pinna, and penis.

What are different types of lipoma?

Lipoma can be encapsulated or it can be diffuse lipoma without any capsule.

Lipoma can be solitary or multiple. Multiple lipomas occurring all over the body are also known as Dercum's disease in which case they are painful and tender.

What are different anatomical planes where lipoma can occur?

a. *Subcutaneous*: Commonly found on shoulder and back.

b. *Subfascial*: Subfascial lipoma can occur deep to palmer or plantar fascia or deep to epicranial aponeurosis. Subepicranial lipoma of long standing duration can cause erosion of underlying bone with palpable bony depression when lipoma is pushed to one side.

c. *Intramuscular lipoma*: These arise from collection of fat around the nutrient vessel entering the muscle or in loose areolar tissue separating different group of muscles. It is felt or seen as lump appearing during exercise and interfering with the functions of muscle. The lump may change its size and shape as the muscle contracts.

d. *Sub-synovial lipoma*: They are common in knee joint and arise from fatty padding around the joint. It can be mistaken for Baker's cyst.

e. *Intra-glandular*: They occur in the pancreas or under renal capsule.

f. *Sub-mucous*: They occur in the tongue or in intestine. In the gut they can act as a lead point for intussusceptions.

g. *Intra-auricular*: It consists of fat-filled pedunculated villi with branches hanging in the clear fluid in the affected joint just like seaweed hanging in a pond. It is also known as lipoma arborescens.

h. *Perosteal*: Lipoma occurring under the periosteum of bone.
i. *Extradural*: They occur in the spinal canal. As there is no fat in the skull intracranial lipomas do not occur.
j. Mediastinal
k. Lipoma of spermatic cord.

Discuss the significance of lipoma at various sites.

a. Lipoma in femoral region can be confused with femoral hernia.
b. Lipoma in lumbosacral region usually overlie the site of spina bifida.
c. Paravertebral lipoma can be confused with cold abscess.
d. Lipoma in the epigastric is usually associated with epigastric hernia.
e. Lipoma in submandibual region may look like an enlarged submandibual gland.

What is the differential diagnosis of lipoma?

- Epidermoid cyst
- Subcutaneous tumours
- Nodular fasciitis
- Liposarcoma
- Metastatic disease
- Erythema nodosum
- Nodular subcutaneous fat necrosis
- Weber-Christian panniculitis

What is the etiology of lipoma?

a. Congenital lipomas have been observed in children.
b. Some lipomas are believed to have developed following blunt trauma.
c. While solitary lipomas are more common in women, multiple tumours (referred to as lipomatosis) are more common in men.
d. Hereditary multiple lipomatosis, an autosomal dominant condition also found most frequently in men, is characterized by widespread symmetric lipomas appearing most often over the extremities and trunk.
e. Lipomatosis may also be associated with Gardner's syndrome, an autosomal dominant condition involving intestinal polyposis, cysts, and osteomas.
f. Term Madelung's disease, or benign symmetric lipomatosis, refers to lipomatosis of the head, neck, shoulders, and proximal upper extremities. Persons with Madelung's disease, often men who consume alcohol, may present with the characteristic "horse collar" cervical appearance. Rarely, these patients experience swallowing difficulties, respiratory obstruction, and even sudden death.
g. A rare clinical consideration is Dercum's disease, or adiposis dolorosa, which is characterized by the presence of irregular painful lipomas most often found on the trunk, shoulders, arms, forearms, and legs. Dercum's disease is five times more common in women, is often found in middle age, and has asthenia and psychic disturbances as other prominent features.

What are clinical features of subcutaneous lipoma?

a. Present as slow growing painless swelling.
b. Dull aching sensation can be present due to repeated trauma, fat necrosis or due to location.
c. Usually spherical or hemispherical in shape.
d. Have a well defined edge.
e. Swelling is freely mobile in both axis.
f. *Slip sign is positive*: As subcutaneous lipoma is freely mobile, the edge of the swelling tends to slip away from palpating finger and a dimple may appear on the surface (due to fibrous septa attached to skin and traversing through lipoma).
g. The surface is either smooth or lobulated.
h. The swelling is free from overlying structures.
i. Firm to soft in consistency.
j. Large lipoma may become pedunculated by gravity when the growth is massive but usually sessile.
k. Transillumination is negative
l. No regional lymph nodes are enlarged.

What are complications which can occur in lipoma?

a. Myxomatous degeneration
b. Saponification (traumatic fat necrosis when it becomes hard)
c. Calcification
d. *Malignant change to liposarcoma*: Malignant change commonly occurs in retroperitoneal lipoma, large lipoma in thigh particularly the intramuscular type, and lipoma of shoulder region.

What is the histopathology of lipoma?

Microscopically, lipomas are composed of mature adipocytes arranged in lobules, many of which are surrounded by a fibrous capsule. Occasionally, a nonencapsulated lipoma infiltrates into muscle, in which case it is referred to as an infiltrating lipoma.

Four other types of lipomas may be noted on a biopsy specimen:

a. Angiolipomas are a variant with co-existing vascular proliferation. Angiolipomas may be painful and usually arise shortly after puberty.

b. Pleomorphic lipomas are another variant in which bizarre, multinucleated giant cells are admixed with normal adipocytes. Pleomorphic lipomas' presentation is similar to that of other lipomas, but they occur predominantly in men between 50 and 70 years of age.

c. A third variant, spindle cell lipomas, has slender spindle cells admixed in a localized portion of regular-appearing adipocytes.

d. A newly described variant of superficial lipoma, adenolipoma, is characterized by the presence of eccrine sweat glands in the fatty tumour; this type is often located on the proximal parts of the limbs.

What is the treatment of lipoma?

Nonexcisional Techniques

a. Steroid injection results in local fat atrophy and shrinking but rarely eliminates it. They are best suitable for lipomas less than one inch. Injection of triamcinolone acetate is used in the strength of 10 mg per ml. Injection is given in the centre of lipoma. 1 to 3 ml of solution is injected and can be repeated at monthly interval.

b. Liposuction can be used for lipomatous growths at position where large scars need to be avoided. Complete elimination cannot be achieved with this. It is an office procedure using 16 gauge needle and a 50 to 100 cc syringe.

Liposuction can be used to remove small or large lipomatous growths, particularly those in locations where large scars should be avoided. Complete elimination of the growth is difficult to achieve with liposuction. Office procedures using a 16-gauge needle and a large syringe may be safer than large-cannula liposuction. Diluted lidocaine usually provides adequate anesthesia for office liposuction.

Excision of Lipoma is the Gold Standard:

Majority of time excision can be done under local anesthesia. For a subcutaneous lipoma excision, a skin incision is deepened through the overlying fat until the capsule of the lipoma is reached. It can be differentiated from the surrounding fat by larger fat globules, color, and a fine capsule. The lesion can often be enucleated after incision of its fine capsule, but larger lesions may need sharp dissection. If a lipoma is adherent to the underlying muscle, it should not be removed under local anesthetic as there may be deep extensions between muscle bellies, with involvement of neurovascular bundles. If a deeper lesion is suspected or if the lesion is more than 5 cm in diameter, a CT or MRI scan is indicated for accurate anatomical delineation.

MALIGNANT MELANOMA

What are the considerations in history in a patient with suspected malignant melanoma?

In patient with melanoma important to take a history of risk factors like sun exposure. Also ask about changes in the colour size shape regularity and secondary changes like it bleeding itching and inflammation at a previous mole as this may indicate a malignant change in a benign nevus. Enquire about any other associated swelling that may indicate enlargement of lymph nodes. Examination has to be done very carefully after exposing the patient completely to look for malignant neavi. Look for the size colour border pigmentation elevation and surrounding lesions apart from any enlarged lymph nodes also look for signs of metastasis like liver nodules and ascites. Auscultation of the chest for pleural effusion must also be done.

What are the important differential diagnoses of a malignant melanoma?

Important differential include pigmented basal cell carcinoma warts, old hemangioma junctional nevus and thrombosed angiomas.

What is Melanoma?

Melanoma is a malignant cutaneous tumour that originates from the melanocytes which are derived from the neural ectoderm. These melanocytes further migrate to the epidermis, meninges, ectodermal mucosa and the uveal tissue in the eye. In the skin these cells produce melanin pigment which absorbs ultraviolet radiation preventing damage and is responsible for the color of skin.

Malignancy may arise during the process of absorbing the radiation and both Ultraviolet A and B can induce malignant change in the genetically predisposed patient. Skin is the most common site of melanoma but it can also involve other mucosal surfaces and lymph nodes. Its incidence is on a rise and whites are more commonly affected than blacks (up to 20 times). Males have a slightly higher preponderance with most lesions arising on the back or the chest while it is more common on the limbs in females. The disease affects patients in the old age usually the 6th–7th decade of life.

What are the risk factors for malignant melanoma?

Exposure of unprotected skin to UVA (320–400 nm) and UVB (290–320 nm) light predisposes to development of melanoma. Presence of nevi such as dysplastic naevi, large number of naevi, positive family history, and immunosuppression also increase the risk. A typical naevi are also a precursor lesion for melanoma. As the number of atypical and dysplastic naevi increases, the risk of melanoma also increases.

What are the various types of melanoma?

There are four subtypes of melanoma:

1. *Superficial spreading melanoma*: Superficially spreading melanomas are the most common subtypes of melanoma with an incidence of 70%. These lesions occur in the older age group with peak incidence in the 50s. It commonly develops on the upper back of both sexes and on the legs of women. It spreads laterally (radial growth) for a considerable period before it becomes invasive.

2. *Lentigo maligna melanoma*: Occurs on the face or sun exposed areas of the upper limbs in the elderly. It may arise from its precursor lesion lentigomaligna.

3. *Nodular melanoma*: These variants do not have a radial growth phase and are polypoidal, nodular and often pedunculated. It accounts for 15–20% of all melanomas. It is more common in older males.

4. Acral lentigenous melanoma. It commonly occurs in palms, roles and terminal phalanges. More commonly occurs in blacks.

How does one approach a case of Melanoma?

Patients with melanoma are diagnosed confirmatively only after biopsy of the suspicious lesion. Excisional biopsy is preferred for diagnosis but in areas where excision is not feasible, incisional biopsy may be performed. Alternatively punch biopsy may also be performed. Biopsy is suggested in the presence of the commonly stated ABCDE criteria.

- A: Asymmetry
- B: Border irregularity or bleeding
- C: Color change/variation
- D: Diameter larger than 6 mm
- E: Elevation (sometimes also designated as evolution)

These triggers for biopsy are not absolute and the clinician must keep a lower threshold for excisional biopsy if melanoma is suspected as up to 5% of melanomas are amelanotic and usually many melanomas are smaller than 5 mm. Presence of bleeding and itching is an important trigger to do excisional biopsy.

Once the diagnosis of melanoma is confirmed based on histopathology, the following parameters are assessed to stage the disease and plan management:

- Clark's level: Clark's level indicates depth of invasion of malignant melanoma in to different layers of skin. Level I is when the tumour is confined to epidermis. Level II is when the malignant tumour invades papillary dermis, but does not reach up to reticular dermis. Level III is when malignant melanoma reaches up to reticular dermis but does not invade it.
  In level IV tumour invades through reticular dermis. In level IV tumour invades subcutaneous fat.
- Breslow's thickness: Indicates tumour thickness in millimeters. The cut off points are 1, 2, 4 mm
- Mitotic rate
- Status of margins
- Status of ulceration
- Microsatellitosis (presence of tumour nests >0.05 mm separated from principal invasive tumour by at least 0.3 mm of normal tissue)
- Pure desmoplasia.

How does melanoma commonly spread?

Melanoma first spreads through lymphatic system forming satellite lesions and in-transit metastasis and then it involves region lymph nodes. Satellite lesions represent intralymphatic extension of the tumour and occur in skin and subcutaneous tissue within 2 cm of the primary tumour. In-transit metastasis are defined as lesions that are more than 2 cm from the primary tumour.

What are the laboratory investigations indicated in a patient with melanoma?

Initial screening after diagnosis is using chest X-ray and serum LDH levels apart from routine haematology, blood sugar and kidney function tests. Patients with node positive disease should undergo cross-sectional imaging in the form of a CT scan. If positive, alkaline phosphatase, CT of the chest abdomen and pelvis and MRI of the brain are also indicated. Bone scan may be performed if clinically indicated based on presence of symptoms.

What is the clinical staging of malignant melanoma?

- TX   Primary tumour cannot be assessed (i.e. curettaged or severely regressed melanoma)
- T0   No evidence of primary tumour
- Tis   Melanoma *in situ*
- T1   Melanoma ≤ 1.0 mm in thickness
  - T1a: Without ulceration and mitoses $<1/mm^2$
  - T1b: With ulceration or mitoses $\geq 1/mm^2$
- T2   Melanomas 1.01–2.0 mm in thickness
  - T2a: Without ulceration
  - T2b: With ulceration
- T3   Melanomas 2.01–4.0 mm in thickness
  - T3a: Without ulceration
  - T3b: With ulceration
- T4   Melanomas > 4.0 mm in thickness
  - T4a: Without ulceration
  - T4b: With ulceration

Regional lymph nodes (N)
- NX   Patients in whom the regional nodes cannot be assessed (i.e. previously removed for another reason)
- N0   No regional metastases detected
- N1–3 Regional metastases based upon number of metastatic nodes and presence or absence of intra-lymphatic metastases (in transit or satellite metastases)
- N1   1 lymph node
  - N1a: Micrometastases
  - N1b: Macrometastases

- N2   2 or 3 lymph nodes
  - N2a: Micrometastases
  - N2b: Macrometastases
  - N2c: In-transit met(s)/satellite(s) without metastatic lymph nodes
- N3   ≥4 metastatic lymph nodes, or matted lymph nodes, or in-transit met(s)/satellite(s) with metastatic lymph node(s)

Distant metastasis (M)
- M0   No detectable evidence of distant metastases
- M1a Metastases to skin, subcutaneous, or distant lymph nodes, normal serum lactate dehydrogenase (LDH) level
- M1b Lung metastases, normal LDH level
- M1c Metastases to all other visceral sites or distant metastases to any site combined with an elevated serum LDH level

Clinical staging

Stage	T	N	M
0	Tis	N0	M0
IA	T1a	N0	M0
IB	T1b	N0	M0
	T2a	N0	M0
IIA	T2b	N0	M0
	T3a	N0	M0
IIB	T3b	N0	M0
	T4a	N0	M0
IIC	T4b	N0	M0
III	Any T	N1, N2, or N3	M0
IV	Any T	Any N	M1

What are the recommended margins for performing wide local excision?

For *in situ* carcinomas a gross margin of 0.5 to 1 cm at excision is considered adequate. For lesion with less than 1 mm depth, the minimum margin should be 1 cm for a lesion with tumour thickness between 1 and 2 cm, a 1–2 cm margin must be taken and if the thickness is more than 2 mm, then a 2 cm margin is needed. Thick melanomas are rare and account for approximately only 10% of the cases, hence the adequate surgical margins for these lesions have not been described. During wide local excision for melanomas margins can be modified based on anatomical and functional requirements. For example, melanomas that present in the subungual region may require distal digital amputation to achieve a suitable margin.

What is the status of lymphadenectomy in patients with melanoma?

Malignant melanoma spread through lymphatic route, haematogenous route, and direct extension to the surrounding tissues. Lymph nodes are often involved and require aggressive management. It was traditionally considered that apart from the area bearing the malignancy all draining lymph nodes must be removed along with surrounding soft tissue that contains the lymphatics. However, elective removal of all lymph nodes has failed to show any benefit in terms of survival. With the advent of sentinel node biopsy, elective lymph node excision is not practised at most centres. Sentinel node, as discussed in the chapter on breast cancer, is the first node to which the lymphatics from an affected area of the skin drain. Lymphatic spread of melanoma is predictable and involvement of sentinel node is predictive of the metastatic status to other drainage nodes. Sentinel node biopsy is done using isosulphan blue and radiocolloid (Tc 99m based sulphur colloid) which is detected using a gamma probe. For lesions in the extremities sentinel node biopsy is predictable but in lesions of the head and neck usually spread occurs to multiple nodes and drainage areas. Nodal involvement is the single most important prognostic factor in melanoma and can direct the further treatment. The indications of sentinel node biopsy are:

- Melanoma > 1 mm in depth
- Melanoma > 0.75 mm in depth with ulceration
- Melanoma > 0.75 mm in depth with Clark level IV/V
- Incompletely biopsied lesions with unknown depth

If the sentinel lymph node is positive, therapeutic lymphadenectomy is performed. In this surgery regional lymph nodes are removed completely.

What is isolated limb perfusion and when is it indicated?

Isolated limb perfusion is a surgical technique to deliver cytotoxic chemotherapy to the extremity while avoiding toxicity to the rest of the body. In this procedure hyperthermic agent is perfused through the isolated artery and recovered through the veins (HILP). This therapy is confined at present to palliation of an affected limb and lesions associated with high risk of recurrence (limb with more than four lesions). Occasionally when complete isolation is not achieved the cytotoxic drugs may leak into the circulation and cause severe toxicity. Side effects of HILP include limb oedema, skin changes, erythema, neuropathy, myopathy, thrombosis and embolism. The agents which are commonly used at 42°C inflow hyperthermia are melphalan, TNF, IFN α, phenylalanine mustard, and actinomycin D.

When should radiation be given to patients with melanoma?

Radiation may be considered in the following situations:

- Locally recurrent disease
- Extensive nerve involvement
- Deep desmoplastic melanoma with narrow and inadequate free margin
- Adjuvant treatment in presence of positive nodes and extranodal tumour extension with LDH < 1.5 times normal
- For palliation in nodal, in transit or satellite lesion that cannot be resected
- For symptomatic bony or soft tissue lesions or brain metastases.

What are the chemotherapeutic agents used in management of metastatic melanoma?

The preferred regimens for systemic therapy in patients with metastatic melanoma include ipilimumab, dabrafenib with trametinib or enrolment in a clinical trial. Some other agents that are active against metastatic melanoma include albumin bound paclitaxel, high dose IL-2, imatinib, paclitaxel and dacarbazine.

BASAL CELL CARCINOMA

What is basal cell carcinoma?

Basal cell cancer is the most common type of skin malignancy that is a locally invasive cancer that rarely metastasizes. Basal cell carcinoma arises from the epithelial cells of the basal cells of the epidermis and the hair follicles. Basal cell carcinoma is also called rodent ulcer as it is a very slowly growing tumour that causes local destruction of the surrounding tissue leading to a raised and rolled out edge. It is found in sun exposed areas, and men are more commonly affected than women. UVB spectrum of light, UVA radiation, exposure to arsenic hydrocarbons, polyaromatic hydrocarbons, coal tar, inherited carcinoma syndrome such as Grolin's syndrome also known as nevoid basal cell carcinoma syndrome is caused by mutations in the PTCH gene with loss of heterozygosity and in activation of the p53 gene. The adverse prognostic factors include large size presence of tumour necrosis and angiogenesis.

How is nevoid basal cell carcinoma syndrome (NBCCS) diagnosed?

NBCCS is diagnosed if two major and one minor criterion or one major and three minor criteria are positive. These criteria include:

Major features:
- Multiple basal cell skin cancers
- Increased calcium deposits in the cranium (seen on an X-ray)
- Jaw cyst(s)
- Two or more pits on the palms of the hands or soles of the feet
- A parent, sibling, or child with NBCCS

Minor features:
- Medulloblastoma in childhood
- Increased head size
- Cleft lip or palate
- Abnormal shape of the ribs or spinal bones
- Polydactyly
- Eye problems
- Fibromas (benign fibrous tumours) of the ovaries or heart
- Abdominal cysts.

What are the presenting features of Basal Cell Carcinoma?

Basal cell tumours have the tendency to grow in the path of least resistance like embryonic fusion planes. They present as an ulcerated lesion with characteristic rolled out edges that may be pearly in appearance. The ulcer is usually covered with a scab. Perineural spread is seen in recurrent and aggressive lesions and may present as tingling and numbness in the limbs along with pain and weakness. Basal cell carcinomas should be differentiated from keratocanthomas, squamous cell cancers, malignant melanomas and basal cell papillomas (seborrhoeic keratosis).

What are the various types of basal cell carcinoma?

Basal cell carcinomas are divided clinically into low risk and high risk tumours. Tumours of the head and neck and those greater than 2 cm in largest dimension or tumours in immuno-compromised patients or those who have received prior radiotherapy are considered high-risk tumours.

The clinic-pathological variants of BCC include:
- *Nodular variety*: Nodular variety is the most common form of BCC. It may be cystic, pigmented or keratotic. This variant presents as a round, pearly, pink to skin-coloured papule with dilated vessels.
- *Infiltrative variety*: Infiltrative variety of BCC has poorly defined margins.
- *Micronodular*: Micronodular variant of BCC presents as multiple small firm whitish nodules with well-defined borders.
- *Morpheaform*: Morphaeform variant presents as an irregular fibrotic and firm plaque
- *Superficial*: Superficial variants also presents are a scaly erythematous plaque

As per WHO 2006 classification of BCC, it can be divided into nodular, superficial, infiltrating, micronodular, fibroepithelial, basosquamous, keratotic, and BCC with adnexal differentiation. Other variants as described by Paterson (2006) and Rosai (2004) include pigmented, infundibulocystic, sclerosin, metatypical, basosebaceous, and mixed variants.

How are patients with basal cell carcinoma managed?

Any suspected lesion must be biopsied and subjected to histopathological examination. For deeper lesions deep reticular dermis should also be included. If the tumour is large and extensive underlying spread is suspected on clinical examination imaging should be done to see the depth of involvement.

In low risk disease excision of tumour should be done. Postoperatively margins of tumour should be assessed and if positive re-excision may be required. Alternative Mohs micrographic surgery may be done with complete circumferential peripheral and deep margin assessment (CCPDMA). In patients who do not want surgery or repeat surgery, radiotherapy can be offered.

In patients with high-risk basal cell cancer, primary resection with at least 10 mm margin must be performed followed by postoperative margin assessment. Alternatively Mohs' micrographic surgery with CCPDMA can be performed. In unwilling patients radiotherapy can be given. If perineural invasion is present in specimen, adjuvant radiotherapy should be considered.

What are the risk factors for recurrence in basal cell carcinoma?

Patients with large area of tumour with poorly defined borders, recurrent tumours, and history of prior radiotherapy or immunocompromised status are at high risk for recurrence. Presence of aggressive growth pattern and perineural invasion are also risk factors of recurrence.

How are patients with basal cell carcinoma followed up?

Low risk patients are followed with annual clinical visit and advised regular self-examination and use of sun protection. In an event of local recurrence repeat surgery and radiotherapy can be offered. In event of distant metastatic tumour cisplatin or carboplatin based combination chemotherapy needs to be administered preferably after tumour board consultation.

What is Mohs' micrographic surgery?

Mohs' micrographic surgery was developed in the 1930s by Dr Frederic Mohs'. This procedure allows a careful dissection of cancer tissue and is used in treatment of basal cell carcinoma, squamous cell carcinoma, melanoma *in situ*, dermatofibrosarcomaprotuberans, Merkel cell carcinoma, microcystic adnexal carcinoma, atypical fibroxanthoma, and sebaceous carcinoma. When initially done 20% zinc chloride paste was used *in vitro* to fix the tumour before slicing. Subsequently frozen section was used to assess free tumour margin. Modifications by Dr Tromovitch of using fresh tissue with chemical fixative have made MMS a day care procedure.

In this micrographic surgery after infiltration with local anaesthetic agent, the tumour is removed grossly. After this stage two sections are taken. The usual depth of these sections is 2–3 mm. It is necessary that the depth of this specimen is adequately represented in the staged sections. To maintain the orientation of the specimen, different types of inks are used and map is created on paper in two-dimensions. It is necessary to have an experienced frozen section pathologist to be able to perform the surgery. If the section is found to be positive, then again at 2 to 3 mm margin is taken and analysed using frozen section after mapping the section. This process continues until a negative margin is achieved. Mohs' micrographic surgery provides excellent tumour control in the range of 90 to 100%.

What are the indications of MMS?

1. Aggressive tumours
2. Recurrent tumours
3. Large tumours
4. Ill-defined borders
5. Presence of perineural invasion
6. Tumours at sites of higher recurrence
7. Tumours at sites of prior radiotherapy
8. Tumours at embryonic fusion planes
9. Tumours in immunocompromised subjects

What are the only other procedures that can be performed for management of basal cell carcinoma?

Apart from surgical excision, resection using lasers, 5-fluorouracil, cryotherapy and radiotherapy can be used for management of these tumours. Minimally invasive procedures have lower rates of control compared to excision surgery and Mohs micrographic surgery. Radiotherapy is an attractive option for patients who do not want surgery but it is associated with complications like scarring, ectropion, fibrosis, haemorrhage, erythema, ulceration and breakdown of skin.

Squamous cell carcinoma of the skin: After basal cell carcinoma, squamous cell carcinoma is the most common tumour of the skin that arises from the malphigian or spindle cell layer of the skin. Exposure to the sun is the most common predisposing factor. Most commonly affected regions of the body are the lower lip, ears and the scalp. This tumour may also arise insights of chronic injury orientation like scars sinuses and fistulas. Squamous cell carcinomas are also common in certain genetic disorders like xerodermapigmentosum, vitiligo and albinism. These tumours usually affect the older age and present as shallow ulcers. The skin surrounding is erythematous due to actinic damage. Squamous cell carcinoma is more common in immunocompromised patients such as those after transplant.

What are the predisposing factors for squamous cell carcinoma?

The various recognised predisposing factors include:

- Ultraviolet B radiation
- Ultraviolet A radiation
- Radiation therapy
- Exposure to smoking
- Exposure to arsenic
- Occupational exposure to coal tar
- Aromatic hydrocarbons
- Human papillomavirus.

What is Unitarian theory of squamous cell carcinoma?

A number of lesions that arise from common pathogenic factors have been grouped together as morphological expressions of squamous cell carcinoma. These lesions include solar keratosis, Bowen's disease, giant condyloma, keratocanthoma, and tricholemmal cysts. These lesions should be regarded as squamous cell carcinoma and not as premalignant lesions.

What is verrucous carcinoma?

Verrucous carcinoma is a distinctive variant of squamous cell carcinoma. It is characterised by slow growth that is locally destructive and invades the contiguous structures. Plantar lesions are most common form. Verrucous carcinoma rarely metastasizes. Verrucous carcinoma is caused by human papillomavirus. Management is by surgical excision and Mohs micrographic surgery. Occasionally these tumours may grow explosively after long period of slow growth. These tumours have very low mitotic activity and are confined to the basal layer of the skin. The papillary variant of squamous cell carcinoma is an important differential diagnosis of verrucous carcinoma.

What are the various other variants of squamous cell carcinoma?

The other variants of squamous cell carcinoma are spindle cell squamous carcinoma, adenoid squamous cell carcinoma, pseudo-vascular squamous cell carcinoma, clear cell carcinoma, signet cell carcinoma, pigmented variant, inflammatory squamous cell carcinoma, pseudo-hyperplastic variant, follicular squamous cell carcinoma, basaloid variant, infiltrative variant and others.

What are the premalignant lesions of the skin?

The lesions which are considered premalignant include:

- Bowen's disease
- Radiodermatosis
- Solar keratosis
- Leukoplakia
- Xerooderma pigmentosum
- Erythroplasia of Queyrat
- Pseudoepitheliomatous hyperplasia

What is a keratoacanthoma?

Keratoacanthoma is a solitary pink, dome-shaped nodule that has a central keratin plug. It is seen in sun exposed skin in the elderly patients. It often develops into a large lesion within a small span of time. This lesion heals spontaneously. Occasionally this lesion may cause local destruction of nearby surrounding tissue due to which excision is often recommended. When healed it leaves a moon shaped scar. Most often it arises over the face but it can also involve the arms, hands and the lower limbs. These lesions are usually less than 2 cm in diameter. Larger than this they are referred to as giant keratoacanthoma.

How is a patient with suspected squamous cell carcinoma worked up?

Squamous cell carcinoma has to be differentiated from other differential diagnosis like basal cell carcinoma malignant melanoma, infected warts, keratoacanthoma and other lesions. For this purpose of wedge biopsy has to be performed prior to definitive therapy. If the biopsies taken from the centre of the lesion, then it may only show necrotic tissue therefore a margin of the lesion with surrounding normal tissue must be taken. Once the diagnosis has been confirmed by histopathological examination, the patient may be managed using surgery, radiotherapy or a combination of the two.

What is the TNM classification of basal and Squamous cell tumours of the skin?

Tx	Tumour primary cannot be assessed
T0	No evidence of primary tumour
Tis	Carcinoma *in situ*
T1	<2 cm tumour with less than two high risk features

T2	Tumour > 2 cm or two or more high risk features	N3	Metastasis in lymph node more than 6 cm in greatest dimension
T3	Invasion into maxilla, mandible, orbit or temporal bone	M0	No distant metastasis
		M1	Distant metastasis

T4   Invasion into skeleton or perineural invasion of skull base

NX   Nodes cannot be assessed

N0   No regional lymph node metastasis

N1   <3 cm ipsilateral single node

N2   Metastasis in a single ipsilateral lymph node more than 3 cm but not more than 6 cm in greatest dimension; or in multiple ipsilateral lymph nodes none more than 6 cm in greatest dimension; or in bilateral contra-lateral lymph nodes, none more than 6 cm in greatest dimension.

N2a   Metastasis in a single ipsilateral lymph node more than 3 cm but not more than 6 cm in greatest dimension

N2b   Multiple ipsilateral lymph nodes none more than 6 cm in greatest dimension

N2c   Bilateral contralateral lymph nodes, none more than 6 cm in greatest dimension

High risk features for the primary tumour staging include:

- Depth of invasion more than 2 mm thickness, Clark's level more than or equal to IV
- Perineural invasion
- Primary site on ear or non-hair bearing lip
- Poor differentiation.

What are the treatment options in the patient with squamous cell carcinoma?

Treatment of squamous cell carcinoma is on the same lines as basal cell carcinoma. Wide local excision of the tumour is the preferred with a margin of 1 cm but prophylactic lymph node dissection is not advocated. Amputation may be done for tumours on the limbs. Only when the lymph nodes are positive that lymphadenectomy is done. Radiotherapy can be given when the patient is not willing for surgery, areas where function needs to be preserved or in case of recurrence.

30

Incisional Hernia

What is incisional hernia?

Incisional hernia is defined as visible or palpable bulge at the site of previous surgical intervention which becomes more apparent during erect position or during coughing, lifting heavy weights and straining.

What is the incidence of incisional hernia?

Incisional hernia is a common complication after abdominal surgery and occurs in 11–20% of patients undergoing laparotomy. The incidence of these hernias has not gone down in spite of advances in techniques in wound closure.

When do the incisional hernias appear?

About 2/3rd of incisional hernia appears within 5 years after laparotomy. Remaining 1/3rd appear within 5–10 years after initial laparotomy. With aging and weakening of tissues postoperative hernia may appear even after 10 years of initial operation. The early onset incisional hernias are generally due to technical failure. Late hernias are generally due to tissue failure or collagen abnormality.

Why incisional hernias should be repaired?

Incisional hernias can cause following serious complications:

1. Irreducibility, obstruction or incarceration of gut
2. Strangulation in 2 percent of cases. Strangulated gut rapidly becomes ischemic, necrotic and perforates if hernia is not repaired.
3. Many patients who are suffering from large incisional hernia are forced to change their life style or give up their gainful employment leading to major social and economic implications.
4. The gradual enlargement leads to relative loss of abdominal domain with adverse effects on postural maintenance, respiration, defecation with profound effect on patients overall physical capacity and quality of life.

What are the indications for surgical intervention in incisional hernia?

1. Symptomatic hernias
2. Enlarging hernias
3. Hernia with a small fascial defect and a large sac with incarcerated contents
4. Irreducible hernia
5. Cosmetic concerns.

What is the classification of incisional hernia?

Incisional hernias may be classified as:

- Small (if the defect is less than 5 cm) in diameter
- Medium (if the defect is between 5 and 10 cm),
- Large or giant (if the defect is more than 10 cm).

What are the risk factors for formation and recurrence after repair?

1. *Obesity*: In obese patients, increases in abdominal pressure and weight of pannus place the fascial closure under tension leading to break down of sutures and recurrence of hernia formation. In obese patients the incisional hernia rate of 15–20% have been noted.
2. Co-morbidities related to obesity, such as diabetes, coronary disease, renal disorders.
3. Patients on steroids.

4. Large fascial defects have more chances of recurrence.

5. Postoperative wound infection is very important independent risk factor in the development of incisional hernia. There is 23 percent risk of incisional hernia formation in patients who develop postoperative wound infection.

6. Postoperative haematoma formation.

7. Postoperative abdominal distension.

8. Chronic pulmonary disease.

9. Advanced age.

10. *Size of hernia*: If the hernia defect is large, there are more chances of recurrence.

11. *Type of repair*: There is reduction in incidence of incisional hernia reduction from 18 to 10% with the use of double stranded no. 1 PDS placed in a continuous fashion and no. 1 Ethibond placed in an interrupted figure of eight fashion. Suture repair carries more chances of recurrence.

12. Incisional hernia following surgery for abdominal aortic aneurysm: Recurrence rate of incisional hernia repair was much high in patients who had surgery for aortic aneurysm possibly due to inherent defect in healing due to defects in collagen and elastin cross-linkages. There is 28% incidence of incisional hernia formation in patients undergoing surgery for aortic aneurysm repair. Defect in collagen metabolism with a decreased ratio of type 1 to type 111 pro-collagen may play a role.

13. The local technical factors and methods in abdominal closure are more important than patient related factors in the development of incisional hernia.

What are the different presentations of incisional hernia?

a. First sign is asymptomatic bulge directly over the operative site or lateral to the previous scar.

b. The hernia becomes more obvious when patient stands.

c. The pain is not an early complaint but sometimes occur before the occurrence of bulge during heavy weight lifting or vigorous activity.

d. More than 50 percent of incisional hernia occur within two years of primary operation but significant number occurs years after primary surgery.

e. Dragging pain with movement, coughing and straining becomes more apparent in long standing hernia.

f. The presence of vomiting, severe pain or constipation indicates incarceration or strangulation of gut.

g. The dull aching abdominal pain and nausea are because of stretching of bowel mesentery as it protrudes through the defect.

h. With long-standing hernia in patients who refuse to undergo surgery can lose their abdominal domain with time and become severely disabled.

i. Patient can develop bowel obstruction due to incarceration, but more often caused by twisting of bowel loop around adhesions at the lateral margin of the hernia defect.

j. The disruption of the linea alba which hold and acts as midline anchor of rectus sheath aponeurosis insertions leads to gradual enlargement of hernia defects due to unopposed lateral contraction of the oblique musculature.

k. With widening hernia defects, significant physiological derangements occur as task dependent functions of abdominal wall musculature are lost. There is a loss of synergy with abdominal wall with paradoxical respiratory movements in large ventral hernia. Normally there is synergy between diaphragm and abdominal wall musculature as internal oblique and transverses musculature receive neural impulses from central expiratory neurons. The transverses abdominis muscle is a major contributor to the generation of expiratory force.

l. Patients with large incisional hernia often have significant lumbar lordosis and severe back ache as abdominal wall plays an important role in posture maintainer and support of lumbar spine. There is counterbalancing effect of abdominal wall muscles with back musculature. The lateral pull of internal oblique and transverses abdominis musculature on the lumbo-dorsal fascia is responsible for a reduction in inter-vertebral joint space. There is relief of back pain after repair of large incisional hernia by restoration of midline myofascial continuity possibly due to restoration of counterbalancing effect of abdominal wall musculature with the back musculature.

m. The expulsive functions are also compromised in large incisional hernia because contraction of abdominal wall musculature and generation of intra-abdominal pressure are important in functions such as coughing, micturition, and defecation.

n. Dermatological changes may occur over the skin of the hernia sac as it enlarges as stretching of skin with atrophy of subcutaneous tissue occurs with resultant ulceration and infection.

When imaging is required for incisional hernia?

In morbid obese individual or in patients with who have undergone multiple operations clinical detection of incisional hernia may be difficult. In these patients CT of abdomen, ultrasonography or contrast gastrointestinal series may be used to evaluate these cases.

What conditions can mimic incisional hernia?

Rectus diastasis or abdominal wall laxity due to nerve injuries or congenital conditions like prune belly syndrome can cause confusion.

What are the goals of incisional hernia repair?

The goals of incisional hernia repair are:
a. Prevention of visceral eventration.
b. Incorporation of the remaining abdominal wall in the repair.
c. Provisional of dynamic muscular support.
d. Restoration of abdominal wall continuity (midline myofascial continuity) in a tension-free manner.

What are different techniques of incisional hernia repair?

Incisional hernia can be repaired by open methods or laparoscopic technique.

Different open methods of incisional hernia repair are:

Primary suture repair: It should be used only for small hernia (<5 cm) if the repair is oriented horizontally. Only non-absorbable monofilament suture should be used with a suture to wound length ratio of 4:1. In order to reduce tension on primary repair relaxing incisions can be used.

This repair is suitable when the patient has adequate muscle tone. Muscle tone is considered adequate if the defect does not remain open on straining. Either transverse or vertical elliptical skin incision is given incorporating previous scar. Hernia sac is dissected up to the lateral edge of the defect and opened. Contents are reduced after

releasing any adhesions between sac and contents. Lateral margins of defects are approximated to each other using continuous or interrupted no. 1 monofilament suture or a loop suture. One should take care that bites should be taken al least 2 cm from margin and distance between two suture bites should not be more than 2 cm.

Cardiff Repair

Sac is excised and peritoneum is closed by polyglactin suture. Abdominal wall closure is performed by interrupted non-absorbable suture using "Cardiff far and near" technique. Placement of far and near sutures reduces tension on abdominal wall and there are less chances of sutures getting cut through. This technique is suitable for defects up to 5 cm.

Keel's Operation

This operation is named Keel operation because appearance of repair is like inverted beam of the old ship or boat in bottom.

Essential steps of Keel repair are:
• Vertical skin incision is made encircling old scar and sac.
• Scar is excised and sac is dissected beyond the margins of the defect.
• Sac is gradually inverted inside peritoneal cavity by pleating by application of continuous or interrupted sutures one over another till the margins of defects get approximated to each other.
• Opposed margins are stitched together by interrupted sutures.

Nuttall's Repair

This operation is done for lower mid-line incisional hernia. Attachments of rectus muscles are detached.

Two rectus muscles are crossed over each other and are reattached to opposite pubic bones to create a firm abdominal wall support by crossed rectus muscles.

Open Mesh Repair

Mesh repair has largely replaced open suture repair because these repairs carry less recurrence rates. Usher in 1963 introduced monofilament knitted polypropylene mesh in clinical practice. Polypropylene mesh and expanded polytetrafluoroethylene (ePTFE) mesh are two most commonly used mesh in hernia repair. Recurrence rate after mesh repair is significantly less than open suture repair (less than 10%). Repair is without tension. Polypropylene mesh induces an inflammatory response which in turn leads to synthesis of collagen over the mesh because fibroblast gets trapped in the pores of mesh and lay down collagen there. The mesh can be placed in following positions.

Onlay Mesh

In this technique mesh is placed over the anterior-rectus sheath after the fascial defect has been closed primarily. Drawback of this technique is that repair is under tension and there are more chances of mesh infection if the surgical wound gets infected.

Inlay Mesh

Hernia sac is excised and fascial margins are identified around the hernia defect. Polypropylene or ePTFE mesh is sutured around fascial defect circumferentially. If polypropylene mesh is used, omentum should be placed between mesh and intestine to reduce the incidence of fistula and adhesions formations. If omentum is not available, ePTFE mesh should be used.

Extra-peritoneal or Subfascial (Rive's Stoppa Repair)

Mesh is placed in between peritoneum and rectus muscle in infra-umbilical region and in between posterior rectus sheath and rectus muscle in supra-umbilical region. This technique is also known as retrorectus mesh repair or Rive's Stoppa repair.

Steps of this repair are:

Operation is done under general anaesthesia

Old scar is excised and hernia sac is dissected till the margins of hernial ring.

Sac is opened and contents are reduced into peritoneal cavity after freeing intestinal contents and omentum from sac. Excessive sac is excised.

Peritoneum is closed with running polyglactin sutures.

A space is created between the rectus anteriorly and posterior rectus sheath posteriorly.

A large polypropylene mesh is kept in the preperitoneal space which has been created. Mesh should be large enough so that mesh extends 2–3 inches beyond the defects.

Polypropylene mesh is fixed to anterior rectus sheath by interrupted sutures. Medial margins of anterior rectus sheath are stitched together using polypropylene sutures.

Suction drain is put and skin closed.

Technical Tips for Mesh Repair of Incisional Hernia

1. Mesh should be placed in extra-peritoneal position to avoid contact of mesh with gut thus reducing incidence of fistula formation, adhesions formation and intestinal obstruction.

2. Mesh should overlap abdominal defect by at least 3 cm so that ingrowths of connective tissue can occur on a large surface area of mesh on lateral aspect which helps in more secure and permanent fixation of mesh to underlying abdominal tissue. This wide overlapping of mesh reduces the incidence of recurrence of hernia at the lateral margin of defect and permits postoperative shrinkage of mesh without creating tension in it. Polypropylene mesh has been shown to shrink by 33% in post-operative period.

3. Postoperative seroma and haematoma formation should be prevented and use of suction drains is thought to decrease incidence of haematoma. If there is a soiling or contamination of wound during surgery due to any reason, use of mesh should be avoided because there are high chances of mesh getting infected in these situations leading to need for removal of mesh.

What are the problems faced during repair of giant incisional hernia?

As the adequate abdominal domain or cavity is not available due to its gradual loss, patients are likely to develop abdominal compartment syndrome and respiratory complications due to elevation of diaphragm. These patients may require prolonged mechanical ventilation. This problem can be overcome by placement of intra-peritoneal catheter and repeated insufflations of air in peritoneal cavity to increase its capacity. Use of tissue expanders and relaxing incisions has been described to overcome this problem.

31

Adult Groin Hernia

What is hernia?

The hernia can be defined as the protrusion of a viscus or part of the viscus through an opening or weakness in the wall of the cavity containing that viscus.

What is groin hernia?

Groin is a hernia in which the bulge of the abdominal contents occurs through inguinal or femoral canal.

What are the basic presentations of inguinal hernia?

Inguinal hernias have four basic presentations:
- Symptomatic or painful groin swelling
- Asymptomatic groin swelling
- Inguinoscrotal swelling (Fig. 31.1)
- Acute surgical emergency due to complications.

Clinical features in the history to be elicited:

1. Bulge in the groin which increases in size with passage of time.

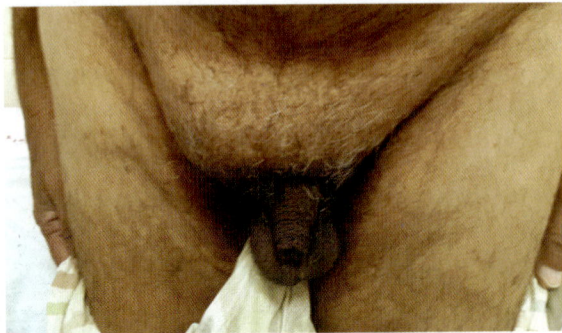

Fig. 31.1: Clinical picture of right incomplete Indirect inguinal hernia

2. Bulge or swelling increases in size on standing, on doing any activity like coughing or lifting heavyweights which entails increase of intra-abdominal pressure.

3. The swelling reduces or decreases in size on lying down position.

4. Large hernias may limit physical activity.

5. With increase in size they may become painful due to dragging sensation caused by large contents or due to stretch at the root of mesentery. This pain is dull aching in nature with mild to moderate in intensity.

6. Increase in size predisposes to increase risk of complications.

7. Groin hernia also causes negative effect on patient well-being and productivity as many of them are manual workers. Due to presence of hernia, there is limited daily activity.

8. The patient can present in the emergency with complications like irreducibility, obstruction or strangulation. The presence of complications increases the risk of mortality and morbidity.

9. History suggestive of predisposing factors like chronic cough, smoking, chronic constipation, lifting heavyweights, history of lower abdominal surgery or history of lower urinary symptoms (LUTS). If any of these factors is present, it should be taken care of before hernia surgery to avoid recurrence.

10. History of irreducibility with sudden development of colicky pain, abdominal distension, absence of cough impulse over hernia swelling and constipation indicates obstructed hernia.

11. Development of local tenderness over hernia site with fever and change of nature of pain from colicky to severe continuous in the setting of obstructed hernia indicates progression to strangulation.

12. Presence of diarrhea instead of constipation in a setting of obstructed hernia indicate that hernia is Richter's hernia involving part of the circumference of the wall of the gut.

Examination of Groin Hernia Case

Aims of examination in a groin hernia are the following:

a. Find out the type of hernia, i.e. inguinal versus femoral.

b. To find out if the hernia is reducible or irreducible.

c. If the hernia is irreducible, then the features of obstruction or strangulation to be noted.

d. In inguinal hernia one should aim to find out the type of inguinal hernia, i.e. direct or indirect.

e. In an indirect hernia, one should determine the extent of hernia, i.e. complete hernia reaching up to scrotum or incomplete hernia confined to inguinal region (Fig. 31.2).

f. What is the content of inguinal hernia? It can be omentum or intestine. It contents are intestine, first part is difficult to reduce and contents reduce with gurgling sound. If the sac contains omentum, the last portion is difficult to reduce and the contents have doughy feeling.

Describe scheme of examination.

The patient is first examined in standing position with clothes removed from below umbilicus.

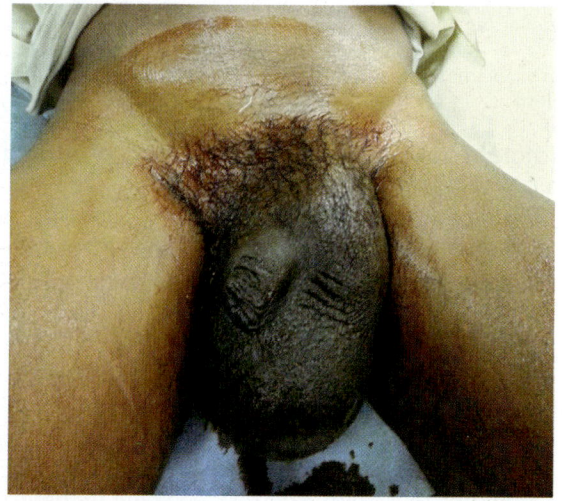

Fig. 31.2: Clinical picture of incomplete left inguinal hernia

Inspection

Exposure is very important—ensure that clinician can see from umbilicus to knees at least!

- Look in the groin for evidence of a swelling—if one can't see one, ask the patient which side they have noticed a lump.
- Look for evidence of previous hernia surgery— oblique scar often well hidden in pubic hairline
- Any other obvious skin changes, swellings, lumps that may be relevant.
- Ask the patient to look over their shoulder and cough (so they don't cough into your face!)
- As they cough, look at the lump to see if there is a cough impulse.

  Any visible swelling which is noticed in the groin is described including extent of swelling downwards, overlying skin, any visible peristalsis and cough impulse.

Palpation

a. *Relation of swelling to pubic tubercle:* If the neck of the swelling is below and laterals to pubic tubercle, it is femoral hernia. If the swelling is above and medial to pubic tubercle, it is inguinal hernia.

b. *To differentiate between purely scrotal and inguinal-scrotal swelling:* If one is able to get above the swelling at the root of the scrotum, it is purely scrotal swelling. The index finger is placed behind the neck of scrotum and thumb in front. If one is able palpate cord structures between thumb and fingers, it is a purely scrotal swelling.

c. Three finger test or Ziemann's test (three finger test) is done to differentiate between direct, and indirect or femoral hernia. The examiner stands on the side of hernia puts index middle and ring over deep ring, superficial ring and femoral region. The patient is asked to cough and the cough impulse is felt (Figs 31.3 and 31.4).

d. *Deep ring occlusion test:* This test is done to differentiate between direct and indirect hernia. The patient is asked to lie down and reduce the hernia. If the patient is not able to reduce, the examiner reduces it. While reduction of hernia, the examiner should be gentle and makes sure that no force is being used. After reduction of hernia, the surface marking for the deep ring is identified. The deep ring lies about 1.25 cm above the midpoint of inguinal ligament (midpoint between anterior-superior iliac spine

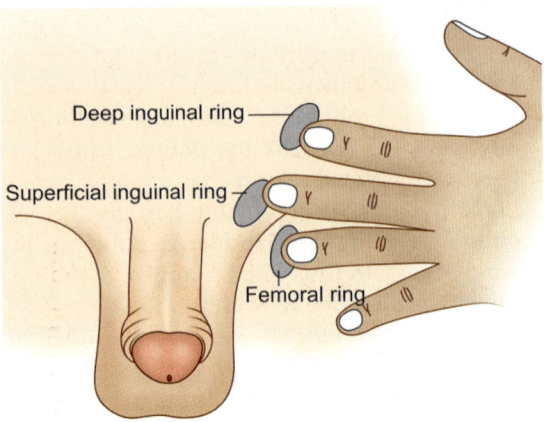

Fig. 31.3: Diagram depicting technique of Ziemann's test

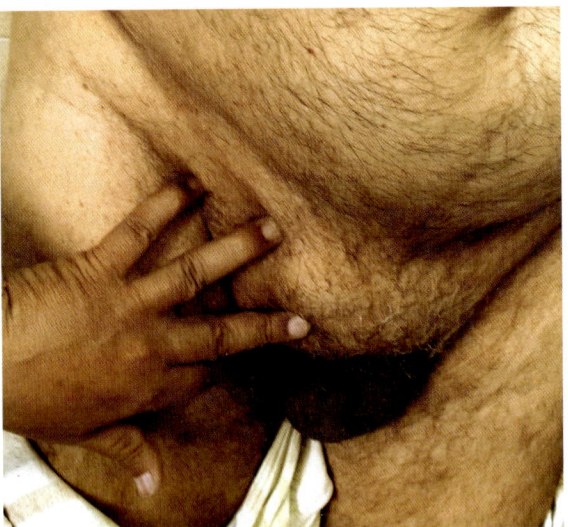

Fig. 31.4: Clincal picture of Ziemann's test

and pubic tubercle). In obese patients, when it is difficult to feel the pubic tubercle, one can follow the tendon of adductor longus which will lead to pubic tubercle as it is attached there. The thumb is placed at the site of deep ring and the patient is asked to cough. If one is able to control the hernia, it is an indirect hernia. If the hernia appears on coughing while the pressure is maintained on deep ring, it is a direct hernia. It is not required to tell the patient to stand while maintain a pressure on deep ring. If the swelling does not appear on coughing in supine position, then only it is required to ask the patient to stand and cough while maintaining pressure on deep ring.

What are the fallacies of deep ring occlusion test?

a. Too wide deep ring and it is not possible to occlude it completely by thumb.

b. Presence of Pantaloon hernia (both direct and indirect elements).

What other necessary examinations are to be done in groin hernia case?

1. Abdominal examination:
   a. Previous scar
   b. Other hernia sites epigastric or umbilical
   c. The tone of abdominal musculature
   d. Any abdominal lump or free fluid in the abdomen.
2. Per rectal examination for prostate enlargement.

What are the differences between indirect and inguinal hernia?

Direct inguinal hernia	Indirect inguinal hernia
Occurs in middle age and old persons	Occurs in young males
Due to weakness of abdominal musculature	Due to presence of patent processes vaginalis
The hernia sac is medial to deep ring and bulges through posterior wall of inguinal canal	The hernia is lateral to inferior epigastric artery and passes through deep ring.
The hernia sac is posterior and medial to cord structures	The hernia sac lies anterior and lateral to cord structures
The hernia cannot be controlled by deep ring occlusion test	The hernia can be controlled by deep ring occlusion test.
On coughing in standing position the hernia appears from backward to forward position	On standing position in coughing the hernia appears obliquely and downwards.
Never becomes complete	Can become complete, i.e. can reach up to scrotum
Less incidence of strangulation	Higher incidence of strangulation

Natural Factors Preventing Formation of Hernia in a Normal Individual

a. *Obliquity of inguinal canal:* The inguinal starts at deep ring and ends at superficial ring. The deep ring is more posterior and at a deeper plane than external ring. Due to this obliquity of inguinal canal, it tends to get closed during contraction of abdominal musculature.

b. Plugging action of spermatic cord due to contraction of cremesteric muscle.

c. *Shutter like mechanism of conjoint muscle:* The conjoint muscle during relaxed stage is convex in shape with convexity upwards. When this muscle get contracted, it becomes straight and comes near the inguinal ligament hereby reinforcing fascia transversalis and preventing direct hernia.

d. *Sliding mechanism of transverses fascial sling*: This mechanism prevents indirect hernia. The transverses fascial sling is the thickened superior and medial margin of deep ring which is inverted U-shaped. The transverses fascial sling attaches the deep ring to under surface of transverses abdominal muscle. When the transverses abdominal muscle contracts, it will slide the deep ring under its deep surface, hence prevents indirect hernia.

What investigations are required in a case of groin hernia?

In the presence of obvious hernia, no investigation is needed to confirm the diagnosis. The only investigations needed are for fitness of patient for anesthesia.

If the no swelling or bulge is palpable and the clinical suspicion is very high, the following investigations can be performed:

a. Ultrasonography (USG) of the groin can be done as it is noninvasive and dynamic. The specificity of ultrasound in relation to surgical exploration is 81–100%.

b. Magnetic resonance imaging (MRI) has a role in the diagnosis of groin hernia if the ultrasound done is nondiagnostic. MRI is especially useful for patients who present with pain that may be related to sports pathologies and for soft tissue differentiation of tumour or inflammation. Furthermore, MRI allows for scanning to be done in any plane and dynamically during straining for further accuracy.

c. The role of computed tomography (CT) is limited in the nonacute setting even. The role of CT may be useful in the rare case of involvement of the urinary bladder and for the evaluation of intra-abdominal pathologies that may cause increased intra-abdominal pressure causing hernia formation.

d. Herniography has been touted as a safe, sensitive (100%) and specific (98–100%) in the diagnosis of the occult hernia. However, it is not widely used secondary to its invasive nature and risk of complications including contrast

allergy, intestinal perforation, abdominal wall haematoma and pain.

e. If the patient gives history suggestive of LUTS, bladder outlet obstruction (BOO) should be ruled out by uroflowmetry and USG of kidney-ureter-bladder (KUB) region and prostate. If peak flow rate is more than 15 mL per second and the postvoid residual urine is less than 60 mL, the BOO is ruled out.

What is modern classification of groin hernia?

It is classified intraoperatively based on functional and anatomical defects. It is designed to choose the appropriate repair. It was originally devised by Gilbert in 1988; but, later modified by Rutkow and Robins in 1993.

Type 1: Hernia with normal internal ring which does not admit tip of index finger

Type 2: Indirect hernia with a moderately enlarged internal ring less than 4 cm in diameter

Type 3: Indirect hernia with internal ring with 4 cm in diameter or larger

Type 4: Normal internal ring direct hernia with a diffuse bulge or defect in the posterior wall of inguinal canal

Type 5: Localized defect less than 2 cm in the posterior wall of inguinal canal

Types 6 and 7 were added by Rutkow and Robins

Type 6: Pantaloon hernia

Type 7: All femoral hernias.

What are the known risk factors for occurrence of hernia?

Known risk factors associated with hernia occurrence are:

1. Smoking
2. Positive family history
3. Patent processus vaginalis
4. Collagen disease
5. Previous appendicectomy (open) and prostatectomy
6. Patients with ascites
7. Peritoneal dialysis
8. After long-term heavy work
9. Chronic obstructive pulmonary disease (COPD).

Indications of hernia repair: All symptomatic groin hernia should be repaired to avoid complications. Watchful waiting for asymptomatic hernia should only be adopted if the patients have free access to medical services. The incidence of hernia accidents in asymptomatic patients is 1.8 per thousand patients followed for 4–5 years.

The objectives of hernia management are:
a. To relieve symptoms
b. To avoid deformity
c. To prevent complications.

What are the essential components of groin hernia repair?

The essential components of a hernia repair by any approach are following:
a. Isolation of hernia sac from cord structures completely by meticulous careful dissection taking care not to damage the vas and testicular vessels.
b. Complete reduction of the contents of the hernia sac.
c. After reduction of contents, the sac can be pushed back in peritoneal cavity or divided at the neck and remaining portion removed. During laparoscopic TEP repair, the sac is pulled back in peritoneal cavity completely. If sac is large or hernia is complete, effort is made to pull the sac in peritoneal cavity as much as possible and then sac divided at deep ring. The same principal is applied in open repair.
d. Strengthening of the posterior wall of inguinal canal by locally available tissue (herniorraphy) or mesh (hernioplasty).
   Steps a, b and c combined together are known as herniotomy. Herniotomy alone is indicated in type 1 hernia as per Gilbert classification.

Other indications of doing herniotomy are:
a. Congenital hydrocele
b. During orchidopexy for undescended testis, as hernia sac is present in 80% of cases in these cases.

What are different methods of repair of inguinal hernia?

Essentially repair methods can be considered under broad categories as given below:

1. *Open*:
   A. *Tissue repair by suture based (herniorraphy)*:

a. *Bassini repair*: In this repair, posterior wall of inguinal is strengthened by approximation of conjoint muscle or tendon towards the inturned portion of inguinal ligament by interrupted nonabsorbable sutures. To avoid tension suture, bites are taken at different levels and thickness in the muscle so that when tied knots do not lie at the same lines and tension gets distributed. To avoid further tension, Tanner slide incision can be given in the anterior rectus sheath above the conjoint muscle so that lateral leaf of incised anterior rectus sheath moves down towards inguinal ligament. If the deep ring is widened, it can be narrowed by one or two sutures. This is known as Lytle's repair.

b. *McVay*: In this repair, the conjoint tendon is sutured to Cooper's ligament medial to femoral vein.

c. *Shouldice*: It is a four-layered repair developed at Shouldice clinic, Toronto, Canada. It is the modifications of Bassini repair. The first two layers involve double-breasting of fascia transversalis. The third layer involves suturing the conjoint tendon to inguinal ligament as in Bassini repair. The fourth layer involves double-breasting of external oblique aponeurosis.

In these repairs, strengthening of posterior wall of inguinal canal is done by locally available tissue. These repairs are under tension and have high recurrence rates.

These repairs still have place in following circumstances in modern hernia surgery:

a. During emergency repair of obstructed or strangulated inguinal hernia.

b. If the patient gives history of known allergy to mesh material.

c. In a young patient with bilateral inguinal hernia with suboptimal sperm count and the patient has not completed the family. The mesh is known to induce intense fibrosis which can entrap the vas leading to its occlusion. Some clinical and experimental studies have shown that mesh may cause male infertility due to constriction of the vas deference. Some authors have even proposed that young male patients who undergo inguinal herniorrhaphy using polypropylene mesh need to cryopreserve their sperm for future fertility.

B. *Mesh based*:

i. *Anterior approach*: The mesh is placed over the fascia transversalis

    a. Lichtenstein also known as tension free mesh repair: In this technique, the posterior wall of inguinal canal is strengthened by 10 × 15 cm polypropylene mesh.

    b. The plug and patch: This approach uses a cone-shaped plug made up of two layers of polypropylene which is inserted into the deep ring along with a placement of patch over posterior wall of inguinal canal.

    c. Kugel: It is performed through groin incision and specially designed mesh is is placed below the fascia transversalis in the preperitoneal space. It uses an anterior approach, but the mesh is placed in preperitoneal space.

ii. *Posterior approach*: The mesh is placed below the fascia transversalis

    • *Stoppa*: It is used for large complex or bilateral hernia. It utilizes vertical midline subumbilical incision or a low horizontal skin incision. The midline fascial layers are divided and preperitoneal space entered and further developed by blunt dissection. The hernia sacs are reduced by gentle traction. Indirect sacs should be isolated from cord structures gently and it should make sure that contents have been reduced. A large piece of chevron-shaped mesh, 24 × 18 cm is placed in the preperitoneal space. No attempt is made to fix the mesh.

iii. The combined anterior and posterior approach: Prolene hernia system (PHS) is used.

2. *Laparoscopic*:

    a. *Total extraperitoneal (TEP)*: Split mesh, rectangular mesh, preformed mesh, three-dimensional (3D) mesh are used.

    b. Transabdominal preperitoneal (TAPP).

What is the biological response to mesh?

a. Immediately after implantation, the mesh absorbs protein and a coagulum forms around it.

b. The coagulum consists of various substances like albumin, fibrinogen, plasminogen, complement factors and immunoglobulin.

c. The platelet gets adhered to this coagulum and release chemoattractants which attract fibroblasts, smooth muscle cells and macrophages.

d. The fibroblasts and macrophages secrete type 3 collagen for 21 days.

e. This immature type 3 collagen gets converted into type 1 collagen.

f. There is also a cross-linking of fibers to increase strength.

g. The overall strength of this collagen increases for 6 months.

A classification of prosthetic materials used in inguinal hernia repairs:

A. Synthetic meshes

    1. Heavyweight: The mesh is more than 90 gm per square meter:

        a. Polypropylene

        b. Polyester

    2. Lightweight is between 35 gm and 50 gm per square meter. Mesh which weigh less than 35 gm per square meter are known as ultra-light weight mesh.

        a. Nonabsorbable mesh

            i. Plain polypropylene

            ii. Coated polypropylene

        b. Partially absorbable mesh

            i. Polypropylene + polyglactine

            ii. Polypropylene + polyglecaprone

B. Biologic meshes: Recently, biological mesh derived from porcine intestinal submucosa revealed promising results after Lichtenstein repair.

What is the pore size of mesh?

The optimum pore size should be between 600 micron and 800 micron to induce optimum and sufficient net of fibrosis.

What are the features of an ideal mesh?

a. It should have good handling characteristics in the operation room.

b. It should invoke a favorable host response.

c. It should be strong enough to prevent recurrence

d. It should not place any restriction on post-placement function

e. Should perform well in the presence of infection.

f. Should resist shrinkage or degradation over time.

g. Make no restrictions on future access

h. Should be inexpensive and easy to manufacture.

Polypropylene mesh is most commonly used mesh. It was developed and polymerized by an Italian scientist Giolo Natta. The propylene is an ethylene with an attached methyl group. In the polymer, the methyl groups are on the same of polymeric chain and add strength to polymer. The properties of this polymer are:

a. It is hydrophobic

b. It is electrostatically neutral

c. Resistant to significant biological degradation.

d. The biological reactivates induce by it depends upon weight, density, pore size, architecture and individual host response.

Drawbacks of mesh:

1. Direct contact of polypropylene mesh with viscera can lead adhesion formation and fistula formation of gut.

2. The scar tissue at mesh tissue interface can cause chronic pain, adhesions and entrapment of vas in fibrous tissue leading to its occlusion.

Polypropylene meshes is nonabsorbable, strong enough to prevent recurrent, cheap and widely available but it can cause foreign body sensation and chronic pain.

Polyester mesh can cause less foreign body sensation and degrade in the presence of infection.

Polypropylene mesh can be light or heavy weight. Heavyweight meshes weigh are more than 90 gm per square meter, but lightweight are meshes weigh between 35 gm and 50 gm per square meter.

Lightweight meshes may improve patient comfort and causes less foreign body sensation and chronic postoperative pain.

Partially absorbable mesh comprises polypropylene and either polyglactine or polyglecaprone in 50:50 ratio.

Polypropylene nonabsorbable part does not lose its strength at all. The other half is absorbed within 12 weeks.

Possible indications for partially absorbable lightweight meshes in inguinal hernia repair are:

- Small indirect hernia
- Female patient
- Inguinal hernia with severe pubic pain
- Preperitoneal repair
- Sportsman hernia
- Patient preference
- Patients concern about male infertility.

What is femoral hernia?

- It is the protrusion of extraperitoneal fat and peritoneum through the femoral ring and canal.
- It is the most common hernia to get strangulated.

What is the incidence of femoral hernia?

- It is the second most common abdominal wall hernia
- It makes up 10% of all hernias
- It is more common in females (4:1) due to different configuration of the feminine pelvis and the musculoaponeurotic attachment.

From where the sac enters and from where it comes out?

- The sac enters the femoral canal through femoral opening and comes out through saphenous opening into subcutaneous tissue.

Describe the anatomy of femoral canal.

- The femoral canal is 2 cm long funnel-shaped with wider mouth downwards.
- Upper opening is formed by femoral ring which is covered by septum femorale (condensation of extraperitoneal fat).
- Lower opening of femoral canal is saphenous opening (fossa ovalis) covered by cribriform fascia.
- Upper margin of saphenous opening is firm and unyielding and to the lower margin superficial fascia of thigh is attached.

What are the boundaries of femoral ring?

- Anterior: Inguinal ligament
- Posterior: Fascia over pectineus muscle and copper's ligament.
- Medial: Concave sharp edge of lacunar ligament.
- Lateral: Femoral vein.

What is path or course taken by femoral hernia?

- While in femoral canal, it runs downwards.
- On coming out of saphenous opening, it changes its direction and turns upwards and can reach up to inguinal ligament.
- It lies in the subcutaneous tissue of groin after coming out of saphenous opening.

Why femoral hernia turns upwards in subcutaneous tissue after coming out from saphenous opening?

- Firm attachment of superficial fascia of thigh to the lower margin of saphenous opening.
- Firm unyielding nature of the upper margin of fossa ovalis.
- Forward curvature of femoral canal.
- Repeated flexion of the thigh.

Why is it important to diagnose and treat femoral hernia early?

- According to Bendavid: Femoral hernias have not received the respect they deserve as a surgical entity. Diagnosis and treatment are often delayed.
- It has high propensity for incarceration/strangulation.
- Incidence of strangulation is 10 times more frequent than inguinal hernias.
- The probability of strangulation is 22% in the first 3 months and 45% at nearly 2 years after diagnosis.
- Therefore, early repair is mandatory.

What is the etiology of femoral hernia?

- Incidence of femoral hernia in infancy/childhood less than 0.5%.
- Most of the time, it is acquired secondary to an expanded femoral ring from natural loss of tissue strength and elasticity (primary etiology).
- It may be secondary to an increased intra-abdominal pressure.

What are the clinical presentations of femoral hernia?

- Small bulge just below the medial groin crease
- Often difficult to reduce on initial presentation
- Extends caudad as the sac increases in size.

Describe special types of femoral hernia.

- *Lacunar hernia*: Hernia through small defect in the lacunar ligament (Laugier hernia).
- *Prevascular hernia*: Hernia sac behind the femoral vessels.
- May be associated with congenital dislocation of hip (Narath hernia).
- *Cloquet hernia*: Hernia passes between the pectineus muscle and its fascia.
- *Hesselbach hernia*: Hernia lateral to femoral vessels.

What is the differential diagnosis of femoral hernia?

- Femoral lymphadenopathy
- Femoral artery aneurysm
- Groin lipoma
- Psoas abscess
- Benign or malignant soft tissue mass
- Saphena varix
- Inguinal hernia
- Psoas bursa.

What are different surgical procedures available for femoral hernia?

- Femoral hernia can be repaired using:
  - Open procedures
  - Laparoscopic approach.

What are open operations?

- Low operation of Lockwood
- Inguinal operation
- High operation of McEvedy
- Henry approach: Low midline approach for bilateral hernia.

Low approach:
- Incision directly over swelling in thigh
- Hernia sac dissected
- Sac ligated at the neck and remaining part excised
- Femoral ring obliterated by suturing inguinal ligament to Cooper's ligament
- Used only for uncomplicated hernia
- Strangulated gut cannot be managed by this approach.

Inguinal approach:
- Incision same as for inguinal hernia.
- After opening inguinal canal tranversalis fascia is incised to identify the sac.
- The sac is pulled up in inguinal canal from femoral canal.
- The contents are reduced and the sac is pushed back in peritoneal cavity.
- Femoral-opening closed by approximating conjoint tendon to ileopectinate line.

Combined approach or high operation:
- Vertical incision over the swelling which extends into inguinal region.
- The sac is dissected off from both above and below.

Henry's approach:
- Lower midline incision
- Extraperitoneal approach
- Reserved for bilateral hernia.

What is sliding hernia?

- Any hernia in which part of the sac is formed by wall of a viscus
- Accounts for 8% of all groin hernias
- Incidence increases with age
- The most common viscus involved is the colon or urinary bladder
- Most sliding hernias are a variant of indirect inguinal hernias.
- Sliding hernia is suspected by long standing large hernia which is partially irreducible.

Sliding Hernia Contents

- On right side: Following structures can form part of the sac.
  - Cecum
  - Ascending colon
  - Appendix
- On left side: Following structures can form part of the sac.
  - Sigmoid colon
  - On both sides
  - Uterus
  - Fallopian tube
  - Ovary
  - Urinary bladder
- Sliding component usually found on posterior lateral side sac
- Opening sac risks damage to sliding contents
- Avoid opening the sac
- The sliding hernia contents are reduced and excess hernia sac ligated and divided
- After reduction repair of the inguinal hernia is done as usual
- Laparoscopic hernia repair is a relative contra-indication for sliding hernia.

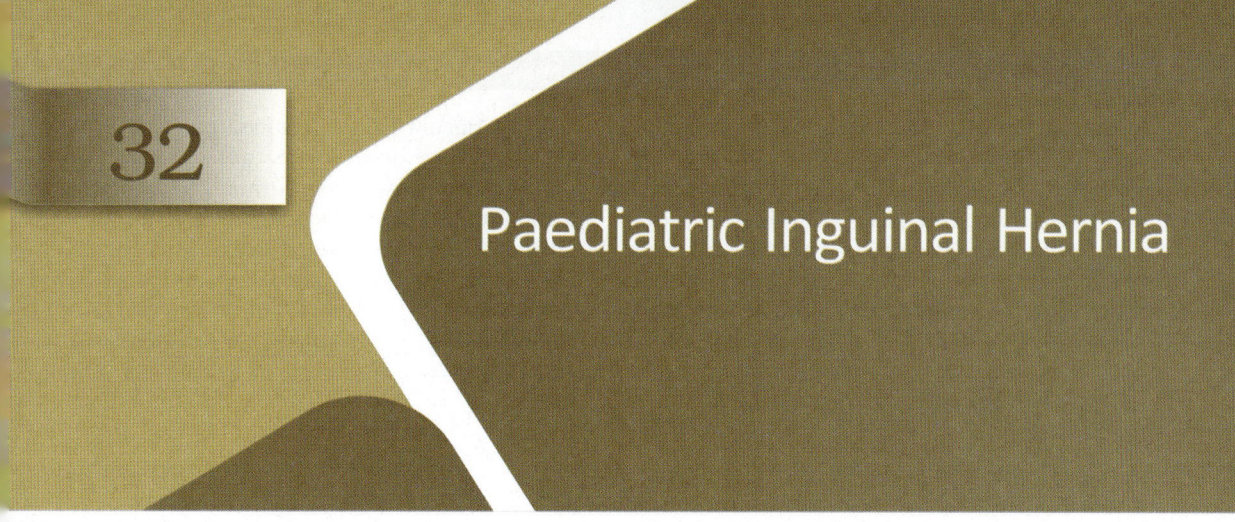

32

Paediatric Inguinal Hernia

What is an inguinal hernia?

A hernia is the abnormal protrusion of the contents of the abdominal viscera or part of the viscera outside its fascial boundaries. It is classified according to the site of the defect. The inguinal hernia occurs when the abdominal contents protrude through the inguinal canal.

What is the incidence of inguinal hernia in paediatric age group?

Overall the incidence of inguinal hernia is 0.8% to 4.4%. About one-third of these appear in first 6 months of life. The premature infants have a higher incidence—about 16–25%. It occurs more commonly in boys than girls (3:1 to 10:1). About 11.5% have family history of inguinal hernia.

Which side is the inguinal hernia more common?

Inguinal hernia is more common on right side (3:2) with 10% being bilateral. The higher incidence is presumably related to the later descend of testis on the right side.

Describe the embryogenesis of the congenital hernia.

The intra-abdominal testis descends into the scrotum through the processus vaginalis. The processus appears in the third month of intra-uterine life. It may be due to increased intra-abdominal pressure or an active process. The testis descends into the scrotum in seventh to ninth month of gestation. As the testis descends, the processus vaginalis obliterates. The exact timing of the closure is not known. It is suggested that 80–100% newborns have patent processus vaginalis. The processus vaginalis obliterates later,

maximum does it in first 6 months of life. Failure of the processus to obliterate results in "PPV". If intra-abdominal contents come into the PPV, it is called inguinal hernia. Mere presence of fluid in the sac results in "congenital hydrocele".

The obliteration of the PPV is probably guided by androgens or by Calcitonin Gen-Related Peptide (CGRP) released by genitofemoral nerve.

Enlist the risk factors for development of inguinal hernia.

- Congenital—weak abdominal wall
  - Urogenital
    - Undescended testis
    - Exstrophy of bladder
  - Connective tissue disorder
    - Ehlers-Danlos syndrome
    - Hunter-Hurler syndrome
    - Marfan's syndrome
    - Mucopolysaccharidosis
- Increased intraabdominal pressure
  - Repair of exomphalos or gastroschisis
  - Severe ascites (like chylous ascites)
  - Meconium peritonitis
  - Increased peritoneal fluid
    - Ascites
    - Ventriculoperitoneal shunt
    - Peritoneal dialysis
  - Chronic respiratory disease
    - Cystic fibrosis.

How a child with an inguinal hernia will present to you?

A child will have complaint of a bulge appearing intermittently in one or both groins, noted by parents at time of bath or otherwise or by paedia-trician while doing routine clinical examination of a well baby. The lump is usually asymptomatic. But, an older child may have dragging sensation during exercise. The hernia (PPV) is present since birth, but may be noted later. A child may present first time with a complication without any prior history.

What are the complications of an inguinal hernia?

A hernia may be complicated by incarceration, obstruction (Fig. 32.1) or strangulation. The contents of a hernia usually reduce spontaneously. If they fail to do so and become stuck in the hernia sac, it results in an incarcerated hernia. The patient has pain and irreducible swelling. The level of incarceration is debated, but usually, it happens at the level of internal ring.

The bowel in the hernia sac may get obstructed due to narrow neck and result in obstructed hernia. The patient may present with symptoms and signs of small bowel obstruction, namely abdominal distension, bilious vomiting and obstipation. The history of hernia may not be provided by the parents. So, it is mandatory to examine the groin in every patient presenting with bowel obstruction.

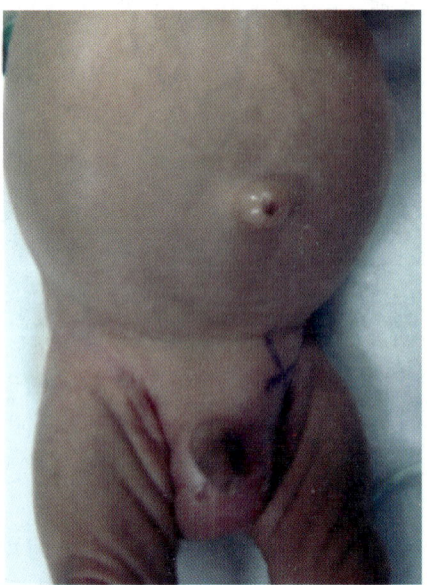

Fig. 32.1: Clinical picture obstructed left inguinal hernia in a newborn

If the hernia is not reduced early, the blood supply of the bowel may get compromised, resulting in strangulated hernia. The venous and lymphatic drainage gets affected first and arterial supply gets compromised later. This results in bowel gangrene and perforation and may result in peritonitis.

The incarcerated hernia may compress on testicular vessels and cause testicular gangrene or atrophy.

Most of the complications occur when the child is less than 6 months old (28–31%) and is infrequent after the age of 5 years (overall 12–17%). The incidence is lesser in premature infants, probably because of wider ring and weak muscles.

What are the differential diagnoses of inguinal hernia?

- Congenital hydrocele
- Undescended testis
- Retractile testis
- Inguinal lymphadenopathy

How will you confirm hernia on clinical examination?

The child is examined undressed in a warm room. The hands of the examiner must be warm. On inspection, differential bulge in both the groins is seen. If the bulge is not seen in supine position, the child may be asked to stand and do Valsalva maneuver or cough or strain or cry. Both the testes should be confirmed in the scrotum. If the hernia is still not demonstrated, the cord is gently palpated with tip of index finger over the pubic tubercle. The cord with a hernia sac will be bulky, and the examiner may be able to elicit "silk sign" (feeling rubbing two pieces of silk together) or "plastic baggie sign" (sensation of a plastic bag with a few drops of water in it).

What is the role of radiological investigations in diagnosis/management of hernia?

Hernia is mainly a clinical diagnosis. However, various investigators have described procedures like herniography and ultrasound for the diagnosis of hernia with a doubtful history and to diagnose contralateral hernia in unilateral clinical hernia.

Herniography is done by inserting a needle infraumbilically and injecting water soluble contrast near deep ring. Serial radiographs are taken after putting the patient in supine position. A PPV can be demonstrated if the contrast flows into the labioscrotal fold. The test will be negative in incarcerated hernia and carries a risk of bowel perforation, intramural haematoma and allergic reaction to contrast.

Ultrasound is a noninvasive and safe investigation. The studies have concentrated on correlating the diameter of inguinal canal with the presence of hernia sac. Clinical hernia had diameter of 7.2 ± 2.0 mm, subclinical PPV had a diameter of 4.9 ± 1.1 mm and normal findings were seen in patients with inguinal canal diameter of 3.6 ± 0.8 mm.

What are the indications of surgery in a patient with inguinal hernia?

Any hernia will need surgical correction to avoid complications. The hernia with complication need to be operated urgently as the progress to strangulation can be rapid, and bowel gangrene may occur within 2 hours. All hernias should be operated within 1 month of diagnosis to avoid the complication. In a few centres, all premature infants are operated before discharge as the risk of operating in emergency is much more than if operated in routine on uncomplicated hernia.

When should a patient with reducible inguinal hernia be operated?

The patient with a reducible inguinal hernia is always at risk of the hernia becoming incarcerated and subsequently obstruction and strangulation. The risk is higher in infants, and more so in neonates. Thus, it is suggested that a patient with reducible inguinal hernia be operated as early as possible. On the other hand, the emergency surgery entails the risk of anaesthetic complications like aspiration, apnea and bradycardia. Thus, the general consensus suggests that the patient be operated in "next available routine OT".

In preterm neonates the risk of postoperative apnea and bradycardia is higher than term neonates, so many pediatric surgeons do wait till the postconceptual week 60 if the baby is under observation in nursery. But, it is generally believed that the baby be operated before discharge for the risk of complications is higher for emergency surgery.

Is "Herniotomy is a day care surgery"?

With availability of safe anaesthesia and potent analgesics of pain control, the hernia surgery can be done on a day care basis. However, in premature infants, the risk of postoperative apnea and bradycardia precludes day care surgery. All patients with postconceptional age less than 60 weeks should be admitted overnight for observation. The surgical techniques of laparoscopy or open repair are safe and allow day care procedures.

Describe the surgery for inguinal hernia in a male child.

Modified Ferguson technique is used for high ligation of sac (herniotomy) after opening external oblique aponeurosis. Earlier, Mitchell Blanks technique was used in which high ligation of sac was done through the external inguinal ring without opening the external oblique muscle.

The child is positioned supine on operation table. The procedure is done under general or regional anaesthesia. After cleaning and draping, an incision is placed. The incision is given in inguinal crease, starting just above and lateral to pubic tubercle (overlying superficial inguinal ring) extending to midinguinal point (overlying deep inguinal ring). The incision is deepened with scissors to divide fascia of Camper and Scarpa, taking care to avoid injury to superficial epigastric vessels. The fat overlying the external oblique aponeurosis is cleared till inguinal ligament. The external oblique is opened with blade and scissors in the line of fibres. The two edges are grasped with hemostats to aid in dissection and retraction. The underlying structures are cleared to identify the conjoint tendon and inguinal ligament, taking care to preserve ilioinguinal and genitofemoral nerves. The spermatic cord is identified and opened in the line of cremasteric fibres. A slight traction on testis may help in the identification. The sac is picked up by a hemostat. The cord structures including the vas and testicular vessels are gently teased off the sac using a dissecting forceps. The sac is palpated for any contents. The sac is divided after putting clamps. The distal sac is left after achieving hemostasis. The proximal sac is dissected till deep inguinal ring. The sac is twisted on itself for complete reduction of any contents. The sac is divided after high ligation using absorbable suture. The wound is closed in layers using absorbable sutures.

How is the technique in a female child different from that in a male child?

In a female child, the inguinal canal does not contain the vas deferens or testicular vessels that need to be preserved. So, the dissection is easier. Also, the deep ring is closed after complete ligation making the recurrence rare. Some surgeons do fix the round ligament after herniotomy to provide support to the uterus (Bastionelli Maneuver).

Also, in females, up to 40% children will have a sliding component with ovary, fallopian tube or uterus in the sac. The sac needs to be opened and examined before dividing it.

A phenotypic female with testis in the hernia sac may be the presentation of a female pseuo-hermaphrodite.

What is the minimally invasive approach to dealing with inguinal hernia?

Laparoscopy has been accepted for hernia repair in adults. However, in children the beneficial effects are yet to be established for wider acceptance. The small incision (cosmesis) and minimal pain (early return to activity) in open surgery have led many paediatric surgeons to avoid laparoscopic approach for hernia repair. The potential benefits for use of laparoscopy in herniotomy are simultaneous repair of bilateral hernia, especially if subclinical PPV and repair of recurrent hernia. The potential for injury to vas and testicular vessels, longer learning curve, high cost and high recurrence rate (when an absorbable suture is used for ligation of sac) make laparoscopic repair less preferred.

In boys, the laparoscopic hernia repair is done by placing a purse string suture at deep inguinal ring using a nonabsorbable suture with or without incision of peritoneum all around. The suture may be placed using intracorporeal suturing (requiring two instruments in bilateral flanks) or using extracorporeal suturing through a stab inguinal incision under vision of laparoscope.

In girls, the laparoscopic inversion ligation (LIL) technique may be used where the sac is inverted into the peritoneal cavity and ligated at deep ring using preformed loops, as there is no vas to preserve.

What are the indications for contralateral exploration in a child presenting with unilateral inguinal hernia?

The incidence of contralateral hernia developing in a child presenting with unilateral inguinal hernia is not exactly known. The incidence of contralateral PPV in such a patient has been widely studied with variable results. It is generally believed that 60–80% of infants, and 40% of older children have PPV while only 20% will eventually develop a clinical hernia ever. The incidence of contralateral hernia is more in premature infants, females and those with left sided inguinal hernia. These may be candidates for routine contralateral exploration or use of ultrasound or laparoscopy to diagnose contralateral hernia. Goldstein test has been described as creation of pneumoperitoneum using abdominal needle and palpation for crepitus in the contralateral spermatic cord.

How will you deal with an incarcerated hernia?

The inguinal hernia that does not reduce is called irreducible hernia. It is at risk of obstruction and strangulation and thus be dealt with emergently. If there are no features of strangulation, the *taxis* can be performed to reduce the contents. It is done with the child calmed down, may be with help of sedatives. The baby is placed in supine position with legs elevated. The ipsilateral scrotum is held with hand and mild traction is given to align the long axis of the hernial sac with that on inguinal canal. With support to neck of the sac with finger and thumb of one hand, gentle pressure is given with the other hand to reduce the hernia.

If the *taxis* fails or there are signs of strangulation, the emergency surgery should be performed. The inguinal exploration may be done either through standard inguinal incision, preperitoneal approach, Pfannensteil incision or laparoscopy.

Inguinal approach: The standard inguinal incision is used although longer. The external ring is opened. The sac is opened to visualize the contents and access viability. If viable, the contents are reduced and herniotomy performed. If the contents are of doubtful viability, the bowel is placed in warm sponges and the viability reassessed. If gangrenous, the nonviable bowel is resected and then reduced through the same incision. However, sometimes the procedure may need counterincision in transversalis fascia (La Roque maneuver) or separate abdominal incision.

Preperitoneal approach: Initially described by Cheatle, a grid-iron incision is made at the level of anterior-superior iliac spine. The preperitoneal space is dissected till deep inguinal ring. The peritoneum is incised, and contents reduced. The contents are dealt as per viability and the herniotomy performed. Pfannensteil incision has been used and claimed to have better cosmesis.

Laparoscopic approach: Various surgeons prefer the laparoscopic approach for reduction of contents and visualization of bowel for viability. This is particularly helpful when the hernia reduces before the contents are visualized for viability (on induction of general anaesthesia or opening the external inguinal ring).

What are the complications of herniotomy?

- *Hydrocele*: If fluid collects in the distal sac, it results in hydrocele. It is self-limiting and usually does not reappear after aspiration. Higher incidence is seen after laparoscopic stitch as the continuity of peritoneum is not broken.
- *Scrotal haematoma*: It occurs after excision of distal sac.
- *Iatrogenic undescended testis*: 0.2% of patients will have testis at a higher position than normal after herniotomy. This is due to entrapment of cord structures in fibrosis. Surgeon should always ensure the dependent position of the testis after the procedure. Correction needs surgical intervention.
- *Recurrence*: Reported incidence of recurrence is 0–0.8% in uncomplicated herniotomy. Most of the recurrences are indirect type due to:
  - Tearing of frail sac
  - Failure to dissect complete sac
  - Slippage of ligature
  - Failure to ligate the sac high enough
  - False recurrence—missed direct or femoral hernia in first surgery
  A higher incidence is seen in:
  - Prematurity—2–15% recurrence rate due to weak muscles.
  - Incarceration—20% recurrence rate due to difficult dissection and weakened muscles.
  - After laparoscopic suture technique— 2.7–3.4% recurrence rate, probably due to incomplete suture or dissolving of absorbable suture.

- *Injury to vas deferens*: Reported incidence between 0.16% and 1.6%. The Müllerian structures may be seen in the excised sac even without vas injury. In a study, it was demonstrated in rats that holding the vas with mosquito hemostats, nontoothed forceps, bulldog clamps and even stretch caused vassal injury and only finger holding was safe. The higher magnification and identification of vas may improve the vas injury rate in laparoscopy.
- *Infertility*: The incidence of infertility is difficult to assess. The possible mechanisms of infertility after hernia surgery are:
  - Injury to vas
  - Injury to testicular vessels by incarceration or surgery
  - Blockage of testicular lymphatics due to partial injury to vas and resulting breach of blood-testis barrier and production of anti-sperm antibodies.
- *Testicular atrophy*: Overall 1% incidence. More often seen in incarcerated hernia (2.6–5%). The underlying cause is injury to testicular vessels due to pressure by incarcerated bowel or injury during surgery. It is recommended to use magnification loops for identification of testicular vessels and preserving them.
- *Ovarian gangrene*: Herniated ovary may get gangrenous due to incarceration or torsion in the hernia sac.
- *Intestinal injury*: Zero to 1.4% incidence of need for resection of small bowel as a result of bowel gangrene has been reported.
- *Respiratory compromise*: Premature infants are at risk of apnea and respiratory failure after general anaesthesia. Small babies are also at risk of respiratory failure due to increased abdominal pressure after large amount of small bowel is repositioned inside the abdominal cavity from a large or bilateral inguinal hernia. It is suggested that large bilateral hernia may be done in staged manner to reduce the risk.

How will you diagnose and manage sliding hernia?

An inguinal hernia is called "sliding" if its wall comprises retroperitoneal organ. The organ may be fallopian tube or urinary bladder on either side, caecum and appendix on right side or sigmoid colon on left side. As the fallopian tube is present in the wall of sac in up to 40% female hernia, it is recommended that the sac be opened and the tube looked for before ligation. Otherwise, thick contents at the base of sac should prompt the diagnosis of sliding hernia.

The sliding hernia is managed by flap procedure (Goldstein and Pott) or simply by ligating the sac above the level of sliding component, repositioning the contents through deep inguinal ring and tightening the deep inguinal ring (Bevan's procedure).

What gonadal anomalies can be present that the surgeon operating on inguinal hernia must be aware of?

- *Absent vas deferens*: Seen in 0.5–1% of general population. It is associated with cystic fibrosis and ipsilateral renal agenesis. Thus, absent vas deferens should make surgeon evaluate for upper tract anomalies or cystic fibrosis.

- *Intersex*: In a phenotypic female, the surgeon may find testis or ovotestis in testicular feminization syndrome or true hermaphrodite respectively. If there is doubt of ovotestis, bipolar biopsies should be taken for confirmation.

- *Splenogonadal fusion*: Splenic tissue may be adherent to testis or ovary. It presents as inguinal or abdominal mass. Diagnosis is made by laparoscopy or frozen section biopsy. It is managed by excising the splenic component while preserving the gonad.

How is management of congenital hydrocele different from that of inguinal hernia?

Congenital hydrocele is the condition where the PPV contains only fluid and an inguinal hernia is a condition when the PPV contains intraabdominal contents like bowel or omentum.

The diagnosis of hydrocele is made clinically when the contents of the sac are fluid, the neck narrow and swelling transilluminant, whereas in inguinal hernia, the contents are bowel or omentum, neck wide, reducible, non-transilluminant swelling. Hydrocele must be differentiated from incarcerated hernia where the fluid in sac distal to incarceration may appear like a hydrocele.

The hydrocele sac may get obliterated, typically during first 2 years of life. Thus, the surgery is not recommended till age of 2 years except if there is doubtful hernia or if the sac is so tense as to cause discomfort. The hydrocele that persists beyond 2 years or that appears after 2 years needs high ligation of sac. The distal sac should be opened, drained and left as such to continue drainage.

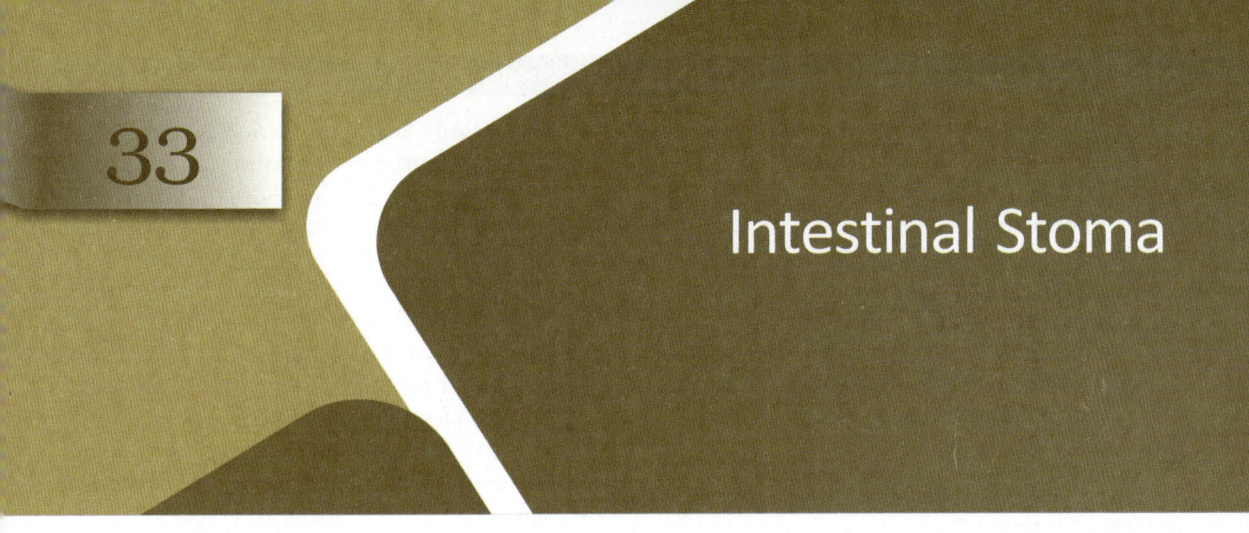

33

Intestinal Stoma

"As the lips of the intestines, so wounded, would sometimes quite unexpectedly adhere to the wound of the abdomen; and therefore, it seemed no reason why we should not take hints from nature."   **—Heiste**

Describe important landmarks to the history of stoma creation.

Lorenz Heister in 1757 first recommended the creation of stoma for the treatment of abdominal trauma. In 1710, Alexis Littre suggested creation of an abdominal stoma for the treatment of imperforate anus, however, first sigmoid colostomy was created in 1793 by Duret, a Naval surgeon for the treatment of imperforate anus. In 1907 Mayo first described right transverse colostomy for the treatment of diverticulitis.

The first diverting ileostomy was performed by Bauncea, Germany, for the treatment of right colon cancer.

How do you define stoma?

An ostomy or intestinal stoma can be defined as an artificial opening of the intestinal or urinary tract on the abdominal wall created surgically. A patient with an intestinal stoma is common in the surgical ward. If such patients are encountered the goal of history and examination is to determine three basic answers. The first question relates to why the stoma was created. The next question is the nature of stoma that has been created and how it is presently functioning. All the associated complications of stoma need to be investigated for. Lastly based on the above two answers, the fate of the stoma is to be decided. To answer these questions and interact with the patient, a thorough understanding of indications, types and complications of stoma are needed. Experienced surgeons realize that this exchange of information is equally important for the surgeon as well. A patient with stoma has a different way of life and in many indigenous ways the patient tries to fit into the everyday life.

Focused History and Examination of a Stoma Patient

History

- General patient data
- Presenting complaint (may be a complication associated with the stoma or the patient may be scheduled for the closure of stoma)
- History and events of the illness leading to stoma formation (should be directed to define the likely pathology due to which the primary surgery was undertaken)
- History pertaining to the functioning of the stoma
- Negative history of all the associated complications of intestinal stoma
- Past and personal medical history (drug therapy and allergies in particular).

Examination

- Vitals and general physical examination
- Abdominal examination
- Examination specific to the stoma (after removal of stoma appliance) (Fig. 33.1) associated figure
  - Site
  - Type
  - Part of intestine involved

– Color (red, purple or dusky or congested, pale or anemia, black or necrotic)
– Peristomal skin
– Type of appliance used
– Length of pouting of stoma
– Mucocutaneous interface
– Cough impulse around stoma to rule out parastomal hernia
– Palpate for tenderness and cough impulse over scar and around stoma
– Auscultate bowel sounds.

What are salient features of history taking for a patient with stoma?

The history of a stoma patient starts from the illnesses that lead to the creation of the stoma and includes the eventual course of life ever since the stoma. Another school of thought is to begin the history since the time the stoma was made and mention the likely causative factors in the past history. Since the stoma is a continuum of the illness that lead to its formation and the closure is guided by the initial pathology in question, we recommend that the history begin from the initial complaints.

It must mention when the patient was apparently well and systematically describe the symptoms and sequence of events that resulted in the stoma. Subsequent to that history must be sought on how the patient is managing with the stoma. Questions that must be definitely included are the description of the contents produced by the stoma, the daily output from the stoma, variation in output on a daily basis, its relation with diet and how often the patient has to replace the appliance. History of any other symptoms that the patient has must also be sought. Ask if the patient passes stools per rectum and if there has been any abnormal discharge per rectum. It is common for patients to occasionally pass mucus and it indicates patency of the lower tract.

Once the normal stoma function has been enquired about, focus on whether the patient has had any complications which include:

- *Diarrhea*: Enquire about the frequency, causative factors and management done
- *Constipation*: Enquire about the frequency, causative factors and management done
- *Obstruction*: Partial or complete, how was it managed, was any imaging performed
- *Dehydration*: Frequency, management and routine measures taken for prevention
- *Retraction*: Duration since when stoma is retracted, peristomal infection, herniation
- *Bleeding*: Frequency, location, character of blood whether fresh or semidigested, causative factors (trauma or constitutional), management
- *Peristomal varices*: Location, duration and whether there has been an episode of bleeding
- *Parastomal hernia*: Duration, location and associated problems (obstipation, pain, etc.)
- *Skin changes*: Burning or itching or bleeding and how the patient is managing the problem
- *Prolapse*: Duration and associated symptoms
- Stenosis.

Before closure is planned it is necessary to ensure that the patient has complied with the treatment of primary pathology so that there is no chance of recurrence, and that the distal segment of intestine is patent. Fitness for surgery in the form of associated comorbidities and symptoms must be asked about and problem rectified.

Examination pattern remains the same apart from the fact that the patient needs to be taken into confidence and the appliance inspected and removed to thoroughly examine for the characteristics of the stoma and its contents apart from above-mentioned complications. A per rectal examination must be done to rule out any approachable distal pathologies before restoring bowel continuity if the stoma is temporary.

Describe classification of stoma.

It is essential to be acquainted with the various classification systems of stoma to understand the intricacies and problems associated with management of stoma. These classification systems when used together will allow the examinee to systematically approach a case of stoma.

Classification of ostomy based on duration:

- *Permanent*: Required in carcinoma and severe inflammation with necrosis where there is permanent removal of structures and continuity of the bowel cannot be restored, e.g. total colectomy in severe ulcerative colitis.
- *Temporary*: Ostomy is created to bridge a small period, usually months to a couple of years after which is the continuity of bowel is restored. This type of ostomy is usually made after surgery or trauma or in the presence of severe inflammation or infection to bypass the affected portion and give time for the gut to heal.

Classification based on structure and construction of ostomy:

- *End ostomy*: In the end ostomy, a single ostomy is created and this ostomy is in continuity with the proximal portion of gut. The ostomy discharges digested or semidigested food whose characteristics vary based on the segment of intestine which has been brought out as the stoma. It is made in situations where the distal end of the bowel has to be removed in its entirety or the leftover portion of the distal bowel too small to be brought to the anterior abdominal wall. In the Hartmann's procedure the distal aspect of the large gut is left *in situ*. The proximal part is brought out as an end ostomy.

- *Loop ostomy*: In loop ostomy a loop of bowel is brought out of the abdomen and partially transected such that the continuity is maintained. In this scenario there are two openings visible externally, one of which generates bowel contents in the form of processed or semi-processed faeces and the other end is in continuity with the distal part of the gut. This stoma usually drains mucus and is also referred to as the distal mucous fistula.

  Another form of the loop ostomy is the double barrel ostomy where the two ends are not contiguous with each other and are brought out through a common opening in the abdominal wall.

- *End loop ostomy*: End loop ostomy is a combination of loop and end ostomy wherein a small loop of intestine is brought out of the abdominal wall while the distal aspect is not in continuity with the rest of the gut. This is a rarely used type of ostomy which is preferred in patients with a short mesentery (patients who have undergone multiple surgeries earlier) or obese patients with a thick abdominal wall. The loop allows a rod to be placed for a couple of weeks that prevents the retraction of stoma.

Classification based on function:

- *Decompression*: Decompressive stoma is created to bridge the gap between definitive surgery and conservative therapy and useful in conditions associated with massive dilatation of bowel resulting from obstruction, toxic mega-colon and other functional causes of obstruction. This stoma is contraindicated in presence of distal perforation but useful to prevent impending perforation due to dilatation and ischaemic necrosis. Both tube cecostomy and Blow Hole stoma are commonly employed forms of decompressive stoma.

- *Diversion*: Diverting stoma is created to provide diversion of intestinal or urinary content. Most stomas are created for the purpose of diversion.

Classification based on continence:

- *Continent ostomy*: The ostomy drains out contents only when it is deliberately emptied using a catheter. It is common to employ continent ostomy in urinary diversion. A number of such pouches have been designed using the small gut, large gut or its combination. For drainage of fecal contents the Koch's pouch is a commonly used continent ostomy. The continent ostomy consists of four parts: (1) the stoma, (2) the nipple valve continence mechanism, (3) the pouch that stores the contents and (4) the efferent limb that produces and delivers the contents into the pouch.

- *Noncontinent ostomy*: Ostomy that drains contents as soon as they are delivered is referred to as noncontinent ostomy. It is a more frequently employed ostomy that requires an external appliance to store the contents delivered.

Classification based on the drained contents:

- *Urostomy*: This stoma drains urine.
- *Enterostomy*: This stoma drains fecal matter.

Classification based on the anatomical location:

- Ostomies in the digestive tract
  - Gastrostomy
  - Jejunostomy
  - Duodenostomy
  - Ileostomy (Fig. 33.1)
  - Colostomy (Fig. 33.2)
- Cecostomy
- Ascending
- Transverse
- Descending
- Sigmoid
- Ostomies in the urinary tract
  - Ureterostomy
  - Ileal or colonic conduit
  - Vesicostomy
  - Continent internal reservoir.

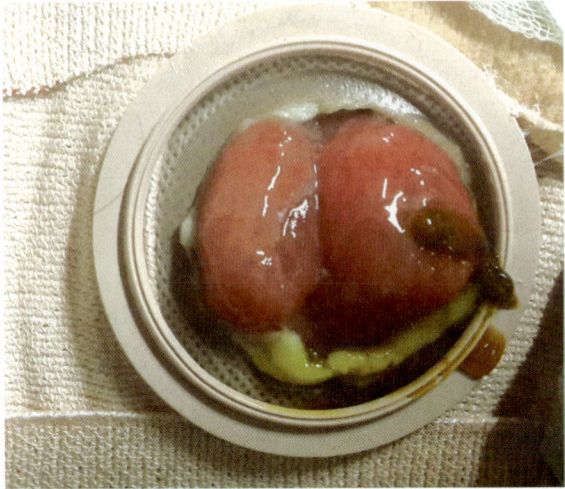

Fig. 33.1: Clinical picture of ileostomy

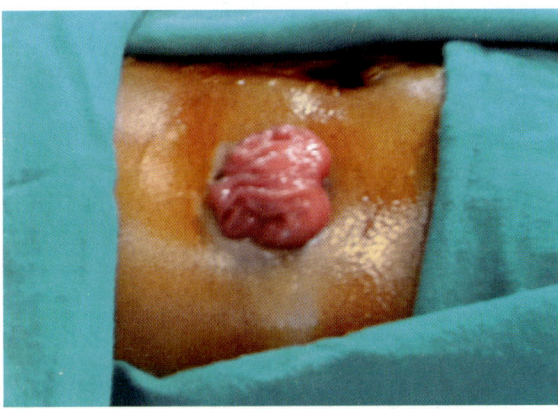

Fig. 33.2: Clinical picture of colostomy

What are the indications of creation of stoma?

- Surgically created stoma
  - Gastrostomy created mainly for providing enteral nutrition in patients who cannot be fed orally due to conditions like:
    - Severe stomatitis
    - Dysphagia resulting from advanced esophageal carcinoma
    - Malignancy related tracheoesophageal fistula
    - Comatose patients requiring enteral nutrition (avoids respiratory complications associated with Ryle's tube/mesogastric tube like aspiration and subsequent pneumonitis)
  - Jejunostomy (created for enteral nutrition with same indications as a gastrostomy)

- Additional indications may include malignancy related gastric outlet obstruction
  - Ileostomy
    - Perforation of small bowel resulting from:
      - *Infective causes*: Tuberculosis, enteric fever
      - *Inflammatory causes*: Ulcerative colitis, Crohn's disease, radiation enteritis
      - Malignancy of the small distal gut or large gut
    - Intestinal obstruction resulting from:
      - Infective causes
      - Inflammatory causes
      - Malignancy of the gut, retroperitoneum, mesentery
    - Carcinoma urinary bladder (for diversion of urine)
    - Following pelvic exenteration for locally advanced pelvic and gynaecological tumours (for diversion of both bowel and diversion of urine)
    - Other causes: Diversion of a distal anastomosis
  - Appendicostomy:
    - Drainage of urinary neobladder
    - Drainage of normal bladder in cases of severe outlet obstruction like complicated urethral strictures
  - Cecostomy:
    - Decompression
  - Colostomy:
    - Obstruction: Carcinoma of distal gut, volvulus, extraluminal compression by tumours, bands, adhesions
    - Perforation:
      - Traumatic
      - Infective: Amoebiasis, tuberculosis, diverticulitis
      - Inflammatory: Ulcerative colitis, Crohn's disease, radiation
    - Intractable fecal incontinence resulting from trauma, surgery or disease
    - Other causes: Diversion of a distal anastomosis, imperforate anus or anorectal malformation, rectourethral or vesical fisula, rectovaginal fistula, perianal sepsis
  - Vesicostomy: Usually performed in children
    - Bladder outlet obstruction commonly posterior urethral valve, stricture urethra.

How to differentiate a colostomy from ileostomy?

	Colostomy	Ileostomy
Site	Right upper abdomen for transverse colostomy	Right iliac fossa
	Left iliac fossa for sigmoid colostomy	
Discharge	Formed faeces or semi-solid stool	Liquid in nature
Colour of discharge	Brownish, blackish	Greenish, yellowish
Odour of discharge	Very offensive (excessive gases)	Less offensive
Stoma	Large lumen and usually constructed flush or slightly elevated from the skin	Small lumen and constructed as nipple like projection above the skin
Reaction of surrounding skin	Surrounding skin usually normal	Surrounding skin red, excoriated, oedematoid from enzymatic digestion

How to chose a stoma site?

As we have already seen earlier various parts of the intestines can be used to divert urine and faeces. The decision of creating a stoma is often life changing for the patient and this issue requires adequate preoperative counseling and special therapists and nursing care. Although the type of stoma needed can be decided finally only intra-operatively, there are a number of preoperative considerations that must be taken into account while creating a stoma.

- The stoma site must be chosen in such a way that it is visible and accessible to the patient in all positions; supine, sitting and standing.
- The site must be marked preoperatively using a permanent mark or dye.
- Avoid any bony prominences, scars, creases of skin, drain sites, infective lesions and belt lines while choosing the stoma site
- It is important to assess the following functions in a patient before constructing the stoma:
  - Ocular function or vision and manual dexterity
  - Hand tremors, paralysis, cerebrovascular accident (CVA) or arthritis
  - Functional status (Karnofsky/ECOG)
  - Current medications
  - Recreational hobbies
  - Sexual activity
- Introduction of the stoma care nurse with the patient prior to the procedure is recommended
- Patient must be able to place and change appliance and be aware of usual complications before discharge. Patient is visited by stoma care nurse on a regular basis initially at home.
- It must be emphasized that of all precautions peristomal skin care is the most important aspect.

What are the complications of stomas?

Till date there are conflicting data regarding whether ileostomy is more often associated with complications than a colostomy. In one of the large series on complications of stoma, highest incidence of complications was seen with the loop ileostomy configuration while lowest complication rate was associated with an end transverse colostomy. A large proportion of early complications (occurring within a month were seen with a descending end colostomy). These included peristomal skin irritation, poor stomal location and accessibility. The pathology for which stoma has been created may be a more important factor influencing the outcome and complication rate rather than the type of stoma. Specific complications differ between different types of stoma. Complications like soiling, skin excoriation and leakage are common with ileal stoma and can be attributed to the nature of the effluent.

What are the early complications of different Stomas and Management?

The most common early complications of stoma include peristomal skin irritation, infection, abscess and fistula formation, acute herniation, improper positioning of the stoma, vascular compromise or ischemia, stoma retraction, and early bowel obstruction.

Poor Stoma Site Selection

Poor site selection during surgery is a forbearer of many complications. A stoma at the wrong place makes it inaccessible and poorly compliant with stoma appliances. This leads to a vicious circle of more leaks and more complications. Pouch leakage and peristomal irritation aggravate each other. Costs to the patient are vastly increased apart from a poor quality of life and impairment of self-care.

Infection/Fistula

Stoma may be complicated by peristomal abscess, infected hematoma and fistula formation early in the course of illness and requires timely initiation of antibiotics. Stoma in hair bearing areas may lead to folliculitis. Abscess formation warrants incision and drainage failing which a fistula may form. Later in the course, fistula formation or infection could signify recurrent Crohn's disease. Pyoderma gangrenosum is diagnosed mainly by physical exam (80%) and has the typical "cookie cutter" appearance. Treatment includes systemic therapy, wound debridement and occasionally steroid injections. Fungal infections are also common in the peristomal areas especially in diabetic and immunocompromised patients and managed with topical and occasionally systemic antifungals.

Stoma Ischemia or Necrosis

Stoma necrosis and ischemia is the most serious early postoperative complication. Ischemia ranges from harmless mucosal sloughing to blackening and frank necrosis and identification is crucial for further management. The proximal portion may then retract and complicate the situation. It is usually the result of aggressive stripping of mesentery, or stenotic fascia defect and occasionally extensive tension. It is important to assess the color of the stoma during examination. A health red stoma is the desired finding but it may occasionally be dusky and congested. It is common to have dusky complexion of a freshly constructed stoma. It is a direct result of vigorous handling of the intestinal segment. A darker brown or black color signifies ischemia and the stoma may have to be refashioned on an emergency basis lest the fecal contents may spill intraperitoneally and lead to infection.

Peristomal Skin Irritation

Peristomal skin irritation is common with acidic effluent from the ileostomy. It is less common with colostomy. Skin irritation is often bothersome and the major reason behind poorly fitting stoma appliances. It may range from mild erythema to severe inflammation causing destruction of surrounding skin and necrotizing fasciitis. Occasionally, stomal granulomas and peristomal warts may also develop as a result of metaplastic change.

Pseudoobstruction

Pseudoobstruction involves the large bowel and is also known as Ogilvie syndrome. It is an idiopathic condition that may arise from mechanical handling of bowel and rarely complicates the early postoperative period. It usually occurs within the first 3 days following surgery and affects patients with multiple comorbidities. It presents as abdominal pain in presence of radiographically dilated colon. Decompression in the form of cecostomy or endoscopic decompression is indicated if colonic diameter increases to more than 12–15 cm.

Metabolic Complications

Metabolic complications are more common with urostomy and electrolyte imbalances vary based on type of intestinal segment employed for the reconstruction, the area of bowel exposed to urine and the duration for which urine stays in contact with bowel. Table 33.1 summarizes these complications in brief.

Stomal Diarrhea and Constipation

Diarrhea and constipation are frequent complications which arise as a result of infection or functional causes. It may be related to diet, hygiene and food habits. Often the patient gains insight to what foods suit the stoma and alters diet based on personal experience, at other times support is needed in the form of fluid replacement and antibiotics when diarrhea leads to severe fluid deficit. Mild losses can be managed with intake of

Table 33.1: Metabolic complications of intestinal stoma		
Symptoms	Complications	Segment of bowel used
Weakness and lethargy, respiratory distress, seizures	Metabolic alkalosis, hypochloremia, hypokalemia	Stomach
Nausea, vomiting, dehydration	Hyperkalemia, hypochloremia, acidosis	Jejunum
Weakness, fatigue and lethargy	Hyperchloremia, hypocalcemia acidosis	Ileum
Weakness, fatigue, anorexia and lethargy	Hyperchloremia, hypokalemia metabolic acidosis	Colon

balanced salt solutions and probiotics. At each presentation with diarrhea, hand hygiene should be reemphasized. Constipation is managed by sticking to a high fibre diet and increasing the intake of fluids. Laxatives and suppositories can be used in severe cases. Refractory constipation should be investigated with contrast studies to rule out anatomical obstruction.

What are the late complications of different Stomas and Management?

Retraction

Retraction of the stoma may occur due to excessive traction on the mesentery and inadequate bowel mobilization. Incidence rates are 1–6% for colostomy and 3–17% for ileostomy. Obesity (high body mass index has been directly correlated with its incidence; steroid use and poor wound healing are common risk factors for retraction. It is the most common reason for reoperation and if not managed timely, it can lead to leakage and severe skin problems. Use of a convex stoma plate and protective barrier helps while patient waits for revision surgery.

Prolapse

Stomal prolapse is another important complication that can present both in the late and early phase. Its incidence has been estimated to be 2–26%. Prolapse is commonly seen in transverse loop colostomy (30%) and is often associated with parastomal hernia. It is managed by reduction and supportive care until definitive surgery can be performed. Loop colostomy can be converted to end colostomy if needed to prevent recurrent prolapse.

Bowel Obstruction

Bowel obstruction develops in 4.6–13% of patients in the early postoperative period. Late occurrence of bowel obstruction is associated with parastomal herniation but is rarer in mature stomas. Early obstruction is due to fibrinous adhesions and warrants conservative therapy unless there are clear signs to proceed with surgery. Late bowel obstruction is common in patients with large fascial defects and managed with hernia repair and meshplasty. Fibrous adhesions, internal herniations and bands can also lead to bowel obstruction in the late period. These respond poorly to conservative therapy and often require adhesiolysis.

Parastomal Hernia

As per J Byron Gathright, (1996) "It doesn't matter if God Himself made your ostomy. If you have it long enough, you have a 100% risk of a parastomal hernia". In most series parastomal herniation has been recognized as the most common late complication. Predisposing factors include stoma placement lateral to rectus making a large stoma aperture, obesity, prior abdominal incisions, malnutrition, and wound infection. Minor cases are managed with abdominal binder while symptomatic patients or those presenting with obstruction due to irreducible hernia require hernia repair with mesh.

Subcutaneous Prolapse (Pseudohernia)

Subcutaneous prolapse is a rarely diagnosed complication associated with stoma. It differs from parastomal hernias in that peritoneum does not protrude out. It is analogous to a sliding hernia and the loop of bowel moves out and coils within the subcutaneous tissue. It can lead to symptoms of local discomfort, abdominal distension and cramps and requires high degree of suspicion to diagnose. Management is on similar lines as a parastomal hernia where in the bowel is fixed to the fascia after reducing excess loop into the abdomen.

Stomal Stenosis and Stricture

Stomal stenosis is another rarer complication of ostomy with incidence ranging between 2% and 14%. It is associated with ischemia, infection and retraction. An important aspect of management of stomal stenosis is to rule out recurrent malignancy and Crohn's disease. Surgery involves enlarging the skin incision using a double Z-plasty. Dilatation is associated with recurrence and mucosal injury.

Peristomal Varices or Stomal Bleeding

Bleeding through the stoma may represent bleeding anywhere along with the proximal gut and should be managed aggressively with resuscitation and identification of the cause. At first local causes like varices, mucosal injury, granulomatous lesions and trauma should be ruled out and gentle compression applied if any of these is found. If no local cause is found, endoscopy and further imaging is warranted. Varices around the stoma arise as a late complication taking about 20–36 months to develop. Bleed peristomal varices may be indicators of portal hypertension and must be managed in the same way.

Diversion Colitis

Diversion colitis affects up to 90% patients in varying intensity. The most common complaint is bleeding from rectum often accompanied by mucus discharge. Additional symptoms like tenesmus and abdominal pain may also be present. Colitis is the result of short-chain fatty acid deficiency which is provided to the colon normally by bacterial breakdown of dietary carbohydrates. Endoscopically, the mucosa appears very similar to that seen in inflammatory bowel disease, with an erythematous granular inflamed look. It can be managed by administration of short-chain fatty acids as an enema twice daily for 2–4 weeks.

Late complications unique to urinary diversion: Ureterointestinal obstruction, urine leak, renal calculi, pouch calculi, osteomalacia, pyelonephritis and renal deterioration are some of the late complications unique to intestinal urinary diversion. They are prevented and managed by regular screening of upper tracts and laboratory investigations as advised later in this chapter.

Describe the salient features which should be observed during care of stoma.

Stoma care should include introduction with a stoma care nurse. Patient should be well aware of the complications of the stoma and danger signs for which one should report to the hospital. Skin care is the most important issue which must be emphasized upon. Timely change of stoma appliance, regular cleaning and application of moisturizer and barrier creams, application of only medically permitted adhesives, regular emptying of the bag when half full, keeping stoma site free of hair, early recognition and management of minor complications, participation in stoma support groups, regular visits by a stoma care nurse and follow-up with the treating surgeon are the basic principles of stoma care. It is important to choose correct size of stoma and patient must be aware that the size of stoma may keep on changing. Preventing stoma leakage is of prime concern to prevent subsequent complications related to stomas. Some patients may have a phantom rectum phenomenon where the patient may experience painful rectal sensation even amounting to tenesmus. It is wise to make the patient aware of these complications before surgery after establishing a good repo.

What are the necessary investigations in a Patient with Stoma?

Investigations in a patient with stoma are directed at assessing the nutritional status and electrolyte balance. Megalosblastic anemia may arise as a result of reduced absorption of vitamin B_{12}. Hence basic laboratory investigations are relevant to all patients with stoma. Additional investigations can guide the treating physician regarding the present status of the primary pathology. Deciphering the stage of disease is essential in guiding the definite closure. Many pathologies like inflammatory bowel disease and long-standing inflammatory suppurative and granulomatous diseases should be in the phase of remission before a temporary stoma can be closed and bowel continuity restored. Anatomical imaging to verify the integrity of bowel segments is also needed. A water soluble contrast study is performed to delineate the proximal loop and an enema or loopogram (contrast instilled through the distal loop of bowel) and ascertain the integrity of the distal bowel. Once these studies have been performed and pre-anesthetic checkup is clear one can proceed with surgery.

What are the usual discharge instructions for Patients with Stoma?

Dietary recommendations for patients with stoma include a well-balanced healthy diet with large amounts of water. Many patients prefer small and frequent meals.

Dried fruits, corn, sprouted beans, mushrooms, foods with seeds and excessive raw fruits and vegetables may cause obstruction. Foods like asparagus, cabbage, eggs, fish, onions, dried beans, and beer cause a foul odour and are often avoided by patients. In an event of constipation fruit juices, baked beans and occasionaly spiced foods may cause diarrhea. Bananas, gram, cheese, rice and pastas may thicken stools and help in management of functional diarrhea.

Stoma pouch should not be allowed to fill more than one-third of its capacity. Frequent emptying can prolong the life of the appliance. A two piece system should be regularly cleaned by washing while a one piece system must be irrigated on a regular basis. A bag may last for up to a week after which replacing the bag is recommended.

In the presence of a sigmoid colostomy, the patient may develop a regular schedule of bowel cleaning and it may be possible to irrigate.

The surrounding skin if hairy must be shaved before applying the stoma bag.

Vascular System

Section 6

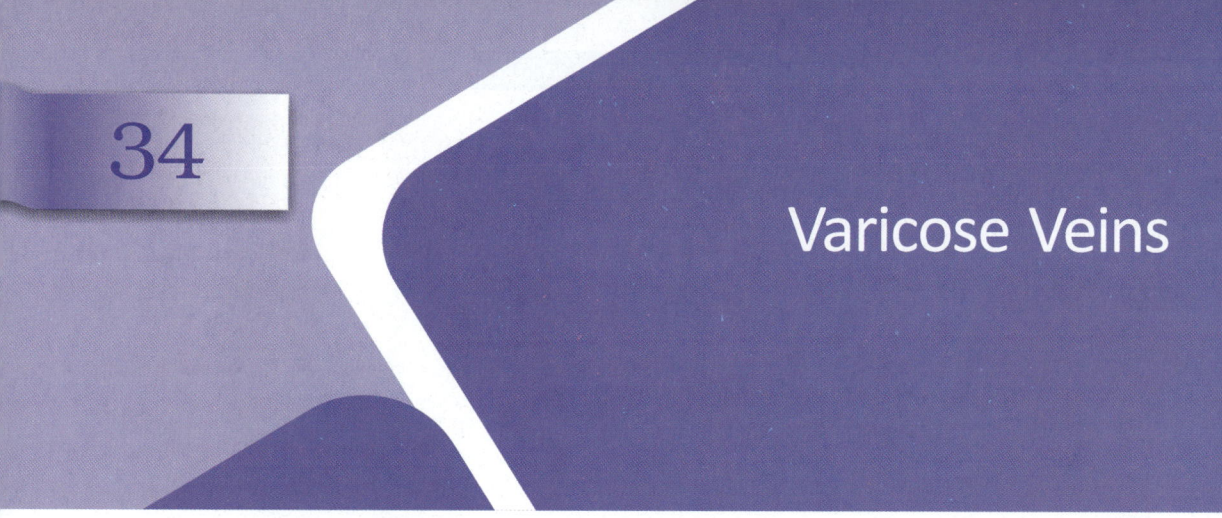

34

Varicose Veins

Describe the anatomy of lower limb veins.

Lower limb veins comprise of:

1. Deep system of veins which lies below the deep fascia.
2. Superficial system of veins which lies outside the deep fascia (carry 10% blood).
3. Perforating veins which pass through the deep fascia joining the superficial to the deep system of veins.

Course of long saphenous vein:

- Originates at the medial border of the foot.
- It passes 1–1.5 inches anterior to the medial malleolus over the distal one-third of the tibia and then alongwith the medial margin of the tibia up to the knee joint.
- It is accompanied by the saphenous nerve below the knee joint.
- At the knee joints it lies 10 cm posterior to the patella.
- Travels close to the deep fascia except at the knee joint where it may become subcuticular.
- In the thigh, it passes anterosuperiorly to reach the saphenous opening which is 3.75 cm below and lateral to the pubic tubercle.

Describe the location of perforators.

Six perforators joining the superficial to deep venous system are located at constant positions which are:

- 2, 4 and 6 inches above the medial malleolus
- Just below the tibial tubercle
- In the adductor (Hunter's) canal of the thigh
- Level of mid-thigh

Course of short saphenous vein:

- Arises on the lateral border of the foot by joining of lateral marginal vein and lateral deep venous arch.
- Passes behind the lateral malleolus
- Runs up in the midline posteriorly in the intra-fascial compartment.
- Pierces the deep fascia in the upper part of the calf, and terminates in the popliteal vein in the midline 4 cm below the popliteal skin crease.
- It is accompanied by the sural nerve, lymphatics and popliteal nerve alongwith its course.
- Derived anatomically from the posterior axial vein of the lower limb.

What factors help in venous return from the lower limb towards heart?

- Negative pressure in the thorax during inspiration of –2 to –6 mm Hg which is transmitted to the great veins.
- Contraction of lower limb muscles compresses the vein and acts as a muscle pump. Normal venous pressure in relaxing phase is 20 mmHg and rises to 80–100 mmHg on muscle contraction.
- Vis a Tergo is produced by arterial pressure which is transmitted to the venous side through the capillary bed.
- Competent valves
- Venae commitantes which lie by the side of the artery are helped by arterial pulsation to propel blood.

Define varicose veins.

The varicose veins are defined as the superficial veins which have permanently lost their valvular mechanism due to resultant venous hypertension and in standing position become dilated, tortuous and thickened.

What are functions of valves in veins?

- Valves prevent the reflux of venous blood from distal to proximal and from deep to superficial venous system.
- They are generally absent above the level of the groin.
- Valves can resist pressure of up to 300 mmHg.

Pathology of varicose veins:
Varicose veins can be primary or secondary:

Secondary	Primary
• Deep vein thrombosis	• Long hours of standing which increase hydrostatic pressure of gravity
• Arteriovenous malformation, e.g. Park-Weber syndrome	• Family history
• Hemangiomatous malformation, e.g. Kippel-Trénaunay syndrome	• Pregnancy
• Pelvic mass or retroperitoneal fibrosis	• Ageing

Clinical presentation:
- Classically described as more common in females compared to males in Western countries, but in India, it is more in males.
- Left limb is more commonly involved than right
- Long saphenous system is affected in two-thirds of the cases.

Points to be taken in history:
- Most common presenting features are:
  1. Dilated and visible veins in lower limb (Fig. 34.1)
  2. The nonhealing ulcer around ankle along with discolouration and thickening of skin (Fig. 34.2)
  3. Pain in the legs
- Associated symptoms, e.g. calf muscle cramps at night, swelling of legs and ankles increasing at the end of the day and resolving or decreasing the next morning
- Bleeding from the dilated veins

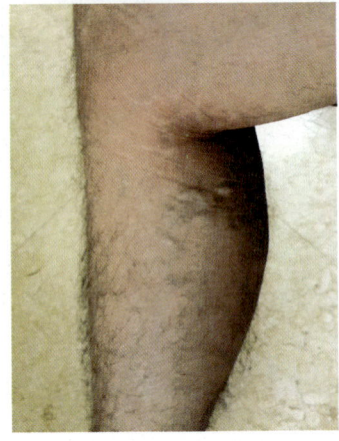

Fig. 34.1: Clinical picture showing dilated and visible veins

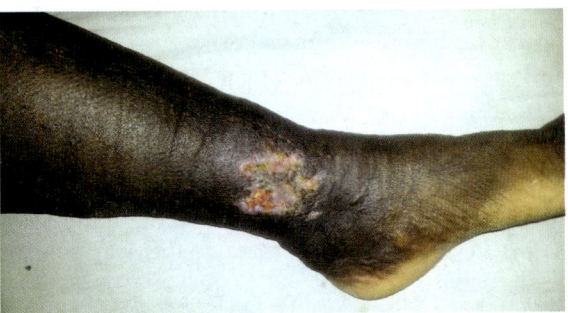

Fig. 34.2: Clinical picture showing incompetent perforator causing varicose veins

- Pain alongwith the dilated veins
- In case of nonhealing wound one must exclude peripheral vascular disease (ask about intermittent claudication, rest pain, previous or present gangrene, smoking)
- History of colour change of skin and itching of lower limb around ankle
- Changes in gait (talipes equines may develop in nonhealing ulcer as the patient preferentially walks on the toes)
- History of pain and redness over the dilated veins may be suggestive of superficial thrombophlebitis
- Any history suggestive of deep vein thrombosis such as acute onset swelling of thigh and calf, pain or any risk factor for the same. Especially in postpartum period in female patients.
- *Occupation* should be mentioned (especially, if the job involves long hours of standing or strenuous exercise, e.g. barbers, conductors, athletes)
- *Family history*: Important in case of congenital conditions such as Klippel-Trénaunay and

Park-Weber syndrome. Suspect if cutaneous hemangiomas or pulsatile veins (arterialization of veins) are present.

- If limb lengthening is present, it suggests associated congenital arteriovenous (AV) malformation.
- The history of trauma to the thigh especially penetrating type suggests traumatic AV fistula formation.
- *Past history*: History of previous varicosities or any intervention for the same.

What are the complications of varicose veins?

- Bleeding
- Thrombophlebitis
- Venous hypertension leading to venous ulcer
- Calcification
- Talipes equinovarus deformity of foot
- Eczematoid dermatitis and pigmentation
- Periostitis of subcutaneous surface of tibia
- Carcinoma in long-standing venous ulcer.

Scheme of examination for varicose veins:
- Finding the system involved
- Extent of involvement
- Skin changes or ulcer around malleolus
- Trendelenburg test for patency of sapheno-femoral junction (SFJ)
- Perthe's test for patency of deep veins

Local Examination

Inspection:
- To be done in standing position
- Describe the location and extent of visible dilated veins present (on the medial or lateral or posterior side) and describe the affected system, i.e. the long saphenous, short saphenous systems or both.
- Any visible swellings or visible cough impulse in the groin (saphena varix).
- Reticular veins or telangiectasias: Reticular veins are subdermal veins up to 5 mm diameter. Telangiectasias are intradermal veins up to 3 mm in diameter.
  - Describe in detail ulcers if any:
    - Scar marks or discoloration

Palpation:
- Elongated, tortuous and palpable veins which are nontender, nonpulsatile or pulsatile. Pulsatile veins suggest AV malformation
- Thickening of skin

- Calf tenderness
- Palpable cough impulse in the groin
- Arterial pulsations
- Measurement of limb length
- *Tourniquet tests*: To rule out SFJ incompetence, perforators in the thigh and deep venous thrombosis (DVT)
- Perform the Fegan's test prior to the tourniquet tests to get an idea about the location of possible perforators.

How to perform Brodie-Trendelenburg test?

- Patient is recumbent
- Raise the legs to empty the veins
- Occlude SFJ by tourniquet or thumb pressure approx 3.75 cm below and lateral to pubic tubercle
- Ask the patient to stand

Three possibilities:
- *Normal/negative test*: Veins fill gradually by capillary inflow over 45–60 seconds.
- *Immediate filling of veins despite sustained pressure*: Denotes perforator incompetence. If the pressure is removed subsequently and the veins become more distended, there is possible SFJ incompetence.
- *Rapid filling after removal of thumb*: SFJ incompetence.

What is three tourniquets test and how is it performed?

For mid-thigh and adductor canal perforators:
- Patient is recumbent
- Raise the legs and empty the veins
- Three tourniquets are tied at the SFJ, just below the mid-thigh and just above the knee
- Ask the patient to stand

Three possibilities:
- *Filling of leg veins*: Implies that the leg perforators are incompetent
- *Lowermost tourniquet opened*: If the segment fills, the adductor canal perforator is incompetent
- *Mid-thigh tourniquet opened*: If the segment fills, the mid-thigh perforator is incompetent
- *Multiple tourniquet test*: It is usually not done as it is quite cumbersome and difficult to perform due to the variable position of the perforators

Modified Perthes' test:
- Patient remains standing

- Tourniquet is tied around the mid-thigh tight enough to occlude the superficial veins (ideally a blood pressure cuff with a width which is two-thirds the circumference of the limb should be used).
- Patient is asked to jump on tiptoes 30 times
- If patient complains of a bursting pain in the calf and there is visible dilatation of the veins, obstruction of the deep venous system is suspected.

(Perthes' test was originally described by the German surgeon, George Perthes. It is also known as the Delbet-Mocquot test. It was modified by Ochsner and Mahorner.)

- **Schwartz test:** It is a palpatory confirmation of valvular incompetence
- One finger is placed over the vein at the maximally dilated point
- Tap with a finger distally
- Feel for a thrill with the proximally placed finger
- Now, reverse the action, tap proximally and feel distally

(The test is positive only when the thrill is felt bidirectionally or from above downwards)

- **Morrissey test:** Indicates incompetent veins between the right atrium and the leg veins and is positive in severe incompetence of the SFJ.
- Patient is recumbent.
- Raise the legs till the varicose veins are empty
- Patient is asked to cough and saphenous opening is watched for an impulse.
- *Auscultation:* Check for any bruit to rule out arterialization.

How to state the diagnosis?

Varicose veins <state the system: GSV/SSV/Both> with Chronic venous insufficiency <state the class according to CEAP classification>

CEAP classification: Classification of chronic lower extremity venous disease

Clinical (C) classification (C 0 to 6)

- Class 0: No visible or palpable signs of venous disease
- Class 1: Telangiectasia or reticular veins
- Class 2: Varicose veins
- Class 3: Edema without skin changes
- Class 4: Skin changes ascribed to venous disease (pigmentation or eczema or lipodermatosclerosis)

- Class 5: Skin changes (i.e. class 4) with *healed ulceration*
- Class 6: Skin changes (i.e. class 4) with *active ulceration*
- *Subcategories:*
  - **A**symptomatic ("a")
  - **S**ymptomatic ("s") (if associated with lower extremity aching or pain or skin irritation).

Etiologic (E) classification

- Congenital E_E
- Primary E_P
- Secondary E_s

Anatomic (A) classification: Segmental classification of CLEVD

- Superficial venous system A_S
- Deep veins A_D
- Perforators A_P

Pathophysiologic (P) classification

- Reflux P_R
- Obstruction P_O
- Reflux and obstruction $P_{R,O}$

What are the investigations needed in a case of varicose veins?

Colour Doppler study of venous system is done:
1. To ensure patency of deep veins
2. To define the site of incompetent perforators.
3. To determine the competency of saphenofemoral junction (SFJ) and saphenopopliteal junction (SPJ).
4. To measure the ankle brachial index (ABI) so that concomitant arterial disease can be ruled out. Normal ABI is equal to more than 1.
5. SFJ or SPJ and incompetent perforators can be marked before surgery.

How are varicose veins managed?

Management can be:
- Conservative
- Sclerotherapy
- Operative management.

Conservative management:

Contraindications	Indications
• Arterial insufficiency	• Refusal for surgery
	• Capillary veins, venous stars (C1)
	• Pregnant patients
	• Waiting for surgery
	• Early cases

Conservative management includes:
- Avoiding prolonged standing.
- Crepe bandaging and elastic stockings from toe to thigh, which decreases edema, venous volume and reflux and increases venous return.
- Limb elevation above the level of heart while lying down.

Sclerotherapy:
- Injection sclerotherapy was first tried by Pravaz in 1851 when he first injected it into an aneurysm.
- In 1853, Chassaignac introduced sclerotherapy in varicose veins.
- Tavel of Berne combined ligation of veins with injection sclerotherapy with carbolic acid 5%.
- Sicard introduced less toxic sclerosant sodium salicylate injection for sclerotherapy in 1922.

Contraindications	Indications
• Deep venous thrombosis	• Varicosity confined below knee and caused by incompetent perforators
• Saphenofemoral incompetence	• Recurrent or residual varicosities postsurgery
• Veins in lower one-third of leg	• Large venous telangiectasia
• Veins on the foot	• Dilated branch veins around the knee following early long saphenous incompetence
• Veins in elderly	
• Veins in fat legs	
• Immobile patient	
• Postthrombotic syndrome	• Refusal for surgery
• Dirty ulcer or extensive eczema	

Method of compression sclerotherapy:
- Patient is made to recline.
- Vein is filled enough for needle to enter by stroking it down towards the needle.
- 0.5 mL of sclerosant is injected slowly into the vein.
- Injection is retained in the short segment of vein by compression by fingers above and below the site for a minute.
- Local compression is applied.
- Patient is asked to immediately walk around.
- Compression is removed after 1 week.

Commonly used agents for injection sclerotherapy are:
- Monoethanolamine 5% with benzyl alcohol 2%
- Sodium tetradecyl sulphate 3% in benzyl alcohol 2%
- Glycerine 25% with phenol 2%

Complications:
- Failure of sclerosis
- Extravenous injection
- Deep vein thrombosis
- Hypersensitivity
- Skin pigmentation
- Gangrene of distal limb.

Ultrasound-Guided Foam Sclerotherapy

This is an alternative to blind sclerotherapy and can be used to treat the main saphenous trunk. A needle is inserted in the vein to be treated under duplex ultrasound guidance and sclerosant is made into foam by air mixing technique using three way tap. Polidocanol is used rather than sodium tetradecyl sulphate. Foam is monitored under ultrasound scanning as it spreads in the vein. Apex of the saphenous opening is compressed by ultrasound probe to prevent the foam entering the deep veins. The leg is also elevated to prevent foam entering the axial deep veins. These techniques can take care of both long saphenous and short saphenous venous system. Up to three sittings may be required to completely obliterate the veins. Extravasation of sclerosing agent in subcutaneous tissue should be avoided as it can lead to cutaneous ulceration. The escape of sclerosing agent in deep veins can lead to deep vein thrombosis. Recurrence rates at present are not known.

Surgery:
- History of attempts at surgery dates back to nearly 2000 years
- In 1891, Trendelenburg advised ligating long saphenous trunk above the large varices in the thigh.
- In 1921, GH Cole of Aberdeen described saphenectomy and high ligation.
- Stripping was reestablished by Linton in 1949.
- In 1954, the flexible stripper was invented by T. Myers.

Contraindications	Indications
• Absence of deep venous system	• Saphenofemoral incompetence with varicosities extending up to the thigh
• Pregnancy	• Chronic venous insufficiency with class 4, 6 or failed conservative management in class 2
• Patient taking oral contraceptives	
• Thrombophlebitis	

Types of surgeries done:
- Flush ligation of SFJ with ligation of all tributaries ending at SFJ.
- Stripping of long saphenous up to the knee joint.
- Flush ligation of short saphenous vein.
- Subfascial ligation of perforators.

Flush ligation of long saphenous vein:
- Patient lies supine with the table tilted head down to an angle of 15°.
- Curved or hockey stick incision is made with the outer half lying in the gutter of the groin and inner half curving towards the thigh.
- Alternatively an oblique incision can also be made parallel to the fold of the groin about 7–8 cm long.
- Incision is carried deeper till the superficial fascia is seen which is then incised.
- Gauze is used to separate the fat and exposes the SFJ.
- Saphena magna is dissected gently using a Mayos tissue cutting scissors.
- Femoral vein is exposed 1 cm above and below the SFJ.
- The six significant veins joining the termination of saphenous vein are defined and ligated.
- The end of the long saphenous vein is ligated with silk and a second ligature is transfixed to avoid haemorrhage. Femoral vein is inspected above and below the junction and long saphenous divided.
- Incision is closed in layers. Biopsy of nodes can be taken if enlarged.

Stripping of long saphenous vein:
- Saphenous vein is exposed and flush ligated as above.
- Small tip is passed into the vein at the groin gently.
- A vertical incision is made just below knee and vein exposed.
- The stripper is extruded from the vein and the acorn firmly tied in the vein.
- The stripper is firmly withdrawn with the vein telescoped over it.
- The track is compressed with a large sterile pad for 3–5 minutes.
- Incision is closed in layers and bandage applied for 7 days.

Flush ligation of the short saphenous vein:
- The patient is made to face down and knee flexed by placing a sandbag.
- Preoperatively junction of short saphenous vein and popliteal vein should be marked as the position of junction is highly variable.
- A 5 cm long transverse incision is made at the level of the knee joint and developed in layers.
- Deep fascia is identified and incised in the line of skin incision.
- Short saphenous vein is located between the two heads of gastrocnemius.
- The vein is lifted by artery forceps and knee flexed further.
- Dissection is done with a gauze swab up to the saphenopopliteal junction.
- All branches are identified and ligated.
- Short saphenous is ligated close to the popliteal vein.
- Incision is closed in layers and compression applied.

Complications of surgery:

Intraoperative complications:
- Hemorrhage from torn varix
- Division or injury to the common femoral vein
- Sural nerve or saphenous nerve injury.

Postoperative complications:
- Haematoma and bruising
- Wound infection
- Neuritis
- Lymphoedema
- Induration of stripper track
- Lymphatoma
- Deep venous thrombosis.

Postoperative care:
- Maintain firm pressure over the limb
- Regular movement of the operated limb
- Limb elevation above heart level to reduce venous pressure
- Removal of primary dressing after 7–10 days

Subfascial endoscopic perforator vein surgery (Fig. 34.3):

Contraindications	Complications
• Secondary varicose veins	• Chronic venous insufficiency (C3,4,5)
• Arterial insufficiency	
• Deep vein thrombosis	

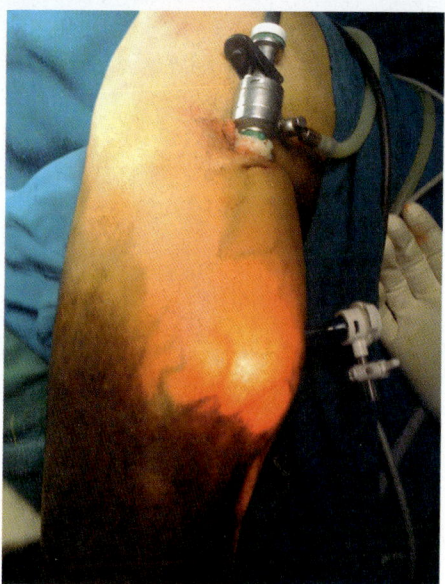

Fig. 34.3: Port placement in SEPS

Operating steps:
- Ten millimeter port is introduced beneath deep fascia 8–10 cm below tibial plateau 2 cm medial to anterior border of tibia. This port is used as camera port and for insufflations of carbon dioxide gas. Zero degree 10 mm telescope is used.
- Pressure is increased up to 30 mmHg. Second 5 mm port is introduced 6–8 cm posterior and inferior to the first port and used as the working port.
- Space is dissected using dissector and perforating veins encountered are clipped and cut. Alternatively electrocautery and ultrasonic shears can also be applied for ligation.

- The incompetent perforators are identified, transected and coagulated under direct vision.
- All venous channels crossing subfascial space from anterior border of tibia till posterior midline and inferiorly till medial malleolus are ligated.
- At the end of the procedure, incompetent SFJ and SPJ are managed accordingly in the same setting.
- Skin incisions are closed with 3–0 nylon sutures.

Radiofrequency closure: The intima of smaller veins can be destroyed by heat generation and denaturation of collagen using a probe consisting of a bipolar heat generator. The procedure is performed under ultrasound guidance and position of the probe is confirmed near the SFJ. With the help of a feedback system, temperature in the range of 80–85°C is attained. The heated probe is gradually retracted down at a constant rate of 2–3 cm/minute. Patient is sedated and local anaesthesia instilled along with the vein. Radiofrequency closure is suitable for smaller and straighter veins. It must be avoided in presence of dilated veins, veins with aneurysms and thrombosed veins.

Endovenous laser therapy (EVLT): It is similar to radiofrequency closure except that it is a painless procedure and employs diode laser for the destruction of endothelial lining of the target vein. The ultrasound guides the location of probe which is placed 2 cm distal to the SFJ. The probe is gradually withdrawn and ablates the lumen as it regresses down the vein by boiling the blood present within the lumen. Another added advantage of the procedure lies in the fact that veins of all sizes can be treated with this procedure.

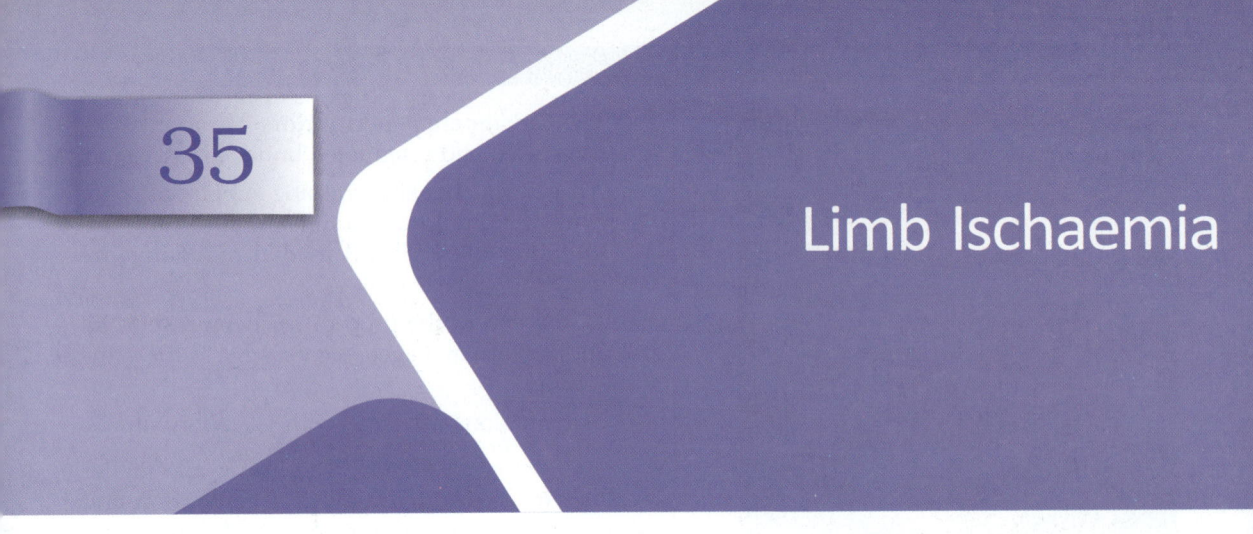

35
Limb Ischaemia

What is the incidence of lower limb ischaemia?

Chronic lower limb ischaemia due to occlusive peripheral arterial disease (PAD) is a common clinical problem. It is said to afflict 10% of western population above 70 years of age. Limb ischaemia cases accounts for 0.9% of all hospital admissions in Indian population.

- Occurs in approximately one-third of patients:
  - Over age 70 years
  - Over age 50 years who smoke or have diabetes mellitus (DM)
- Strong association with coronary artery disease and cerebral vascular disease:
  - Obvious associated risk of stroke, myocardial infarction (MI), cardiovascular death
- Progressive disease in 25% with progressive intermittent claudication/limb threatening ischaemia
- Outcomes:
  - Impaired quality of life
  - Limb loss
  - Premature mortality.

What are risk factors for peripheral vascular disease (PVD)?

Framingham heart study showed:
- Data from the Framingham heart study revealed that the odds ratio for developing intermittent claudication was:
  - 2.6 for DM
  - 1.2 for each 40 mg/dL (1 mmol/L) elevation in the serum cholesterol concentration
  - 1.4 for each 10 cigarettes smoked per day
  - 1.5 for mild and 2.2 for moderate hypertension
  - In addition, diabetic patients had worse arterial disease and a poorer outcome than nondiabetics.

What is the relative risk of developing PVD in smokers?

- Relative risk of PVD in smokers
  - Relative risk (RR) of smoking:
    - Never smoked 1
    - Former smoker 7
    - Current smoker 16.

What is the effect of diabetes on PVD?

- Increased risk of claudication; in men 3.5 times and in women 8.5 times
- Rate of amputation is 7–10 more in the presence of diabetes in PVD.

What is the association between hyperlipidemia and PAD?

- Fifty percent of patients with lower extremity PAD have dyslipidemia
- Increased cholesterol has 2 times more risk of PAD

Increased triglyceride has 1.7 times more risk of PAD
- Best predictor of PAD is high ratio of total cholesterol and high-density lipoprotein (HDL)

Other serum markers for PAD:
- *Fibrinogen*: Edinborough and Rotterdam population studies showed elevated fibrinogen is a predictor of PAD.

- *C reactive protein*: It is a marker for inflammatory state associated with PAD, but no causal connection demonstrated.

Describe the plan of workup of a case of chronic ischaemic limb.

1. Establish that lower limb ischaemia is present
2. Assess the severity of the condition
3. Determine the level of the occlusion or stenosis
4. Find out the possible aetiology.
5. Determine any comorbid conditions from which patient suffer.
6. Evaluate the therapeutic options available.
7. Weigh the risk or benefit ratio of planned therapeutic procedure.

How to establish that lower limb ischaemia is present?

Patient present with the following features:

- *Intermittent claudication*: The word claudication is derived from the Latin and French, claudication and claudico, respectively. These Latin and French words are used to describe a lame horse. Claudication means pain or discomfort in the extremity induced by exertion that is exacerbated with further exercise and relieved with rest. As it occurs intermittently, it is known as intermittent claudication. The patient describes this discomfort as cramping, burning, aching or fatigue and can be felt in both lower and upper extremities. This can be reproduced by performing same amount of exertion, activities like walking or lifting weights or brushing teeth's. The location of discomfort is a clue to the site of greatest stenosis. Symptoms generally occur in the most proximal muscle area with inadequate perfusion. The stenosis in the iliac artery will cause claudication in the thigh or buttock. The narrowing in the superficial femoral or popliteal artery will cause claudication in the calf muscles or in the feet. Relief from discomfort with a specific period of rest is a hallmark of claudication. The relief of pain requires a consistent period of rest on each episode of claudication pain. For relief, the patient might have to sit stand or recline. Pain that is relieved immediately upon stopping is not claudication and not related to inadequate perfusion. Pain, that results from specific positional changes, occurs while lying or can be relieved by activity is not a consequence of PAD and may be neuropathic or musculoskeletal in origin.

The intermittent claudication is due to lack of oxygen in muscle tissues as the blood supply cannot keep pace with the demand while walking. The respiration changes to anaerobic respiration one at the affected site with accumulation of metabolites which cause pain (substance P, and lactic acid).

Grading of intermittent claudication is as follows:

Grade I: Pain appears on walking certain distance but disappears as the mismatch between the demand and supply of muscle is minimal and is taken care by local vasodilatation caused by accumulated substance P and lactic acid.

Grade II: Pain appears on walking but patient can manage to walk with pain.

Grade III: Patient is forced to take rest after walking certain distance due to pain.

Grade IV: Rest pain.

- *Rest pain*: This pain is described as severe, continuous and unremitting in the foot which is worse at night ("night pain"). It is said to be the "cry of the dying ischaemic nerves", and signifies advanced ischaemia as the ischaemia is so severe that even the vasa nervosa, the arteries supplying the nerve, get affected. In contrast to intermittent claudication, it is felt in the forefoot or the entire foot. Rest pain occurs when the perfusion pressure during inactivity is inadequate to meet basal requirements. The pain keeps the patient awake at night. Hanging the leg by the side of the bed may relieve pain. This intense pain is not relieved by commonly used analgesics; regular use of narcotic analgesics may lead to addiction. When perfusion pressure drops low enough to cause rest pain, gravity plays an important role in blood supply. Patients will report more pain at night when the leg is elevated and mitigation of pain with leg dependency as occurs when sitting on the edge of the bed.

- *Non-healing ulcer*: Many patients present with nonhealing ulcers over the toes, foot or distal leg following trivial trauma. These ulcers are usually painful, but may be painless especially there is associated neuropathy as in diabetic foot. The ulcer does not show any evidence of healing in the form of granulation tissue or sloping edges (Fig. 35.1).

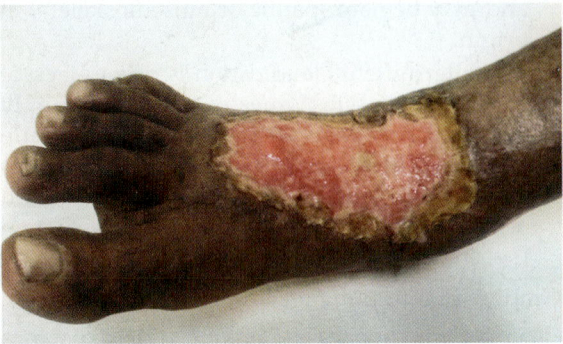

Fig. 35.1: Clinical photograph showing nonhealing ulcer of leg due to ischaemia

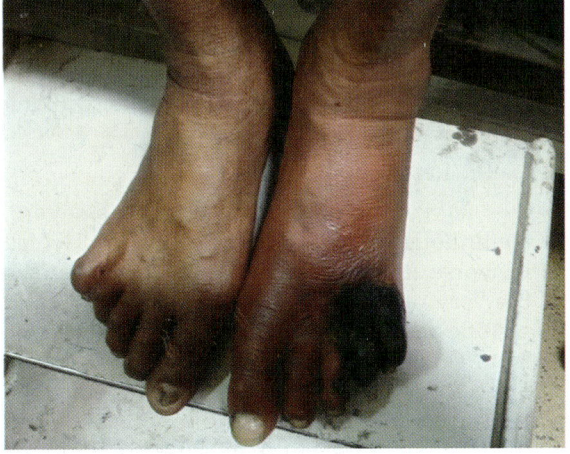

Fig. 35.2: Clinical photograph showing gangrene of toes

- *Gangrene*: The involved area (usually toes or forefoot) becomes black, dry, shriveled and dead with a good line of demarcation. This dry gangrene may be converted to the wet type in the presence of superadded infection (Fig. 35.2).

- *Absent or weak pulses*: All the peripheral pulses should be palpated and compared with opposite side. All the peripheral pulses are palpated against a bony point. The patient should be in a comfortable position to avoid muscle tensing. The examiner should use the fingertips of the hand and avoid the thumb. The thumb pulse may be large enough to transmit sensation cause perception of the patient's false pulse. Palpation should begin lightly and increase in pressure gradually. Pulses may be palpated in the neck, arms, legs and trunk. Subtle changes may be defined by comparing each pulse bilaterally.

- The carotid pulse may be palpated between the trachea and the sternocleidomastoid muscles. Palpation should be performed lightly at first, especially in older patients, for the carotid body may be sensitive and promote bradycardia and hypotension. It is palpated against the carotid tubercle which is the prominent transverse process of 6th cervical vertebrae.

- The subclavian pulse is palpated either in the supraclavicular fossa or between the lateral clavicle and the pectoralis muscle.

- To examine the *brachial artery* in the right arm, the examiner holds the patient's forearm in his left hand with the upper arm abducted, the elbow slightly flexed, and the forearm externally rotated. The examiner's right-hand fingers palpate the artery just medial to the biceps tendon and lateral to the medial epicondyle of the humerus.

- For the *radial artery*, the patient's forearm should be supported in one of the examiner's hands and his other hand used to palpate alongwith the radial volar aspect of the subject's forearm at the wrist. This can best be done by curling the fingers around the distal radius from the dorsal toward the volar aspect with the tips of the first, second, and third fingers aligned longitudinally over the course of the artery.

- The *abdominal aorta* is best palpated by applying firm pressure with the flattened fingers of both hands to indent the epigastrium toward the vertebral column. It is essential that the subject's abdominal muscles be completely relaxed which can be encouraged by having the subject flex the hips and by providing a pillow to support the head. In extremely obese individuals or in those with massive abdominal musculature, it may be impossible to detect aortic pulsation. Auscultation should be performed over the aorta and alongwith both iliac vessels into the lower abdominal quadrants.

- The *common femoral artery* enters into the upper thigh from below the inguinal ligament one-third of the distance from the pubis to the anterior superior iliac spine. It is palpated against head of the femur at a point just below the midinguinal point. For palpation the lower limb of the patient should be abducted and externally rotated so that head of femur comes out. It is best palpated with the examiner standing on the ipsilateral side of the patient and the fingertips of the examining hand pressed firmly into the groin. Auscultation should be performed to hear any bruit (Fig. 35.3).

– *The popliteal artery* travels vertically through the deep portion of the popliteal space just lateral to the midline. It may be difficult or impossible to palpate in obese or very muscular individuals. Generally, this pulse is felt most conveniently with the patient in the supine position and the examiner's hands encircling and supporting the knee from each side. The pulse is detected by pressing deeply into the popliteal space with the supporting fingertips. Since complete relaxation of the muscles is essential to this examination, the patient should be instructed to let the leg "go limp" and to allow the examiner to provide all the support needed. In supine position, it is palpated in the lower half of popliteal fossa over the posterior surface of tibia. In prone position, it is palpated in the upper half of popliteal fossa against posterior aspect of lower end of femur (Figs 35.4 and 35.5).

– The *posterior tibial artery* lies just posterior to the medial malleolus. It is palpated against the calcaneus at a midpoint between achilles tendon and medial malleolus (Fig. 35.6).

– The *dorsalis pedis artery* is examined with the patient in the supine position and the ankle relaxed. The examiner stands at the foot of the examining table and places the fingertips transversely across the dorsum of the fore-foot near the ankle. The artery is palpated lateral to the extensor hallucis tendon in the first metatarsal space against the head of first

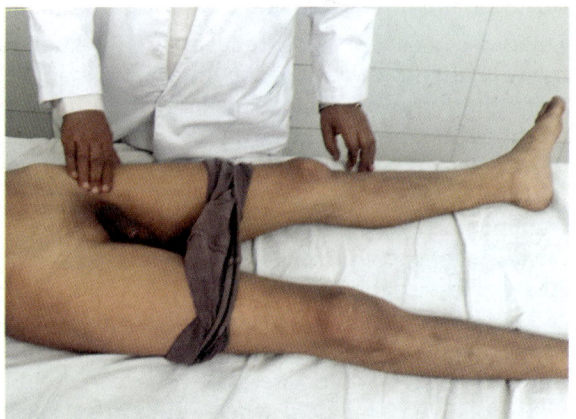

Fig. 35.3: Method of clinical examination of the femoral artery

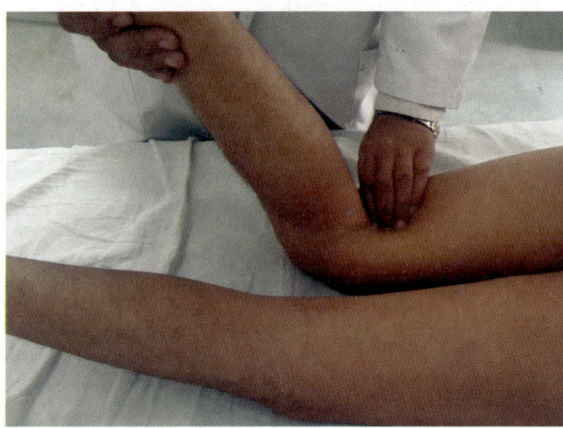

Fig. 35.5: Method of clinical examination of the popliteal artery in prone position

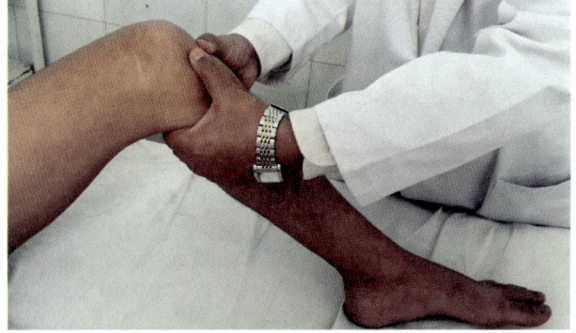

Fig. 35.4: Method of clinical examination of the popliteal artery in supine position

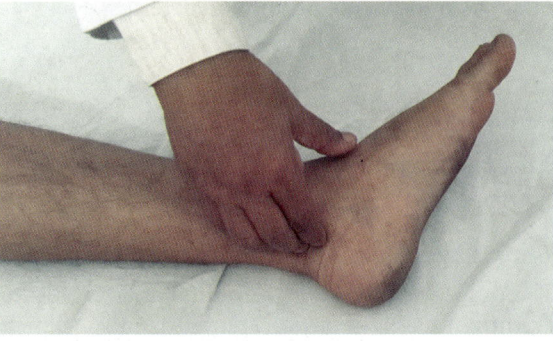

Fig. 35.6: Method of clinical examination of the posterior tibial artery

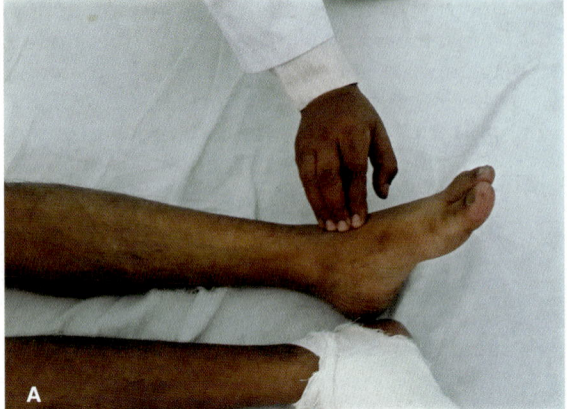

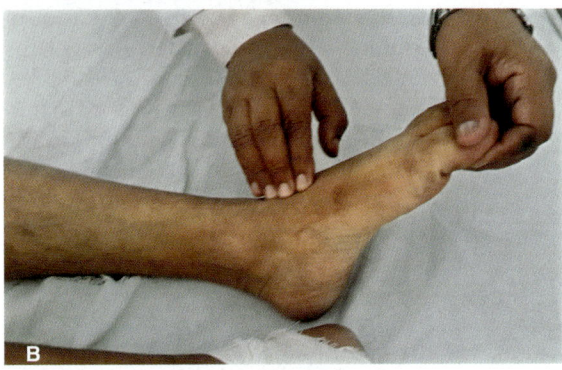

Fig. 35.7A and B: Method of clinical examination of the dorsalis pedis artery

metatarsal. This pulse is congenitally absent in approximately 10–20% of individuals (Fig. 35.7A and B).

What are common causes of reduced or absent pulses?

Reduced or absent arterial pulses are a sign of impaired blood flow. The causes include:

- Congenital abnormalities (coarctation of the aorta, anomalous peripheral arteries)
- Intrinsic arterial disease (atherosclerosis, thrombosis, arteritis)
- Vasospastic disorders (Raynaud's phenomenon)
- Involvement of the vessel by extrinsic compression (thoracic outlet syndrome, trauma, neoplasms).

What is hypokinetic pulse?

The pulse which is of low volume and amplitude is known as *hypokinetic*. This is usually seen in conditions with low cardiac output as in shock or myocardial infarction. Other causes include idiopathic dilated cardiomyopathy, valvular stenosis, pericardial tamponade or constrictive pericarditis.

What is hyperkinetic pulse and in which conditions it is seen?

The large amplitude bounding pulses are known as hyperkinetic pulse.

It can classically occurs in anxiety, exercise, fever, hyperthyroidism, and anemia as in these conditions there is a large left ventricular stroke volume and an otherwise normal cardiovascular system. Hyperkinetic pulses can also occur where there is a rapid peripheral runoff of blood in addition to a large stroke volume from the left ventricle as seen in

- Patent ductus arteriosus with normal pulmonary pressures
- Large arterial venous fistulas
- Severe aortic regurgitation can cause these hyperkinetic pulses.

Describe the pulse of severe aortic regurgitation.

The pulse of severe aortic regurgitation is known as water-hammer and collapsing. Severe aortic regurgitation can also lead feeling of a pulse in the fingernail bed (Quincke's pulse) which is best demonstrated by placing a penlight on the finger pad and seeing casting light through the fingernail from behind. Varying the pressure of the penlight on the finger pad will bring out the Quincke's pulse. A few of these patients have a double systolic pulse called a *bisferiens pulse*. This occurs when some aortic stenosis accompanies the severe aortic regurgitation. These two waves are called the percussion wave followed by a tidal wave—both in systoles. The bisferiens pulse is strongly associated with idiopathic hypertrophic subaortic stenosis.

Describe the nutritional changes in the limb due to ischaemia.

These include:

- Subcutaneous fat loss
- Shiny atrophic skin
- Loss of hair over the affected part
- Transverse ridges over the nail, and interdigital fungal infection
- Pallor of limb on elevation and rubor on dependency is also characteristic (due to loss of vasomotor tone) but may be difficult to detect in dark-skinned people
- Capillary and venous refill time is prolonged.

What is the importance of bruit over the site of narrowing in arteries?

Presence of bruit indicates turbulent flow suggestive of stenosis at a proximal site. Bruits are detected by auscultation over the large and medium-sized arteries (e.g. carotid, brachial, abdominal aorta, femoral) with the diaphragm of the stethoscope using light to moderate pressure. One should listen over the artery after palpation of the artery to avoid overlooking a significant lesion. Frequently the examiner will detect a "thrill" or palpable vibratory sensation over a vessel in which a loud bruit is audible. The thrill is indicative of marked turbulence in local blood flow and suggests significant vascular pathology. If a thrill is noted during examination of the pulses, it should be recorded in the appropriate space on the database.

How is an arterial pulse produced?

The arterial pulse is the abrupt expansion of an artery resulting from the sudden ejection of blood into the aorta and its transmission throughout the arterial system. The impulse that results from left ventricular ejection can be transmitted down the aorta at a velocity 20 times greater than the velocity of the ejected blood bolus. The peak of this arterial pulse is the systolic blood pressure.

What are diagnostic modalities for PAD?

- Ankle brachial index (ABI)
- Noninvasive vascular laboratory
- Angiography: Magnetic resonance angiography (MRA), computed tomography (CT), digital substraction angiography (DSA).

Initial Assessment

- Identifying risk factors and symptoms
- Pulse palpability
- Further assessment relies on functional non-invasive testing and radiological imaging
  - Determine not only the anatomic, but also the physiological aberration of peripheral vascular flow.

Enumerate the PVD Aetiology

- Large arteries
  - Atherosclerosis
  - Thromboembolism
  - Trauma

- Arteritis of various types including
  - Fibromuscular dysplasia
  - Takayasu's disease
- Medium and small vessel occlusions
  - Diabetes
  - Buerger's disease
  - Chronic recurrent trauma
  - Multiple small emboli
  - Collagen vascular diseases
  - Dysproteinemias
  - Polycythemia vera
  - Pseudoxanthoma elasticum
  - Drug reaction
  - Vasospasm
- Specific to certain anatomical sites
  - Cystic adventitial disease of the popliteal artery
  - Popliteal artery entrapment
  - Iliac endofibrosis (seen in cyclists)
- Various neurovascular compression syndromes affecting the upper limb
  - Cervical rib
  - Costoclavicular syndrome
  - Scalenus tunnel syndrome
  - Hyperabduction syndrome
  - Quadrangular space syndrome.

Describe the clinical grading system of chronic ischaemic limb.

Clinical grading systems:
- Fontaine 1954
- Rutherford current.

Fontaine clinical classification:
- Grade 1—Mild claudication
- Grade 2—Severe pain with walking
- Grade 3—Rest pain
- Grade 4—Tissue loss presenter name.

Rutherford classification described in 1997:
- Category 0—Asymptomatic
- Category 1—Mild claudication
- Category 2—Moderate claudication
- Category 3—Severe claudication
- Category 4—Ischaemic rest pain
- Category 5—Minor tissue loss
- Category 6—Major tissue loss presenter name.

What are common features of Lower Limb Ischaemia?

- Intermittent claudication
- Rest pain
- Coldness, numbness, paresthesia, colour changes
- Ulceration or gangrene
- Temperature changes
- Decreased sensation
- Decreased movement or absence of movement
- Pulsation decreased or loss of pulsations
- Bruit
- Venous refilling prolonged.

PVD Differential Diagnosis

- Deep venous thrombosis
- Musculoskeletal disorders
  - Osteoarthritis
  - Restless leg syndrome
- Peripheral neuropathy
- Spinal stenosis (pseudoclaudication)
  - Worse with erect posture (lordosis), better sitting or lying down
  - Can find relief by leaning forward and straightening the spine (pushing a shopping cart or leaning against a wall)

Differential diagnosis of intermittent claudication:

	Neurogenic claudication	*Venous claudication*	*Intermittent claudication*
Quality of pain	Electric shock like	Bursting	Cramping
Onset	Can be immediate, inconsistent	Gradual, can be immediate	Gradual, consistent
Relieved by	Sitting down, bending forward	Elevation of leg	Standing still
Location	Poorly localized, can affect whole leg	Whole leg (buttocks, thigh, calf)	Muscle groups
Legs affected	Often both	Usually one	Usually one

Location of Intermittent Claudication Indicates Site of Obstruction

Buttock or Hip

- Usually indicates aortoiliac occlusive disease (Leriche's syndrome) if bilateral and impotency present.
- Some cases have thigh claudication also.
- Question diagnosis of bilateral disease if erectile dysfunction is not present.

Thigh

- Occlusion of the common femoral artery leads to claudication in the thigh, calf or both.

Calf

- Symptoms in upper two-thirds is usually due to superficial femoral artery.
- Lower one-thirds is due to popliteal disease.

Physical Examination

- *Trophic signs*:
  - Skin atrophy, thickened nails, hair loss, dependent rubor
  - Ulceration, gangrene.

- *Pulse examination*:
  - May miss more than 50% of times.

    The patient should be examined in a warm room with arrangements made so that the patient's pulses can easily be examined from both sides of the bed. A cool environment may cause peripheral vasoconstriction and reduce the peripheral pulse. Palpation should be done using the fingertips and intensity of the pulse graded on a scale of 0 to 4 +

- 0 indicating no palpable pulse
- 1 + indicating a faint, but detectable pulse
- 2 + suggesting a slightly more diminished pulse than normal
- 3 + is a normal pulse;
- 4 + indicating a bounding pulse
- Elevated and dependency test (Buerger's test).

	Venous filling(s)	*Colour return(s)*
Normal	10–15	10
Adequate collaterals	15–30	15–25
Severe ischaemia	>40	>35

Criteria for Critical Limb Ischaemia

- Persistent pain >2 weeks requiring analgesics
- Ulceration or gangrene of toes and ankle systolic BP <50 mmHg
- Toe systolic pressure <30 mmHg
- Transcutaneous O_2 pressure <10 mmHg
- Absence of arterial pulsation in big toe
- Structural or functional changes in skin capillaries of affected area.

What is the differential diagnosis of chronic ischaemia of lower limb?

Differential diagnosis of chronic ischaemia of lower limb includes:

1. Atherosclerosis
2. Buerger's disease
3. Early onset (premature) athersclerosis in homocysteinuria, lipid disease or diabetes mellitus
4. Popliteal artery entrapment syndrome
5. Fibromuscular dysplasia of popliteal artery
6. Persistent sciatic artery
7. Arterial endofibres leading to intimal thickeing of external iliac artery in athletes
8. Drug induced arteripathy due to concave, amphetamine and ergot
9. Cystic adventitial disease of popliteal artery.

What are noninvasive investigations for PAD?

Ankle Brachial Index

- Cornerstone of lower extremity vascular evaluation
  - Blood pressure cuffs or Doppler is used
  - Ankle (dorsalis pedis or posterior tibial) to brachial artery pressure is measured

0.96	Normal
0.50–0.95	Claudication
0.21–0.49	Rest pain
0.20	Tissue loss
0.15 or more	Significant change

Limitations of ABI

- Falsely raised in noncompressible vessels
  - Diabetes
  - Renal failure
- If ABI is >1.5, then use toe-brachial index
  - Normal >0.7
  - Rest pain <0.2.

Segmental Pressures Studies

- Pneumatic cuffs applied at multiple levels:
  - Doppler pressure measured at pedal artery and upwards
  - Drop of >30 mmHg between two levels indicates ischaemia
- Reflects status of artery above drop in pressure
- Inaccurate with calcified vessels.

Duplex (Doppler) Ultrasound

- Noninvasive method of evaluating the blood vessels using sound waves, similar to ultrasonography and echocardiography
- Can obtain both anatomic and hemodynamic information
- *Anatomical detail*:
  - Vessel wall
  - Intraluminal obstructive lesions
  - Perivascular compressive structures
- *Doppler waveform analysis*: Hemodynamic information
  - Sensitivity of 92.6% and specificity of 97% (angiography gold standard)
  - Inaccurate at adductor canal and the aorto-iliac regions
  - Ninety five percent accuracy in the detection of bypass graft stenosis, but can overestimate stenosis
- *Qualitative assessment of waveform analysis*:
  - Simple equipment
  - Not affected by medial calcinosis
  - Supplements segmental pressures.

Radiologic Imaging: MRA and CTA (Fig. 35.8)

- DSA (conventional angiography) remains the gold standard for evaluation of PVD
- Newer modalities that match its accuracy are rapidly evolving
- It is a matter of time before imaging replaces DSA with the invasive angiographic techniques reserved for interventional procedures.

Indications for Angiography

- When decision to intervene is taken on clinical grounds
- Angiography is a road map for surgery if
  - Limb threatened
  - Livelihood threatened
  - Life-style affected.

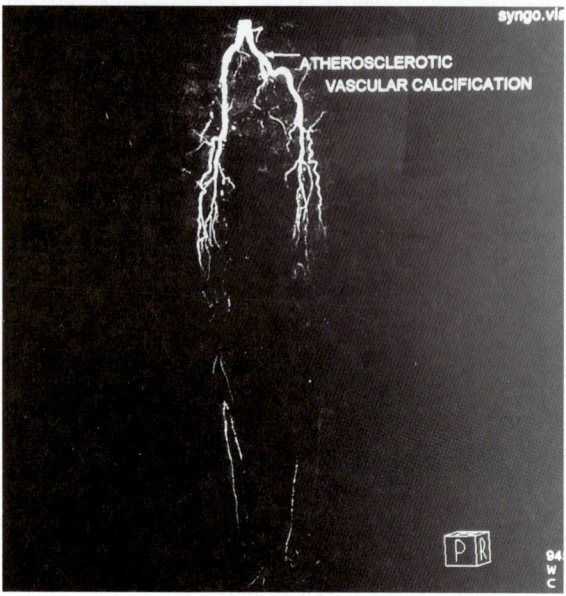

Fig. 35.8: CT angiogram showing narrowing due to atherosclerosis in left femoral artery

Information Extracted from Angiography

- Exact site of obstruction
- Length of obstruction
- Number of obstructions
- Distal run-off.

MRA: Current Technique

- Three-dimensional gradient echo (fast acquisition)
- Gadolinium enhanced
  - 20–40 cc
  - Automated scan delay
- Renal arteries to toes
- Stepping table or bolus chase
- Forty-five minutes examination.

Limitations of MRI

- Uncooperative patient
- Claustrophobia
- Metal artifact
- Pacemakers or implantable cardioverter defibrillators (ICDs)
- Lack of visualization of calcium.

CTA of PVD

- Multidetector CT scanner necessary (4+)
  - Many hospitals now have 64 slice

- Iodinated contrast volume similar to conventional angiography
  - 80–150 cc
  - Automated scan delay
- Renal arteries to ankles
- 20-minute examination
- High power postprocessing software is crucial
- Large volumes of data are generated via CTA studies and displayed in various formats to refine the analysis of study results
  - Maximum intensity projection (MIP) (most common)
  - Shaded surface display
  - Three dimensional volume rendering.

CT Limitations

- With significant and dense calcifications, a false diagnosis of patency can result
- Uncooperative patient
- Pregnancy
- Bad pump
- Inconsistent pedal vessel visualization
- Renal failure or contrast allergy.

Digital Subtraction Angiography

- Gold standard of arterial imaging
  - Has almost totally replaced conventional cut film angiography
- Compares a precontrast image with a postcontrast image using a computer, and "subtracts" elements common to both.
  - Prevents images of objects like bones, etc. from obscuring vascular details
  - Contrast resolution is improved through use of image enhancement software
- Radiation exposure and contrast volumes are lower than conventional angiography
- Images are immediately available for review
- Images are stored in digital format on computerized data storage media
- Interventional procedures can be performed.

Drawbacks Precluding Use as a Screening Modality

- Technique is invasive and expensive
- Requires arterial puncture
- Longer study than CT
- Contrast nephrotoxicity.

Suggested Algorithm for Work-up

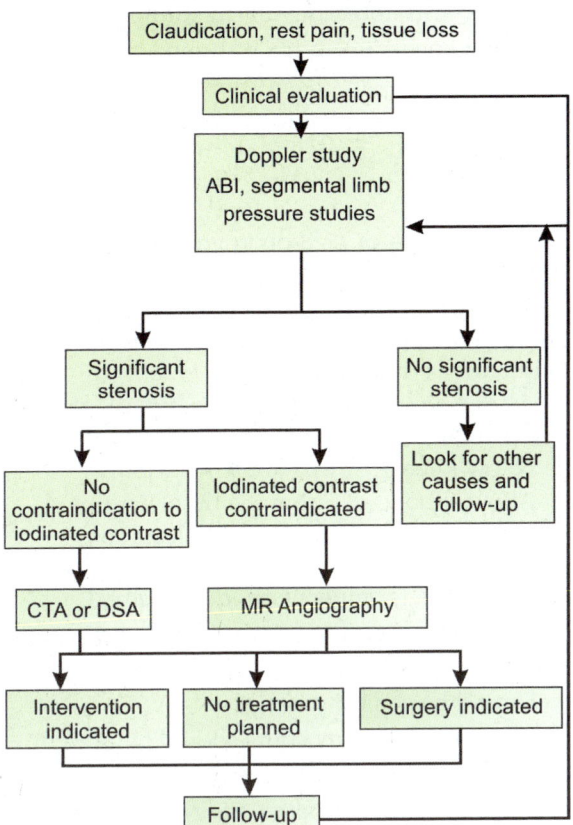

Workup: Summary

- Noninvasive vascular laboratory is the first line evaluation in nonacute patients
- ABI is an easy screening test
- Beware of noncompressible vessels in renal failure and diabetes
- Segmental limb pressures can often be combined with Doppler waveform analysis
- MRA is indicated for intervention planning
  - MRA (gadolinium enhanced) provides excellent renal to pedal imaging
  - It surpasses CT for imaging the foot
  - Overestimation of stenosis in small vessels
  - Limited by metal artefacts, magnetic field, and length of study
- CTA indicated for intervention planning
  - CTA provides excellent renal to ankle imaging
  - Pedal imaging is poor
  - Soft tissues and bones are also imaged
  - Small vessel calcification is a limitation.

Treatment for PVD

- Life style modification
- Risk reduction
- Drugs
- Percutaneous intervention
- Surgery
- Lumbar sympathectomy.

Lifestyle Modification

- Stop smoking
- Exercises just short of pain
- Buerger's position
- Buerger's exercises
- Heel raise
- Weight reduction
- Diet modification.

Risk Reduction

- Control of diabetes
- Correction of abnormal lipid profile
- Control of hypertension or CAD.

Drugs

- *Anti-platelet drugs*: Aspirin or clopidogrel
- Naftidofuryl oxalate can help alter tissue metabolism
- Oxypentafylline
- Prostacyclin.

Percutaneous Interventions

- Balloon angioplasty for iliac vessel disease or vessels of leg, upper limb and renal arteries
- Metal stenting

Operations

- Aorto-femoral bypass
- Femoral-popliteal bypass graft

Materials Used

- Dacron graft
- Autogenous vein graft
- Human umbilical vein

Sutures Used

- Prolene suture

Lumbar Sympathectomy

For limb salvage in:
- Critically ischaemic limb
- Pregangrene stage
- Adjunct to bypass surgery
- Hyperhidrosis.

What is difference between amputation and disarticulation?

The amputation is defined as removal of the extremity or part of the extremity through the bone while removal of the extremity or part of the extremity through the joint is disarticulation.

What is the difference between primary and secondary amputation in a ischaemic limb?

Primary amputation is amputation in an ischaemic limb without attempted revascularization. Secondary amputation is done if revascularization has failed and no further revascularization is possible or there is continued deterioration of a limb despite a patent reconstruction.

What is the indication of amputation of the limb?

Amputation is indicated when the limb is dead, deadly or deformed.

Dead

- Limb destroyed by severe trauma in blunt or crush injuries
- Severe vascular injury of major vessels where reconstruction has failed or not possible
- Gangrene of limb due to severe peripheral vascular disease
- Severe rest pain or critically ischaemic limb where limb cannot be salvaged

Deadly

- Soft tissue sarcoma or bone sarcoma where limb preserving resection is not possible
- Subungual melanoma
- Infected spreading gangrene
- Gas gangrene
- End stage diabetic foot
- Actinomycosis of foot when medical treatment has failed
- Chronic osteomyelitis of foot

Deformed

- Deformed, shortened or unstable lower limb that hampers the day to day life of the patient and patient wants the surgery.

What is the ideal stump length?

The stumps should be of adequate length for fitting the prosthesis. The following guidelines are followed while deciding upon the stump length:

- Hand should be preserved as much as possible
- Upper arm/forearm—20 cm stump
- Below knee—14 cm tibial stump
- Above knee—25–30 cm stump

Amputation through joint is more appropriately called disarticulation and should be avoided.

What is the site of division in various commonly performed amputations?

The site of division varies based on the type of amputation. The distance is measured from a bony landmark as described below:

- Above knee—11″ from the tip of greater trochanter
- Below knee—5–6″ from the knee joint
- Above elbow—8″ from the tip of acromion
- Below elbow—7″ from tip of olecranon

What are the features of an ideal stump?

The ideal stump should have the following features:

- Should be conical in shape
- No projecting bony spurs should be present
- No redundant muscle mass over stump
- Terminal scar should be transverse
- Skin should not be adherent to underlying structures
- Skin should not be loose or thin over the stump
- Free from scar tenderness
- Joint above stump should be fully mobile

Discuss the level of energy expenditure during walking in various levels of amputation.

The energy expenditure during walking is more for proximal amputations. For a below knee amputation with a long stump the patients spends about 10 percent more energy than normal during walking. For below knee amputation with a short stump the extra energy expenditure is about 40 percent. In an above knee amputation energy expenditure above normal during walking is 63 percent.

What are the commonly employed methods of amputation?

Flap and guillotine methods are used to perform amputation.

- *Guillotine method*: This method is used in case of infective pathology, wet gangrene or if line of demarcation is not yet formed. Stump is left open till infection is fully controlled.
- *Flap method*: Stump is closed either by long posterior flap or by skew flap method.

What are the common complications of amputation?

The common complications of amputations are:
- Bleeding
- Infection
- In soft tissue
- In bony stump
- Necrosis of skin flap
- Adherent scar
- Infection
- Suturing of skin
- Necrosis of skin flaps
- Painful stump neuroma
- *Phantom limb*: The patient continue to feel the presence of amputated limb.
- *Causalgia*: Pain, tenderness and redness at the end of stump
- *Jactitation*: Intermittent distressing spasms in the stump
- Stiffness of proximal joint.

36

Buerger's Disease

What is Buerger's disease?

- Buerger's disease is also known as thrombo-angitis oblitrans involves the small and medium-sized arteries and leads to chronic ischemia of lower limbs and upper limbs in young (<45 years of age) in chronic smokers.
- Inflammatory nonatherosclerotic occlusive disease.
- Small and medium-sized arteries involved.
- Involves distal vessel of extremities.

Give historical facts about Buerger's disease.

1879: Felix Von Winiwater first gave description of thromboangitis oblitrans in an amputated limb.

1908: Leo Buerger's published series of 11 cases and gave more detailed description.

What is the epidemiology?

- Affects young males <40 years
- Smokers
- Females affected in only 10% cases
- Tobacco use is a major factor
- Continued smoking leads to high amputation rates approaching 40%.

What genetic factors are involved?

- Increased frequency with HLA (human leuko-cyte antigen) A9, B8 and B40.

Discuss the histopathology.

- *Tunica adventitia*:
  - Increased fibroblast proliferation
  - Endothelial proliferation
- *Tunica media*:
  - Lymphocyte infiltration
  - Intact internal elastic lamina
- *Tunica intima*:
  - Intimal proliferation
  - Intimal cushioning
  - Luminal narrowing
- *Lumen*:
  - Occlusive highly cellular thrombus
  - Microabscesses
  - Multinucleated giant cells.

What are the clinical features of Buerger's disease?

- Chronic ischemia of lower limb:
  - Intermittent claudication
  - Rest pain
  - Nonhealing ulcer of the leg
  - Gangrene of toes or foot
  - Nutritional changes in lower limb
- Raynaud's phenomenon of upper limb
- Migratory superficial thrombophlebitis
- All four limbs may be involved in 43% cases.

What is Olin's diagnostic criteria for Buerger's disease?

- Age of onset less than 45 years
- Current or recent history of smoking
- Distal extremity ischaemia, e.g. claudication, pain at rest, ischaemic ulcer
- Exclusion of autoimmune disease, hyper-coagulable state, diabetes mellitus
- Exclusion of proximal source of embolization by echocardiography or angiography
- Consistent arteriographic findings.

What are typical arteriographic findings?

- Multiple segmental arterial involvement (skip lesion)
- Smooth vessel wall in nonaffected arteries
- Abrupt or smoothly tapered arterial occlusion
- Tortuous corkscrew collaterals
- Direct collaterals (Martorell's sign)
- Normal proximal vessels.

How will you investigate a case of Buerger's disease?

- Erythrocyte sedimentation rate (VDRL), venereal disease research laboratory (ESR), antinuclear antibodies, rheumatoid factor, complement level estimation
- Antithrombin III, antiphospholipid antibodies, protein C and S estimation.
- *Doppler study*: Ankle brachial pressure index (normal >1).

What are the treatment modalities?

- Stop smoking
- Regular graded exercises
- Heel raise
- Medical management:
  - Pentoxyphylline 400 mg BD: Improves microcirculation and reduces blood viscosity
  - Cilostazole 100 mg BD: Improves micro-circulation
  - Low dose aspirin
  - Intravenous iloprost (prostacyclin analog)
  - Prostaglandin E1
- Lumbar sympathectomy: Removal of L1 to L4 ganglion
- Therapeutic angiogenesis:
  - Vascular endothelial growth factor
  - Basic fibroblast growth factor

Omentoplasty: A pedicle of omentum is brought down up to the ankle through a subcutaneous tunnel.

Management of ischaemic foot:
- Protect from mechanical and thermal trauma
- Use proper fitting shoes
- Promptly treat local infection.

37

Vascular Lesions

Vascular lesions can be grossly categorized into:

- Tumours
  - Hemangioma
  - Pyogenic granuloma
  - Kaposiform hemangioendothelioma
  - Other rare tumours
- Malformations (classified based on the predominant channel type)
  - Capillary
  - Lymphatic
  - Venous
  - Arteriovenous
  - Combined

Unlike tumours malformations do not have increased turnover of endothelial cells.

What are the important points in history and examination in patients presenting with a vascular lesion?

History should be carefully sought from parents of a child with hemangioma enquiring how the lesion was first noticed and whether it was present since birth. The evolution of the lesion with regards to its size and secondary characteristics must also be ascertained. Parents must be reassured to reduce anxiety. The number of lesions and their location must be enquired about. Ask about history of trauma at birth and secondary changes within the lesion like ulceration, bleeding, color changes, etc.

On examination, look for the shape, size, number, surface, margins and character of the adjacent skin surrounding the vascular lesion. Note any deformity of the extremities, limitation to any dermatomes, lumbosacral or perineal involvement, ocular defects, active bleeding or ulceration, lengthening of the affected limb, and presence of pulsations. Palpate the swelling and determine whether it is soft or there is evidence of thrombosis. Ascertain the consistency and compress the swelling to see how fast it refills. Auscultate for the presence of any bruit. Also look for the Nicoladoni-Israel-Branham sign by applying pressure on the artery proximal to the swelling (using a tourniquet or blood pressure cuff) and observing whether the swelling diminishes in size, pulse rate returns to normal and bruit disappears. In the general physical examination take vitals carefully and measure the Jugular venous pulse and blood pressure in the other limbs apart from the affected limb. There may be dyspnea resulting from compression of the airway or difficulty in speech. Perform a thorough cardiovascular examination as well.

What are the necessary investigations required in these patients?

Apart from the routine investigations, a duplex ultrasound can be the initial diagnostic test in these patients. It can define the nature of the lesion, the flow, presence or absence of fistula, status of the major and deep vessels and the surrounding viscera. It can also be used to screen for associated hemangioma at other sites like the liver, kidney and spleen. Doppler imaging primarily provides anatomical and haemodynamic information. It can demonstrate arterial and venous components and define the anatomy and extent of the lesion in particular the presence of feeding arteries and draining veins. If there is deeper involvement of anatomical structures such as in the chest, abdomen, pelvis and involvement of long bones, Doppler imaging is limited in its diagnostic potential. Occasionally there may be involvement of the whole limb by the lesion and a skiagram of the affected limb may be useful. Lesions may compress the underlying bone which can be appreciated on the skiagram. An X-ray of the chest may reveal cardiomegaly. ECG should also be done in all patients where a hyperdynamic circulation is suspected. MRI is the most informative imaging to ascertain the nature and size of the lesion. MRI provides the excellent anatomical detail of the extent of the cardiovascular malformations, differentiate between high and low lesions and very useful in the diagnosis of venous malformation. CT scans are valuable for assessment in malformation of bone, the thorax, abdomen and pelvis and in diagnosis of AV malformations.

Simple bone X-ray is indicated where there is limb asymmetry in the presence of vascular—bone syndrome.

What is a hemangioma and what are its various types?

Hemangioma is a developmental anomaly of the blood vessels resulting in various defects. It is characterized by rapid growth and slow involution. It most commonly affects infants presenting within the first 2 weeks of life. The key differential is that hemangiomas arise usually after birth. Hemangiomas keep growing and stabilize usually by the end of the first year, however, some may continue to grow as described later. Based on how long it takes for the hemangiomas to involute they are referred to as rapidly involuting hemangiomas (involute in a few weeks to months) or non-involuting congenital hemangiomas. Males are more commonly affected compared to females. Incidence also increases in prematurely born individuals. These lesions most commonly affect the craniofacial region followed by the trunk and extremities. Usually solitary, the presence of multiple hemangiomas should prompt a search for these lesions at other sites including the viscera.

Hemangioma typically passes through three stages of life, each stage having different clinical and biological features:
- Proliferating phase (0–1 year of age)
  - Actively dividing endothelium with closely spaced endothelial channels
- Involuting phase (1–5 years of age)
  - Increasing apoptosis along with reduced division and replacement of hemangioma with fibrofatty tissue
- Involuted phase (>5 years of age)
  - There is near complete regression of the hemangioma and only fibrofatty tissue along with some feeding vessels remains
  - More than half of these lesions completely disappear but a large part may remain in the form of anetoderma, discoloration, scarring or alopecia.

The various types of hemangiomas include:
- Capillary hemangioma (used to describe superficial hemangiomas)
- Venous or cavernous hemangioma (used to describe deep hemangiomas)
- Arterial or plexiform hemangioma

How are rapidly involuting hemangiomas clinically differentiated from non-involuting hemangiomas?

Rapidly involuting lesions are often coarse, raised and violaceous. They usually involve the torso and the extremities and closely resemble arteriovenous malformations with signs of high flow shunting. Rapidly involuting lesions are associated with superficial ulceration. Non-involuting lesions are usually macular and deep seated leading to a dusky or gray appearance with telangiectasiae.

How are vascular malformations classified according to the Hamburg classification?

Type	Truncular form	Extratruncular form
Arterial	Aplasia or obstruction	Infiltrative
	Dilatation	Limited
Venous	Aplasia or obstruction	Infiltrative
	Dilatation	Limited
Lymphatic	Aplasia or obstruction	Infiltrative
	Dilatation	Limited
Arteriovenous shunt	Deep	Infiltrative
	Superficial	Limited
Combined/mixed	Arterial and venous without shunt	Hemolymphatic
	Hemolymphatic with or without shunt	Infiltrative or limited

Based on the flow type vascular lesions can be classified as:

Slow flow
- Capillary
  - Port wine stain
  - Senile angioma
  - Nevus araneus

- Lymphatic
- Venous

Fast flow
- Arterial

Combined
- Arteriovenous (AVM)
- Capillary–Lymphatic (CLM)
- Capillary–Venous (CVM)
- Lymphatico–Venous (LVM)
- Capillary–Lymphatico–Venous (CLVM)

What is capillary hemangioma (Fig. 37.1)?

Capillary hemangioma results from abnormality in proliferation of capillaries at the stage of canalization. Although it is a misnomer, most of the times it refers to the superficial variety of hemangioma. It leads to abnormal dilatation and telengectasia and presents in the form of:

- *Salmon patch*:
  - Mildine vascular lesion that disappears by the first year of life
- *Portwine stain*:
  - It is characterized by a diffuse dilatation of capillaries that persists throughout life
  - Also referred to as naevus flameus as per the older terminology
  - It is actually an arteriovenous malformation
- *Spider nevus*:
  - Small vascular telengectasia with vessels radiating from the centre.
  - Resolve spontaneously within a variable period of time
  - May be associated with cirrhosis

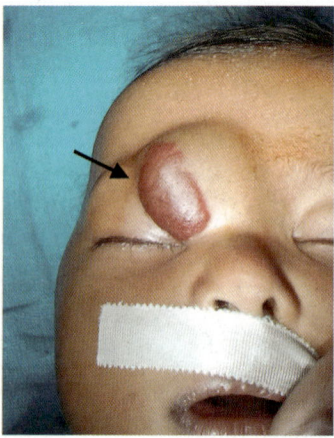

Fig. 37.1: Clinical picture of capillary hemangioma

- *Strawberry angioma*:
  - Behaves characteristically like the hemangioma appearing within the first few weeks of life and increasing in size up to the first year
  - Resolves by itself by the first decade
  - May be associated with secondary changes as described earlier.

What are the features of cavernous hemangioma (Figs 37.2 and 37.3)?

Cavernous hemangioma arises due to duplication of venous channels with abnormal dilatation that increases with passage of time. Cavernous hemangioma is associated with naevo-lipoma and does not involute with time. It is commonly seen in internal viscera as well as the skin and subcutaneous tissues.

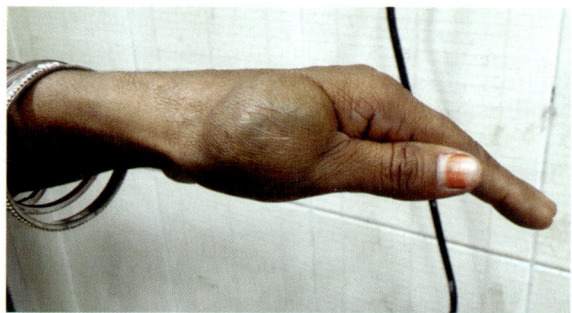

Fig. 37.2: Clinical picture of cavernous hemangioma of the hand

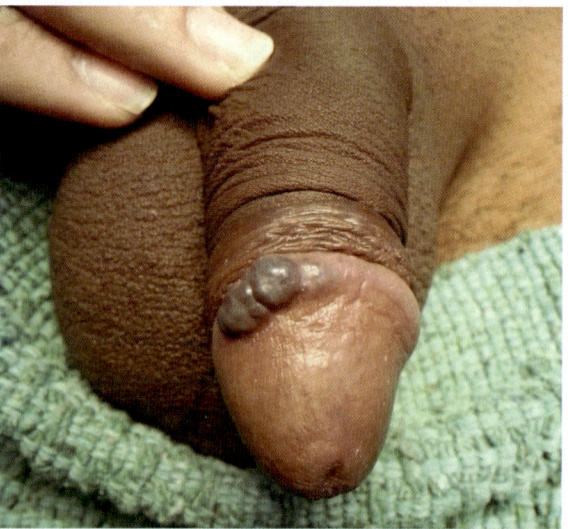

Fig. 37.3: Clinical picture of cavernous hemangioma of the penis

These hemangiomas appear as bluish compressible nodules. Unlike swelling arising from the arterial system, this swelling is non-pulsatile and calcified plaques may arise within the lumen which may become palpable. Sign of emptying is present. (When the swelling is compressed, it diminishes in size and eventually disappears. It slowly refills when the pressure is released.)

What is an arterial hemangioma?

Arterial hemangioma or plexiform hemangioma results from arterialization of the vein in a congenital arteriovenous fistula. This leads to a diffuse swelling which is pulsatile and compressible. Systolic thrill and bruit are also present.

What are the complications that are associated with hemangiomas?

- Bleeding
- KMS
- Ulceration
- Infection
- Obstructive symptoms
  - Stridor
  - Dysphagia
  - Visual disturbances.

What is Kasabach-Merritt Syndrome?

Hemangioma with thrombocytopenia syndrome also known as Kasabach-Merritt syndrome is a rare disease affecting mainly infants and children where platelet trapping within the vascular tumour leads to consumption coagulopathy. Platelets along with coagulation factors are utilized leading to systemic coagulopathy and disseminated intravascular coagulopathy. The syndrome requires early detection and management is directed at sclerosis of excision of the vascular tumour.

What is the management of hemangiomas?

Reassurance is the key to successful management of these lesions. Most of the lesions spontaneously involute and malformations which persist can be managed by a combination of surgeries. The lesions must be timely photographed to follow the course of involution/progression. If the hemangioma is suspected to involve a particular dermatome, consideration must be given to PHACES syndrome (posterior fossa malformation, hemangioma, arterial anomalies, coarctation of aorta and other cardiac defects and eye anomalies.)

Topical or intralesional steroids may be administered at a low pressure. Multiple sittings are required with this approach and the rate of response is similar to that with oral corticosteroids. Triamcinolone is one of the commonly used agents in a dose of 3–5 mg/kg. Systemic corticosteroids are the first line management and prednisone is the preferred oral agent given in a dose of 2–3 mg/kg/day. The course of therapy includes full dose of steroids for 2–4 weeks followed by gradual tapering and continuation up to a year. Second line agents include vincristine and interferon alpha may be used when the primary therapy fails or steroids cannot be given to the patient.

Pulsed dye laser therapy may be useful in hemangiomas that do not respond to the conventional treatment. Surgical excision must be considered in patients presenting with obstruction to the airway or vision or secondary complications like bleeding and ulceration. Whenever feasible resection should be postponed to the involuted phase.

Ulceration which occurs in 5–10% of hemangiomas is managed with daily cleansing and application of a petroleum based jelly or topical antibiotic. It can also be excised along with the lesion if excessive or refractory to conservative therapy.

What is the management of arterio-venous malformations?

Sclerotherapy is an effective therapy for management of arterio-venous malformations. OK-432 can be used for sclerotherapy of macrocystic lymphatic malformations. Intralesional Bleomycin can also be administered in such lesions. For venous malformations sclerotherapy can be performed using conventional agents like ethanol. Multiple sessions are usually required usually at an interval of few weeks as these lesions tend to recanalize. Before surgical resection is performed, the lesions should be shrinked using sclerotherapy. A combination of embolization and surgery is often used in diffuse arteriovenous malformations. Resection can be performed when the child reaches infancy. If the lesion is large, subtotal resection in a stage-wise manner can also be performed.

What are common syndromes associated with arterio-venous malformations?

Parkes-Weber Syndrome: This syndrome is characterized by arteriovenous malformations usually manifesting as Port wine stains or intra-osseous malformations, bone hypertrophy and varicosities.
Klippel-Trénaunay Syndrome: It is associated with low flow arteriovenous malformations that may

be venous or lymphatic and involve the extremities and torso. Involved limb may hypertrophy and varicosities may be seen all over the limb.

Sturge-Weber syndrome: It is associated with intracranial arteriovenous malformations of the meninges, trigeminal area and choroid that manifests with neurological symptoms such as mental retardation, epilepsy, and neurovascular deficits.

Rendu-Osler-Weber syndrome: It is also referred to as hereditary hemorrhagic telangiectasia characterized by punctate angiomas, telangiectasia and gastro-intestinal arteriovenous malformations. It involves mucosal surfaces leading to hematemesis, melena, hematuria, epistaxis and bleeding manifestations that are managed by transfusion and embolization.

Maffucci's syndrome consists of vascular hamartomas with dyschodroplasia involving the extremities. This leads to skeletal defects, fractures and short stature.

What are the various types of arteriovenous fistulas?

Arteriovenous fistulas are grossly divided into the acquired and congenital varieties. Acquired varieties can be post-traumatic or iatrogenic (Brescia-Cimino fistula). Congenital fistulas commonly involve the central nervous system, such as carotid-cavernous fistulas and dural AVFs, pulmonary vascular malformations, coronary artery fistula, intrarenal fistulas and hepatic AVF. These fistulas are associated with a palpable thrill, bruit and vascular compromise distal to the fistula. Fistulas can eventually lead to dilatation of the artery and arterialization of the vein along with sustained venous hypertension. Due to bypass of capillary resistance the circulating volume increases leading to high volume heart failure. Distal arterial ischaemia (steal phenomenon), venous hypertension and high output cardiac failure are indications of surgical correction.

What is the management of arteriovenous fistulas?

Arteriovenous fistulas can be managed by ligation of the artery and vein proximal and distal to the fistula and bypassing the artery with a graft. This is often referred to as quadruple ligation. Often the fistula leads to a large swelling with distal vascular compromise. There may be cardiac failure due to a hyper dynamic circulation that is lethal. In these situations and in cases where prior management has failed a number of times, amputation of the extremity can be considered.

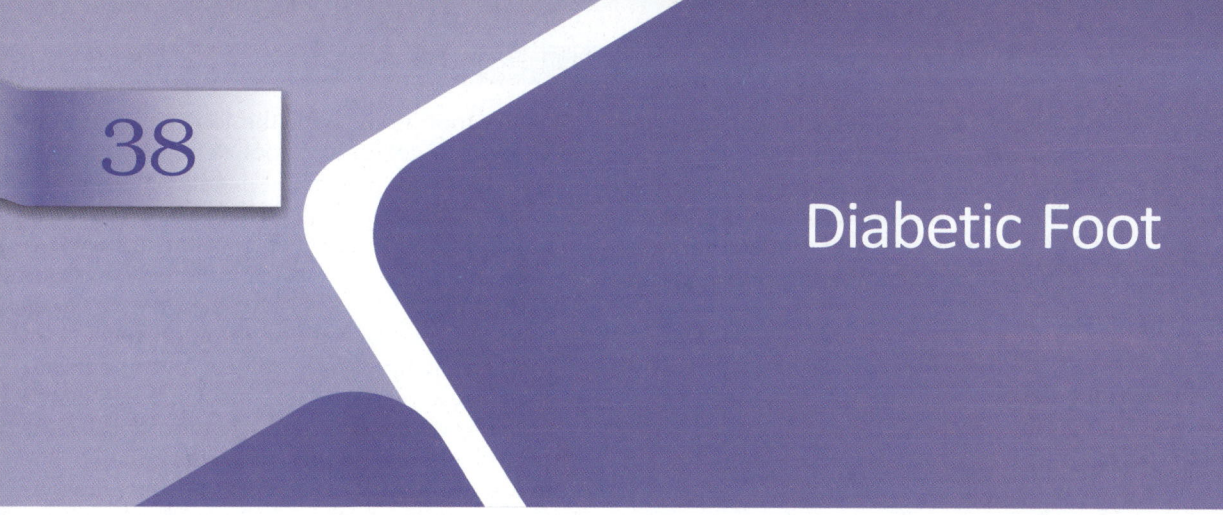

38

Diabetic Foot

Definition

- Spectrum of foot disorders ranging from ulceration to gangrene occurring in diabetics as a result of peripheral neuropathy or ischemia or combination of both.

Incidence

- It is seen in 15–20% of diabetic patients during their lifetime.
- It is more common in 45–65 years of age.
- Patients with diabetes are four times more likely to develop peripheral arterial disease (PAD).
- A diabetic patient has 10–16 times more risk of having lower limb amputation in his or her life-time.
- A patient of diabetes mellitus (DM) with PAD has 70–80% more risk of dying from cardio-vascular disease problem in comparison to patient who has DM alone.

Pathophysiology

Following distinct processes lead to problem of diabetic foot.

- Ischemia due to macroangiopathy or micro-angiopathy
- Neuropathy—sensory, motor and autonomic
- Sepsis—glucose saturated tissue provide a good culture media for bacterial growth
- Immunopathy.

Macroangiopathy

- It is similar to atherosclerotic occlusive disease, except:
  - Diabetics are four to seven times more prone to get atheroscelosis.
  - It occurs at an early age (decade earlier) as the process is accelerated.
  - It involves men and women equally.
  - There is involvement of small vessels below knee (tibial and peroneal) with relative sparing of proximal aortoiliac vessels and the foot vessels. Implication of this is the need for more distal bypass in comparison to non-diabetics.
  - The media of vessels in diabetic patients is excessively calcified in comparison to non-diabetic atherosclerotic vessels, so much that it is visible on plain X-ray or angiography.
  - This calcification increases the impedance of vessels with resultant difficulty in surgery and measurement of ankle branchial index (ABI) becomes difficult as it may not be possible to obliterate the lumen of calcified vessel with Doppler probe.

Microangiopathy

- It is characterised by:
  - Thickening of arteriolar and capillary basement membrane leading to inability of capillaries to dilate in response to injury resulting in functional ischaemia of the skin.
  - The thickening of basement membrane is a part of general abnormality of extracellular matrix component with excessive glycosylation of collagen and proteoglycans.
  - This excessive glycosylation reduces the charge on basement membrane with resultant increase in capillary permeability to highly charged molecules such as albumin.

- The transcapillary movement of leucocytes and macromolecules is affected.
- Basement membrane thickening leads to less migration of white blood cells (WBCs) at the site of injury infection and ulceration and unable to dilate small vessels in response to injury.

What are the risk factors for diabetic foot infections (DFI)?

The significant independent risk factors for DFI included:
a. Wounds that penetrated to bone
b. Wounds with a duration of 30 days
c. Recurrent wounds
d. Wounds with a traumatic etiology
e. The presence of PAD.

Clinical Features

Neuropathic Features

Neuropathy can involve somatic sensory, motor nerves, visceral sensory and autonomic nerves.

What is the cause of neuropathy?

Two theories to explain neuropathy:
a. One related to metabolic factors
b. Other theory related to microvascular disease.
   Metabolic factor theory:
   a. Hyperglycaemia results in increased levels of intraneural sorbitol which may be directly toxic to neural tissue.
   b. Hyperglycaemia reduces the sodium dependent uptake of myoinositol by competitive inhibition. Reduction in the levels of myo-inositol impairs the action of the membrane bound sodium-potassium-dependent ATP-ase which in turn results in the reduction of nerve conduction velocity.

- Extrinsic neuropathy foot ulceration results from somatic sensory disturbances over plantor aspect of the foot lead to neuropathic foot ulceration following trivial trauma. This trauma can result from ill fitting shoe thermal, foreign bodies in the shoe and toe nail cutting. In the absence of sensation, this tissue damage continue and an ulcer get established.
- Intrinsic neuropathic foot ulceration results from somatic motor neuropathy which results in weakness of the intrinsic muscles of the foot resulting in abnormal movement of small bones

of the foot along with the joint subluxation. These changes lead to foot deformity such as claw foot with prominent metatarsal head or a rocker bottom foot with collapse of the longitudinal arch and prominence of tarsal bones. If these subluxated, joints get inflamed Charcot's arthropathy results. These bony changes produce areas of high pressure on the sole of foot, on the tip of toes, on heal and under mid foot. These high pressure areas are associated with ulceration. There is formation of protective callus in these high pressure areas initially. Due to longitudinal shear forces, the subcutaneous tissue between the underlying bone and the callus gets traumatised, resulting in cavities containing serum or blood. These cavities under the callus coalesce and the callus breaks down resulting in ulcer.

- Autonomic dysfunction leads to changes in microvascular blood flow and arteriolar-venous shunting, diminishing the effectiveness of perfusion and elevating skin temperatures. With the loss of sweat and oil gland function, the diabetic foot becomes dry and keratinized which cracks and fissures more easily, leading to a portal for infection.
- Trophic changes
- Plantar ulceration
- Degenerative arthropathy known as "Charcot's Joints" occurs in diabetic foot.
- Neuropathic ulcers are deep and painless. They are present over pressure points, e.g. planter aspect of foot or big toe.
- The most commonly utilized clinical method of objectively diagnosing sensory neuropathy in the foot and ankle setting involves the use of a Semmes-Weinstein 10 gm monofilament to assess for protective sensation and a 128 Hz tuning fork for loss of vibratory sensation. Two nylon monofilaments of 5–10 cm lengths of differing thickness are used. One which will buckle when a load of 80 gm is applied and another which will buckle with a load of 10 gm. Firstly, a 10 gm nylon filament is applied to patient foot skin till it buckles. If patient is unable to feel, it means protective sensation is lost. If patient is unable to feel the 80 gm mono-filament, a severe neuropathy is present.
- Feet are warm
- All pedal pulses are present
- No intermittent claudication.

Ischaemic Features

- Rest pain and history of intermittent claudication
- Feet may be cold
- Reduced or absent pulses
- Ischemic ulcers are painful, present over toes or medial aspect of first or fifth metatarsal.

Sepsis can occur in both neuropathic and ischemic ulcers and can lead to:

- Cellulitis
- Deep tissue abscess
- Osteomyelitis
- Gangrene.

    Usual organisms are *staphylococci, streptococci, E. coli* and anerobic bacteria.

What is the role of immunopathy in the development of diabetic foot?

Immunopathy has been implicated in the diabetic patient's inherent susceptibility to infection as well as the potential to mount a normal inflammatory response.

Impaired host defenses secondary to hyperglycemia include defects in leukocyte function and morphologic changes in macrophages. The leukocyte phagocytosis is significantly reduced in patients with poorly controlled diabetes, and improvement of microbiocidal rates was directly correlated with correction of hyperglycemia. There is decreased chemotaxis of growth factors and cytokines, coupled with excess of metalloproteinases, impede normal wound healing by creating a prolonged inflammatory state.

Fasting hyperglycemia and the presence of an open wound create a catabolic state with negative nitrogen balance occurs secondary to insulin deprivation caused by gluconeogenesis from protein breakdown. This metabolic dysfunction impairs the synthesis of proteins, fibroblasts and collagen, and further systemic deficiencies are propagated which lead to nutritional compromise. Research indicates impairment of the immune system with serum glucose 150 mL/dL. Patients with diabetes tolerate infection poorly and infection adversely affects diabetic control. This repetitive cycle leads to uncontrolled hyperglycemia, further affecting the host's response to infection.

What is Wagner classification system for diabetic foot?

Preulcerative areas without open lesion
1. Superficial ulcer (partial or full thickness)
2. Ulcer deep to tendon, capsule, bone
3. Stage 2 with abscess, osteomyelitis or joint sepsis
4. Localized gangrene
5. Global foot gangrene.

Investigations

- Plain X-ray of the foot to rule out:
  - Osteomyelitis—lytic lesions, periosteum elevation, loss of cortical bone with erosions, new bone formation and bone sclerosis are suggestive of osteomyelitis.
  - The sensitivity of plain X-ray foot in detecting osteomyelitis varies from 25% to 75%.
  - Magnetic resonance imaging (MRI) has 77–100% sensitivity in detecting osteomyelitis and deep-seated soft tissue infections; but it is less specific as cannot differentiate them from fractures.
  - Radiolabelled white cell bone scans have high sensitivity and specificity in detecting osteomyelitis as the normal bone does not absorb radiolabelled white cells.
  - Invasive soft tissue infection suggested by the presence of gas in subcutaneous tissue
- Ankle brachial index
  - Ratio of ankle systolic blood pressure and arm systolic pressure.
    - ≥ 1.0 Normal
    - < 0.5 Claudication
    - < 0.3 Severe ischaemia.
- Due to medial calcification, arteries are relatively incompressible and ABI may be falsely normal.
- Digital blood pressure—30–40 mmHg suggest adequate perfusion.
- Transcutaneous oxygen tension (TcPO$_2$) of skin of foot if >50 mmHg consistent with wound healing. Revascularisation is indicated if the TcPO$_2$ is less than 30 mmHg.
- Angiography to identify the site of block:
  - MR angiography
  - Digital substraction angiography.

Management

Advice for Foot Care

Do's
- Carefully wash and dry feet daily
- Inspect feet daily for injury
- Meticulous care of toenails
- Use antifungal powder on feet daily.

Dont's
- Walk bare footed
- Wear ill-fitted shoes
- Use a hot water bottle
- Ignore any foot injury.

Treatment

Aim is to control of infection and removal of necrotic tissue.

- Braod spectrum antibiotics intravenously in form of vancomycin, flouroquinolines and metronidazole are ideal empirical antibiotics pending culture report. If renal function is impaired, a third generation cephalosporin can be used.

- Wound debridement:
  - Local removal of callus or slough
  - Drainage of abscesses and removal of dead or necrotic tissue
- Control of blood sugar
- Dressings—initially betadine, later on with normal saline, calcium alginate or petroleum gauze dressings.
- If ischaemic disease, arterial bypass using an autogenous saphenous vein grafting may be needed.
- Amputation may be needed with the aim to remove infected and gangrenous tissue and to create a functional foot or stump for weight bearing.
- Toe or transmetatarsal stump usually provides a functional foot for walking.
- Major amputation is needed in cases of extensive tissue loss with failure of wound healing even after revascularisation. Below knee stump is ideal but above knee stump may be needed if there is fixed contracture of knee joint.

39

Aneurysm

How to define aneurysm?

It can be defined as localized dilated sac filled with blood which directly communicates with the lumen of the artery and usually caused by weakness of the wall of the artery.

Discuss the etiology of aneurysm?

a. *Congenital*: It is caused by deficiency of elastic lamina. They occur in cerebral arteries leading to their rupture and subarachnoid hemorrhage.

b. *Acquired*:

   Causes of acquired aneurysm are:

   1. *Traumatic*: The trauma is usually penetrating in nature, but can be blunt trauma. The trauma to artery can also occur due to displaced fracture fragment.
   2. *Degenerative*: It can be due to athero-sclerosis or cystic medial necrosis.
   3. Hypertension
   4. *Infective etiology*: Infective etiology can be due to bacterial infection leading to mycotic aneurysm. It can be a complication of sub-acute bacterial endocarditis in which arterial wall becomes weak either due to abscess formation or due to infected embolus resting upon arterial wall. It can also occur in cases where an artery traverses tubercular cavity in a lung. Rarely, it can be seen an artery located near the base of a peptic ulcer.
   5. The syphilitic infections which are rarely seen these days can also lead to aneurysm.

What are different types of aneurysm?

1. *True aneurysm*: In this variety, there is actual dilatation of artery which can be symmetrical or eccentric.

2. *False aneurysm*: The sac is formed by condensed periarterial fibrous tissue which communicate with the lumen of artery through an opening.
3. Arteriovenous fistula.

Types of True Aneurysm Based on Shape

a. *Fusiform*: There is uniform expansion of entire circumference of arterial wall alongwith the long axis of artery in all directions.
b. *Saccular*: There is expansion of part of the circumference of the arterial wall.
c. *Dissecting aneurysm*: Blood dissects its way along a tunnel between layers of artery.

Discuss Clinical Features of Aneurysm.

a. There is a swelling situated alongwith the course of an artery.
b. The swelling shows an expansile pulsation.
c. If the artery is compressed proximal to swelling, the pulsation ceases and the swelling reduces.
d. A thrill may be palpable over the swelling.
e. A systolic bruit may be audible over the swelling.

What are the effects of aneurysm?

a. Pressure on adjacent structures, e.g. distal edema due to pressure on veins or altered sensation due to pressure on nerves. The underlying bone, e.g. vertebrae may get eroded or underlying tubular structures may get compressed. The overlying skin may get stretched or undergoes necrosis.
b. Thrombosis in the aneurysm
c. Rupture of aneurysm
d. Ischaemia of distal part.

Which investigations are performed?

Computed tomography (CT) or magnetic resonance (MR) angiography is the investigation of choice.

Discuss Treatment.

a. *Arterial ligation*: Simple ligation of an artery immediately above and below the aneurysm prevents embolisation and rupture. The procedure, however, carries the risk of distal ischaemia if sufficient collateral are not present.

b. *Anel's method of ligation*: The ligature is applied just above the sac.

c. *Hunter's method of ligation*: The ligature is applied just proximal to the sac and above the branch of artery.

d. *Brador's ligature*: The ligature is applied below the sac.

e. *Antylus' method*: Two ligatures are applied—one proximal and one distal to the sac.

f. *Aneurysmorrhaphy (matas)*: This is suitable for saccular aneurysm which are small mouthed. The diseased sac is excised and the defect in the artery is closed by lateral suture of healthy arterial wall.

g. *Reinforcement*: The aneurysm is wrapped with fascia or with some synthetic material to strengthen it. This method is used in intra-cranial aneurysm.

h. *Excision of aneurysm* and arterial grafting is the treatment of choice in aortic aneurysm.

Abdominal Aortic Aneurysm

a. Commonest type of large vessel aneurysm
b. Seen in 2% of population at autopsy
c. Ninety five percent are seen below renal artery
d. Ninety five percent are due to atherosclerosis.

Different Presentations of Aneurysm

a. It may be asymptomatic
b. It may cause various symptoms
c. It can present as ruptured aneurysm as life-threatening emergency.

Asymptomatic

1. Mostly, it is an incidental diagnosis.
2. Repair is only done if the diameter is more than 55 mm
3. The incidence of rupture is less than 1% if diameter is less than 55 mm.
4. If diameter is more than 70 mm, chances of rupture increases to more than 20%.

Symptomatic

1. It can present as back or abdominal discomfort.
2. It can present as pain in the thigh or groin due to nerve compression
3. Pressure effects
4. Symptoms due to distal embolization
5. Inflammation of aneurysm wall.

Rupture

The anterior rupture occurs in 20% of cases. Anterior rupture results in free bleeding into peritoneal cavity and only a few patients survive to reach the the hospital.

The posterolateral rupture occurs in 80% of cases. It produces retroperitoneal hematoma. The combination of resistance offered by retro-peritoneum and moderate hypotension stops bleeding for some time. Patient is in great pain, but conscious. If urgent surgery is not performed, the patient will die. Timely surgery can save 50% of patients.

Investigation

CT or MR angiography.

Treatment

1. Open surgical repair
2. Endoluminal procedure.

Index